The Essential Med

For Baillière Tindall

Senior Commissioning Editor: Sarena Wolfaard
Project Development Manager: Mairi McCubbin
Project Manager: Jane Dingwall
Designer: Judith Wright
Illustrations Manager: Bruce Hogarth

The Essential Medical Secretary

Foundations for Good Practice

Edited by

Stephanie J. Green
Formerly Lecturer, Norwich City College of Further and Higher Education, Norwich, UK

Foreword by

Pauline Young MBA MAMS
Chairman of Council, Association of Medical Secretaries, Practice Managers, Administrators and Receptionists

SECOND EDITION

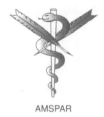

AMSPAR

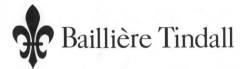
Baillière Tindall

EDINBURGH LONDON NEW YORK OXFORD PHILADELPHIA ST LOUIS SYDNEY TORONTO 2005

BAILLIÈRE TINDALL
An imprint of Elsevier Limited

First edition 1998
Second edition 2005
 Reprinted 2007

ISBN 978 0 7020 2707 9

British Library Cataloguing in Publication Data
A catalogue record for this book is available from the British Library

Library of Congress Cataloging in Publication Data
A catalog record for this book is available from the Library of Congress

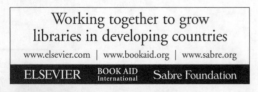

Working together to grow
libraries in developing countries

www.elsevier.com | www.bookaid.org | www.sabre.org

ELSEVIER   BOOK AID
            International   Sabre Foundation

your source for books,
journals and multimedia
in the health sciences
www.elsevierhealth.com

The
publisher's
policy is to use
paper manufactured
from sustainable forests

Printed in China

Contents

Contributors

Ingrid Anstey BA(Hons) Law
Lecturer, Business School, City College of Further and Higher Education, Norwich

Tracy A. Grafton AMSPAR MedSecDip
Personal Assistant to National Director, Cancer Services Collaborative Programme, Cancer Services Collaborative, Leicester

Stephanie J. Green SRN CMB Part 1
Lecturer, Business School, City College of Further and Higher Education, Norwich

Barbara Jones DipPM MAMS
Practice Manager, Pen Y Bont Surgery, St Asaph, Clwyd, Wales

Dilys Jones AAMS CertEd
Lecturer, Business School, City College of Further and Higher Education, Norwich

Sara Ann Ladyman MAMS
Course Director, Talking Medical (Distance Learning), Gawcott, Buckingham

Vincent Leach MA MB ChB DRCOG MAMS LRPS
Formerly Chairman, AMSPAR Education Committee, Tavistock Square, London

Helen Mortimer BA DipHV CertEd RGN RM
Senior Tutor, City College of Further and Higher Education, Norwich

Grizelda Moules MSc RSADipTEFL DipMedSec FETC MAMS
University and College Lecturer, University of Bath, Bath; City of Bath College, Bath; Examiner, University of Cambridge, Cambridge; Trinity College, London

Veeren B. Rambohul BA(Hons) MA IHSM
Lecturer, Business and Finance Department, Crawley College, Crawley

Barbara Sen BA MA MCLIP
Senior Lecturer, Liverpool John Moores University, Liverpool

Foreword

The new edition of Stephanie Green's book has, I know, been eagerly awaited by both medical secretaries and those training to be medical secretaries, and I am very pleased to be asked to write this Foreword.

The role of the medical secretary is a vital and highly specialised one. They have to be fast, efficient and have excellent office skills. In addition they have to be aware of medical ethics and etiquette and act as a link between the clinician and patient, so must be able to translate the language of the medical professional into that of the layman. If that is not enough they must often be a sympathetic listener. As one medical secretary puts it, 'The good bits about the job are being able to make a difference each day, feel that you have actually helped or reassured someone and seen a patient able to return to normal daily living after surgery'. The profession of medical secretary is one that can truly be described as pivotal. Without the input of medical secretaries, much of what is done on a daily basis in the health service wouldn't happen.

Properly trained medical secretaries are always in demand and this excellent book will be of enormous value to those who are undertaking this training.

London, 2005   Pauline Young

THE ASSOCIATION OF MEDICAL SECRETARIES, PRACTICE MANAGERS, ADMINISTRATORS AND RECEPTIONISTS

The Association of Medical Secretaries, Practice Managers, Administrators and Receptionists (AMSPAR) was founded in 1964, initially as the Association of Medical Secretaries. Its primary task at that time was to promote recognition of the valuable role played by those working as medical secretaries, and to establish a nationally recognised professional qualification. Such was the success of the Association that it expanded both its membership and the range of qualifications during the 1970s, resulting in a change of the Association's registered name. A range of AMSPAR qualifications are now available at over 200 centres throughout the United Kingdom.

Today, the Association remains the only nationally recognised awarding body providing specialist qualifications for medical secretaries, receptionists and general practice managers. It has over 6000 individual members from all corners of the United Kingdom and a growing international membership. Further details of the Association's activities and membership opportunities are available from:

AMSPAR
Tavistock House North
Tavistock Square
London WC1H 9LN.

Tel: 0207 387 6005
Fax: 0207 388 2648

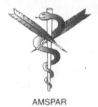

AMSPAR

Introduction

This revised edition of the *Essential Medical Secretary* seeks to update the student with the changes and development made to the NHS under the present government, as far as is possible at the time of going to publication. Needless to say it will always be necessary for students to make a point of reading the press and listening to the news to keep abreast of further change.

As with the first edition, we have concentrated on the knowledge, skills and attitudes needed for the specific role and practice of the medical secretary in what is an ever-changing environment. We remain firm in seeing the team as important in working practice and examine the qualities necessary to be successful as a medical secretary.

The book is divided into four sections. The first gives a background to today's health service. It has been updated in specific areas of NHS organisation and we have extended the sections on Scotland, Wales and Northern Ireland. We look at the impact that the new Health Service organisations have had and at the changes to the organisation of Primary Care. There is also more detail on legislation pertaining to mental health.

Section 2 discusses aspects of practice common to medical secretaries in both hospital and general practice. Where necessary this has been updated, especially in the areas of information technology and the implications this has within medicine as well as in the secretarial role.

Section 3 is specific to work within the hospital environment, with particular attention being paid to the different departments, including admissions, outpatients and medical records. The book looks at the different personnel involved and the functions they all perform to enable care to take place.

Section 4 explains the everyday work in general practice and describes the various changes that have taken place recently, both in the wider organisation and in the development of roles in primary care. The importance of health and safety is specifically mentioned.

Finally, an extensive range of appendices provides useful information for the student to enhance their own learning and to equip them for the next stage when applying for jobs and looking at their own career development.

Should you wish to keep your records electronically, the CD-ROM that accompanies *The Essential Medical Secretary* contains copies of useful forms in two digital formats. The forms are available as PDF files, which can be accessed and updated using Adobe Acrobat Reader. A copy of this software is available on the CD should you need to install it. Alternatively, the forms are also available in Microsoft Word format. Also included are labelled colour illustrations of the main human anatomical structures.

How to use this book

This book has been designed to help readers make the most of their study for qualification and to point out the importance of work experience. Each chapter has clear objectives at the beginning to enable the reader to understand the nature of the content. Chapters will include a variety of challenges to encourage the reader to think more deeply, through the inclusion of reflection and discussion points. Discussion and debate on the various problems and points raised within the text are encouraged. Specific activities may be suggested or the reader may be encouraged to discuss work placement experiences with fellow students or health care workers. There may be documentation to find, websites to search and other reading materials to study. Useful addresses are also included where appropriate. Throughout the book students are encouraged to read other publications and journals and to make a point of being up-to-date with the constant change within the NHS.

The *Essential Medical Secretary* is intended for students studying for medical secretarial diplomas, and will also be a useful reference for those already in practice. We hope that it will also prove to be helpful for those moving from one area of practice to another.

Norwich, 2005   Stephanie J. Green

Acknowledgements

The Editor would like to express grateful appreciation for the support given by many individuals, particularly the contributing authors, whose cooperation and time given is much valued. I would also like to acknowledge the help given by several hard-pressed Norfolk health professionals who have always been ready to provide a listening ear and have made time to make relevant and helpful comments. The staff at Elsevier with whom I have worked have been supportive and responsive – without them nothing would happen! I must not forget the interest and encouragement of many students over the years for this project and, of course, my family, who have lived with it.

SECTION 1

The context of medical secretarial practice

Chapter 1

The development of the welfare state and the National Health Service

Veeren Rambohul

OBJECTIVES

- To explain what is meant by the term welfare state

- To describe the origins of the British welfare state, with particular reference to the development of the health services

- To examine the health and welfare reforms which have had and are having significant impact over the last two decades

- To provide an understanding of the issues facing the welfare state in the 21st century and an appreciation of the direction of recent government policies.

INTRODUCTION

As we move into the third millennium, the British welfare state and the National Health Service (NHS) are over half a century old. However, with the changes introduced in the 1980s and 1990s, and the modernisation programme at the start of the 21st century, it is becoming more and more certain that the British citizens of 2010 can expect a very different form of provision to that received by their forebears in the aftermath of the Second World War in 1948.

As current or potential employees in health care, it is becoming vitally important to be aware of the new environment within which health and social care are being delivered. Medical secretaries will find the history of the development of the NHS and welfare state quite enlightening, especially in seeing how various administrations addressed problems in the management of welfare. The main theme of interest has always been the ever-increasing demand for services and how to satisfy this in the face of new social pressures.

WHAT DO WE MEAN BY THE WELFARE STATE?

The concept of the welfare state has evolved over a long period of time. It was around 1950 that it became acceptable to speak of the United Kingdom as having become a welfare state.

The *Encyclopaedia Britannica* defines the welfare state as follows:

> *A concept of government in which the state plays a role in the protection and promotion of the economic and social well-being of its citizens. It is based on the principles of equality of opportunity, equitable distribution of wealth, and the public responsibility for those unable to avail themselves of the minimum provisions for a good life.*

In 1942 the Report on Social Insurance and Allied Services commissioned by the government was published. This Report (which became known as the Beveridge Report) recommended the provision of comprehensive welfare benefits and services to all citizens. It became the blueprint for the post-war government to follow. It also became the model for a number of countries and thus is a major landmark in the development of the modern welfare state. Sir William Beveridge, the author of the Report, wrote:

> *We should regard Want, Disease, Ignorance, Squalor and Idleness as common enemies of us all, not as enemies with whom each individual may seek a separate peace, escaping himself to personal prosperity, while leaving his fellows in their clutches. This is the meaning of social conscience: that one should refuse to make a separate peace with a social evil.*

One of the main features of the welfare state is the provision of a comprehensive system of welfare by the state. In the UK a series of Acts was passed by Parliament at the time, including:

1944	Education Act
1945	Family Allowances Act
1946	National Health Service Act
1948	National Insurance Act

Thus by 1950 Britain had a comprehensive system of state-run services capable of looking after its citizens from 'cradle to grave'. These services included education, health, housing and social security. These state services brought new emancipation: freedom from anxiety, worry and uncertainty caused by the 'social evils' described so eloquently by Lord Beveridge. The government was engaged in a programme of post-war reconstruction which also ensured full employment, thus combating 'idleness' became part of this programme.

The principle of the welfare state is based on the notion of citizenship rights. In this context rights to welfare should not be based on such qualifications as working in certain industries, living in certain parts of the country, or one's social class or background. It means that *any* citizen has the right to avail himself or herself of the provisions made at the time of his or her need. These provisions are not meant to be charity, but a citizenship entitlement. The state creates these rights through legislation, and establishes obligations on its administration and agencies entrusted with the duty of making these provisions available. Importantly, the welfare state is redistributive in character. It redistributes from the rich to the poor, from one generation to the other, or collects from those in work to compensate those not in work owing to sickness, injury, disability, unemployment or retirement.

Reflection Point 1

- Think about the five social evils referred to by Lord Beveridge. What would you consider as being present day social evils? What might the state do to overcome these?

- Think about why the welfare state was set up. Are the reasons compatible with the aspirations of today's Britain?

- Which benefits would you like to see increased and which decreased or abolished? In considering 'deserving' and 'non-deserving' cases, assess whether your views have changed over time due to your own personal circumstances or to the influence of the media.

Students must guard against the belief that the UK was the first country to become a welfare state. Countries such as Denmark, Sweden and New Zealand are deemed to have attained that status several years before the UK.

In reflecting upon the founding principles of the British welfare state students may find it useful to consider how relevant these are to the needs of twenty-first century Britain.

EVOLUTION OF THE HEALTH SERVICES

Box 1.1 summarises the main stages in the development of the health services until the inception of the NHS in 1948. You may find it interesting to trace how historical circumstances are reflected in the health service we have today.

EVOLUTION OF MEDICAL PRACTICE

The evolution of medical practice in this country can be seen as a three-stage development.

Before the 18th century

The first stage dates from before the 18th century when those providing medical services were physicians, surgeons and apothecaries.

The *physician* was a 'professional man' trained at a university (in those days, Oxford, Cambridge and Edinburgh) who restricted his practice to a small wealthy clientele. An Act passed in 1511 attempted to limit the practise of medicine to qualified persons by controlling the number of 'quacks', who at the time outnumbered those who had any training. This Act empowered bishops to grant licences in their diocese and unlicensed practitioners had to pay a heavy fine. This proved not to be a very satisfactory arrangement, and in 1518 a group of physicians led by Thomas Linacre petitioned Henry VIII. The outcome of this was the granting of a Royal Charter setting up a Royal College of Physicians.

The primary functions of the Royal College of Physicians were to:

- license those qualified to practise
- punish those pretending to be qualified
- punish malpractice.

Although the College was not directly involved in providing pre-qualification training, it arranged lectures and seminars by the elites of the profession. Physicians thus practised as family doctors to those who could afford it and in hospitals, essentially the voluntary hospitals; the distinction between hospital doctors and general practitioners came later.

The *surgeon* was a 'craftsman', trained by apprenticeship. His work was supposed to be limited to surgical procedures, but many surgeons practised midwifery, kept shops and dispensed drugs. In 1461 the Company of Barber-Surgeons was founded, the title reflecting the origins from which the art of surgery has evolved! In 1540 the Company gained royal approval, and certain rights and privileges were conferred, one of which was to be called 'Master'. In time, colloquial use changed it to 'Mister'. Hence in Britain a surgeon is still called 'Mister' and not 'Doctor'.

The Royal College of Surgeons was formed later in 1800, but the social status of surgeons remained lower than that of physicians.

The *apothecary* was a 'tradesman' trained by apprenticeship, who was allowed to charge only for the sale of drugs prescribed by physicians. By the 17th century apothecaries were seeing patients and writing prescriptions, and, without acknowledging it, became the doctors of the middle and poorer classes. In 1617 a Society of Apothecaries was formed. Apothecaries were drawn mostly from lower middle class families and underwent a five-year apprenticeship training in the dispensing of herbs and drugs. In 1815 the Apothecaries Act gave the Society of Apothecaries the power to license and examine in medicine.

From 1700 to 1858

The second stage of development dates from around the 19th century with the development of voluntary hospitals. The status of surgeons improved and some apothecaries began working in hospitals. At the same time it became increasingly important for doctors to hold a hospital appointment. In time this practice led to the distinction between hospital doctors and general practitioners, as more hospitals developed.

After 1858

The third stage of development dates back to the 1858 Medical Act. This prepared the way for the common recruitment, training and registration of doctors, thereby removing the historical distinction

Box 1.1 Early history of the health service

Pre-Tudor times	Monastic orders provided relief and care for the sick. The churches were also the main centres of teaching and learning.
Post-Reformation	Monastic orders were no longer able to provide the same level of support as most of their property was confiscated. Most of the established hospitals came into secular hands. By 1700 there were about a dozen voluntary hospitals, of which half were in London. Voluntary hospitals were managed by their own board of governors, and relied on rich benefactors, funds raised during 'flag' days, and on charges levied. Initially, their aims were the same as the predecessor monastic orders but they soon started to exclude the destitute, sick children, pregnant women, the infectious and the mentally ill. Gradually, sick children and pregnant women came to be cared for in specialist voluntary hospitals. Although there was an expansion of voluntary hospitals in the 18th and 19th centuries, the vast majority of the sick, disabled and mentally ill were left to the care of Poor Law institutions.
Poor Laws	With the implementation of the Elizabethan Poor Laws, some of the workhouses set aside room and facilities for sick paupers. In time, sick paupers in the community could also attend.
1808	The first lunatic asylum for sick paupers was built with public funds. The majority of mental institutions were built in the 19th century on the fringes of centres of population. These were passed to local county control in 1889.
1834	The Poor Law Amendment Act gave a boost to the expansion of Poor Law Infirmaries. With the curtailment of outdoor relief, more families had to enter the workhouses.
1867	An Act of Parliament enabled infirmaries of a better standard to be built by Local Authorities. These soon adopted a similar model to the voluntary hospitals.
1867	Parliament directed Local Authorities to build Fever Hospitals.
1897	Qualified nurses started to be employed in workhouse infirmaries.
1929	The Poor Law Board was abolished. Control of workhouses and workhouse infirmaries was transferred to the County and Borough Councils.
1939	Emergency Medical Services were created as part of the war-time measures.
1946 (Nov)	The National Health Service Act was passed.
1948	The NHS became operational. All hospital services came under a unified service under the Ministry of Health (voluntary hospitals were assimilated). As a compromise to pressure groups, the NHS was established with a tripartite structure:

1. the hospital and specialist services, managed by the hospital management boards and accountable to the Regional Hospital Boards

2. the general practitioner services (including GPs, opticians, dentists and chemists), answerable to Local Executive Committees

3. community services, including district nursing, health visiting and environmental health, provided by Local Authorities.

Box 1.2 Major events in the NHS (1948–1998)

1948	NHS set up (see Box 1.1)
1962	Guillebaud Report. Allayed fears about rising costs. Introduced international comparisons. Percentage of gross national product spent on NHS in the UK significantly less than in other major developed countries.
1974	Reorganisation of the NHS. Introduction of Consensus Management. Local Authorities (LAs) lose responsibility for community services, which are integrated with NHS at the local level. LAs retain responsibility for environmental health. Community Health Councils created for each District (Districts covered a population of approximately 250,000-400,000). Regional Health Authorities (14) created in England, and Area Health Authorities (AHAs) co-terminous with LA boundaries to manage services provided within each District. District management teams responsible for managing services within the District.
1983	Griffiths Report. Introduction of General Management. NHS restructured. AHAs abolished, District Health Authorities (DHAs) created.
1990	NHS and Community Care Act. Creation of the internal market, creation of NHS Trusts and GP fundholding scheme. New GP contract.
1994	Mergers of Regional Health Authorities (RHAs).
1996	Replacement of RHAs by regional outposts of NHS Executive. Mergers of DHAs with FHSAs (Family Health Service Authorities).
1998	*The New NHS – Modern, Dependable* (government White Paper) is launched, indicating the overhaul of GP fundholding, and the abolition of the so-called internal market, to be replaced by a system of integrated care based on a partnership between NHS bodies and other local agencies.
1999	*A First Class Service* (government White Paper) published, outlining the government's proposals for ensuring that quality is addressed, maintained and improved
2000	*The NHS Plan – A Plan for Investment, a Plan for Reform* published. It unveiled the government's detailed plans for investment, reform and improvement programme in health and social care to be implemented over the next ten years.
2002	The 95 Health Authorities in England ceased to exist, as from 1st April, to be replaced by 28 Strategic Health Authorities covering larger areas. Commissioning of local health services devolved to the new Primary Care Trusts and the Primary Care Groups (the last PCG in England ceased to exist in October). As announced in *Shifting the Balance of Power*, the 8 regional offices of the Department of Health are closed, replaced by 4 Regional Directorates of Health and Social Care in England.
2002	Foundation Trusts announced, as part of programme for earned autonomy.

between physicians, surgeons and apothecaries. Apart from the curricula, the shape of medical training has not significantly changed since then.

Physicians had been able to combine working in the community and providing medical supervision to patients in the voluntary hospitals. Initially, the association with voluntary hospitals was more for prestige than for salaries. The association with hospitals was one way of building a reputation and securing a larger clientele outside. The more prestigious the hospital (e.g. teaching hospitals) the better the prospects. Hence the development of Harley Street practices, where consultation surgeries still exist serving rich clients, in close proximity to the major London teaching hospitals.

The freedom to combine private practice with NHS work was a compromise reached after very intensive negotiations between medical interests and health ministers over arrangements for the 1948 NHS.

KEY EVENTS IN THE POST-1948 NHS

Box 1.2 outlines the main developments in the NHS since 1948.

During the 1950s, 1960s and 1970s there was a general consensus that the welfare state should be supported and improved, especially in terms of access to services.

There were also growing concerns about rising costs and how to manage budgets and resources within an increasingly complex system. This became a major issue following the OPEC oil crisis of the mid-1970s. The ensuing recession forced all governments in the West to adopt stringent measures to reduce government spending. In the UK such measures brought the Labour government of the day onto a collision course with the Trade Unions. The frequent strikes and the culmination of these in the notorious 'Winter of Discontent' ushered in Mrs Thatcher at the helm of the new Conservative government with a mandate to control public expenditure and reform public services.

There was a reappraisal of the role of the welfare state and the way that welfare was perceived and delivered, with frequent reference to the need to 'roll back the frontiers of the state', and a distinction being made between the 'wealth-creating' sector of the economy and the public sector. Through the introduction of new management techniques learnt from industry (cash-limited budgeting, general management and competitive tendering, for example) the government put its faith in improving efficiency by market forces. A 'mixed economy' in welfare was encouraged. This meant that a mixture of state and private involvement was encouraged in a number of key areas, for example the private health insurance schemes, private sector hospital service provisions, and especially the private residential and nursing home sector. The voluntary sector was also asked to play a bigger role in the health service, with renewed vigour in fundraising and income-generation schemes.

The most radical concept was the introduction of an 'internal market' where the functions of purchasing/commissioning services and providing services were separated. New organisations were created with these specific purchasing/commissioning duties in mind. With the implementation of the 1990 NHS and Community Care Act, self-governing NHS Trusts (independent of Health Authority control) were set up to be responsible for the delivery of local services.

With its election into office in May 1997, the New Labour government set about undoing the excesses of the internal market. *The New NHS – Modern, Dependable* (1998) announced the redirection of expenditure from bureaucracy to direct patient care, an abandonment of the internal market in favour of collaborative and partnership working between relevant agencies, and a number of initiatives to modernise the NHS.

With its return for a second term in office the New Labour government embarked upon the implementation of its programme of modernisation and reform outlined in *The NHS Plan – A Plan for Investment, A Plan for Reform* (2000).

As usual, both supporters and critics of these reforms have been so vocal as to ensure that their implementation will be within a highly politicised environment, with media and political scrutiny. The main stakeholders – the patients, their relatives and carers, and those working on the front-line on a daily basis attempting to deliver the most appropriate care, treatment and service – will be hoping that real improvements will eventually be achieved following the government's pledge to match reform with new investment rather than continue the underfunding that has hampered the NHS throughout its history.

CHANGES IN RELATED SOCIAL SERVICES

Unlike the NHS, which was set up as a state service funded directly by and accountable directly to central government, the provision of Social Services was the responsibility of local government. Local Authorities were responsible for:

- residential homes for the elderly
- residential homes for long-stay hospital patients who were deemed to be ready for discharge into the community
- day centres for various client groups
- domiciliary services such as home help and meals-on-wheels
- Personal social services, e.g. social work, community incontinence laundry service
- Children's services, e.g. child protection, fostering and residential care (Children's Act 1989)

- Services for the disabled, e.g.adaptation of homes, home help and residential care

In 1974 the community health services (health visiting, district nursing etc.) which in 1948 were also being provided by the Local Authorities were integrated under the control of the Health Areas. With the recognition that Local Authorities and Health Authorities needed to work together in order to benefit their resident population, joint planning was encouraged and some joint finance was made available as an inducement.

The 1980s saw a squeeze on Local Authority funding as well as competitive tendering for all Local Authority services. Consequently, most of the Local Authority residential homes moved out of Local Authority ownership, either through private sales or through management buy-outs.

Reflection Point 2

- 'Care in the community' is an expression that covers a whole range of changes in the way that community services are provided, but what does it conjure up for you? How is it used in the media?

- Try to find out about different agencies which are involved in community care in your area. These will include housing and benefits agencies as well as health-related agencies. Try to distinguish between government-funded agencies and voluntary agencies.

The 1990 NHS and Community Care Act imposed the following obligations on the Social Services:

- lead agency responsibility in community care
- responsibility for assessment of need
- responsibility for care management in the community
- responsibility as from April 1993 for the funding of residential and nursing home places on the application of a means test.

In 1997 the arrival of the New Labour government brought new emphasis on collaboration and partnership working between Local Authority services and the NHS. The Health Act 1999 created more flexibility, enabling the local councils and the NHS to:

- pool budgets
- lead commissioning on the basis that either local authority or the NHS/PCT takes the lead in commissioning services on behalf of both bodies
- integrate and merge service delivery so that Local Authorities and the NHS bodies deliver a one-stop package of care.

ISSUES FACING THE WELFARE STATE IN THE 21ST CENTURY

In its White Paper *A First Class Service* (1999) the government outlined its proposals for ensuring that quality is achieved, maintained and improved via clinical and corporate governance.

Since the 1980s there has been growing emphasis on ensuring that the services generally are sensitive to the needs of users. Customer care is a prevailing motto in private enterprise, out of competitive necessity. Client/patient-centredness remains a major theme in government policies as responsiveness to user/patient demands/needs continue to challenge services in the public sector.

Initiatives in the past have included:

- Setting up Community Health Councils (CHCs) to act as the consumers' watchdog (1974)
- Quality management initiatives such as Quality Circles, Total Quality Management
- Clinical Audit
- Citizens' Charter and Patients' Charter (1992) which became the formalised vehicle for monitoring standards in the 90s.
- Other formal appraisals such as compliance with the British Standards Institute's quality standard (BSI 5750).

With a more discerning and assertively demanding consumer population it is obvious that quality of service and its responsiveness to user needs will continue to be a major issue in the 21st century. Maintaining the right partnerships within a changing environment will be a major challenge to the organisations and individual practitioners. There are likely to be new opportunities created, with new gainers and new losers. At the individual practitioner level there will be new opportunities for those willing and able to work more flexibly. Old job demarcations are being redefined, with nurses being able to take on more of the tasks that were traditionally within the province of the doctor only. Client-centredness is

Reflection Point 3

- As a medical secretary, you must be concerned about customer care. In addition to patients, who else might be regarded as your customers?

forcing practitioners to be more 'holistic' taking into account not only the medical needs of person, but also the psychosocial needs of each individual.

The arrival and availability of modern electronic information technology poses a challenge to organisations and practitioners in ensuring that the potential benefits are realised in the interest of the service users. Evidence-based practice will be at the heart of clinical governance and performance management. Access to this technology will hasten the implementation of standard management and clinical protocols.

At the dawn of the 21st century, the government has embarked on an ambitious programme of reform and modernisation. The challenges facing any administration for the immediate future remain:

- meeting the needs of an ageing population
- increasing health services to keep up with advances in medicine
- reconciling the desire to contain/reduce taxation and to meet increasing demands for services
- ensuring that resources are directed to end-users and not wasted on bureaucracy
- ensuring proper accountability of public expenditure and proper conduct in the management of public funds and services
- ensuring provision of services and assistance in line with the standards of a civilised and just society whilst avoiding abuses and disincentives
- improving quality of services provided in line with the present user demands, and the perceived future needs of the economy and the nation
- attracting additional funding, and the pros and cons of turning to new and varied sources of funding, e.g. state, private and voluntary combined.

CONCLUSIONS

As a medical secretary, it is important that you are aware of policies which affect the organisation you work in. This is true whether you are working in a hospital department or in general practice. Often policy can seem remote, but as a front-line employee in the NHS you are potentially a crucial member of the team in ensuring:

- quality to customers
- essential liaison between different members of health care teams as well as personnel from other agencies
- the provision of effective and efficient administrative support to the clinical team.

All of these are fundamental to the future of the NHS.

Exercises

- Keep up to date with developments in health service policy by reading coverage in national newspapers. Try to obtain copies of the executive summaries of government policy documents. They are available in libraries, from the HMSO and via websites. The further reading suggested below may also be helpful in providing more detailed information about the history and background of the development of the welfare state and the health services.

- Discuss with colleagues what kind of help and advice you might be able to provide to a family who are now responsible for looking after a chronically ill relative in their home. How would you find out about the services of which they will need to be aware?

Further reading

Butterworth E, Holman R 1975 Social welfare in Britain. Fontana, London

DoH 1998 The New NHS – Modern, Dependable. HMSO, London

DoH 1998 A First Class Service. HMSO, London

DoH 2000 The NHS Plan. HMSO, London.

Ham C 1992 Health policy in Britain. Macmillan, London

Ham C 1990 The new NHS. Radcliffe Medical Press, Oxford

Ham C 1994 Management and competition in the new NHS. Radcliffe Medical Press, Oxford

Hutton W 1996 The state we're in. Vintage, London

Johnson N 1990 Reconstructing the Welfare State ... a decade of change 1980-1990. Harvester Wheatsheaf, London

McKeown T, Lowe CR 1974 An introduction to social medicine. Blackwell Scientific Publications, Oxford, London

NHS Confederation 2002 NHS handbook 2001/2002. JMH Publishing, London

Chapter 2

The National Health Service today

Veeren Rambohul

OBJECTIVES

- To explain the management structure of the NHS
- To describe the role of those responsible for managing the NHS
- To explain the arrangements for the delivery of health and related social care
- To examine the main issues facing the NHS.

INTRODUCTION

The National Health Service has been one of the major successes of the British welfare state. It is one of the largest employer organisations in Europe, employing around one million people and spending around six per cent of the UK's gross domestic product. It was designed to provide health care to all UK citizens free at the point of service. The service has undergone five major reorganisations over the last 25 years and some of these are discussed in Chapter 1. Its founding principles of providing access to care to all on the basis of need, not on the ability to pay, remain as relevant as today as in 1948.

As the 21st century began, it was acknowledged that in spite of its undoubted achievements, the NHS had failed to keep up with changes in society. 'Too often patients have to wait too long. There are unacceptable variations in standards across the country. What patients receive depends too much on where they live and the NHS has yet to fulfill the aspiration of a truly national service. Constraints on funding mean that staff often work under great pressure and lack the time and resources they need to offer the best possible service.' *The NHS Plan* (2000) set out the government's plan for reform and investment to address these failings.

As a medical secretary it is very likely that you will work in some part of the NHS or be liaising with it. Therefore it is important that you appreciate how it has been set up and the services it comprises.

BACKGROUND OF PRESENT MANAGEMENT ARRANGEMENTS

The present arrangements for the management and delivery of health services relate back to radical changes brought about in the 1990s and, more recently, through the implementation of *The NHS Plan* (2000).

The 1990 NHS and Community Care Act enabled the following changes to be brought about:

1. The separation of purchaser and provider functions within the NHS
2. The creation of Trust hospitals and other Trust provider units within the NHS
3. New health purchasing powers being given to GPs (under the GP fundholding scheme)
4. The allocation of 'lead agency' responsibility for community care to Local Authority Social Services
5. Streamlining the membership of Health Authorities.

The Act was based on two White Papers, *Working for Patients* and *Caring for People*. These measures were designed to take the quest for greater efficiency and financial management a step further by the introduction of an internal market within the NHS.

The New NHS – Modern, Dependable (1998) and *The NHS Plan* (2000) signaled the abandonment of the internal market and market forces in favour of a more collaborative and inter-agency partnership working between the NHS and its traditional (and some relatively new) partners on the scene. The GP fundholding scheme was stopped, with all GPs services being grouped in Primary Care Groups (which later became Primary Care Trusts). However the concept of a *Primary Care-Led NHS* was reasserted with primary care being given a bigger and more effective role in planning and commissioning services for the local population thereby acting as more effective gatekeepers for the *secondary* and the *tertiary* care sectors.

Shifting the Balance of Power (2002) outlined the different roles expected of the DoH, the Regions, the Health Authorities, Trusts (NHS and Primary Care), and their partner organisations. The vision of the NHS plan has been to redesign the service around the patient: 'a service of high quality and national standards which is fast, convenient and uses modern methods to provide care where and when it is needed.' This meant a shift in organisation and ways of working from a hierarchical monolithic organisation to a devolved system of local networks with collaborative and partnership working.

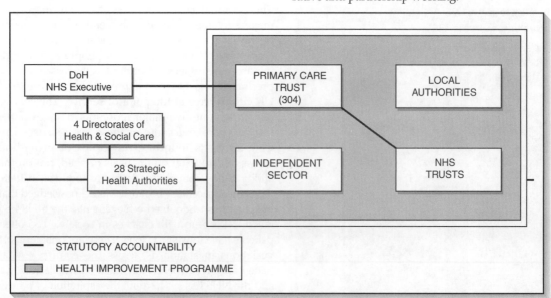

Figure 2.1 The new NHS (NHS England 2003)

Within the United Kingdom there are slight variations in the structure adopted by England, Scotland, Wales and Northern Ireland. The structure of the health and social care services in England is illustrated in Figure 2.1. The organisation for Scotland, Wales and Northern Ireland is as follows.

SCOTLAND

The health service in Scotland has traditionally been managed under Scottish law and the organisation of the service has reflected Scottish local preferences. This has been reinforced since the creation of the Scottish Parliament, which under the devolution of government from the UK government in Westminster, has the power to raise taxes to fund its spending plans.

The Scottish Executive Health Department (SEHD) is responsible for health policy and administration of the NHS in Scotland.

The Chief Executive of the SEHD leads the management at the local level and is accountable to ministers. The Chief Executive heads a Management Team that supervises the work of Health Boards and the NHS Trusts. There are 15 Area Health Boards and 28 NHS Trusts responsible for commissioning and delivery of local services in Scotland. Primary and secondary care have traditionally been integrated under the Health Boards.

Special Health Boards accountable to the SEHD are responsible for the nationally provided health services as well as the national organisations set up to support staff education, training and performance management.

NHS 24 is Scotland's equivalent of NHS Direct. It is a 24-hour telephone advice and information service which was initially set up in Grampian and Greater Glasgow, and will extend to the rest of Scotland by 2004.

The Health Education Board for Scotland is responsible for health promotion, providing focused public health education and enabling the Scottish population to gain better awareness of healthy living.

The NHS Education Board for Scotland was set up in April 2002. It oversees education and training policies for staff in the health service. In particular, it has specific responsibility for post-graduate medical training, training for nurses, midwives and pharmacists.

In January 2003, five bodies joined together to form the Quality Improvement Board for Scotland.

The bodies were:

- The Clinical Resource Audit Group
- The Clinical Standards Board for Scotland
- The Health Technology Board for Scotland
- The Nursing and Midwifery Practice Development Unit
- The Scottish Health Advisory Service.

The Quality Improvement Board for Scotland is now responsible for enabling the Scottish NHS to improve and maintain quality of services.

The Ambulance Service in Scotland is provided from around 150 locations which include ambulance stations and home-based operating points. The Helicopter Emergency Medical Service operates from two dedicated airbases, one in central Glasgow and the other at Inverness Airport.

The SEHD is responsible for high security forensic psychiatric patients at the State Hospital, Carstairs.

The NHS in Scotland has around 132,000 staff, including over 63,000 nurses and midwives and 8,500 hospital doctors. There are also more than 7,000 family practitioners, including GPs, dentists, opticians and community pharmacists.

In 2003 *Partnership for Care,* Scotland's health White Paper, was published outlining proposals for modernising and improving the service. The White Paper places emphasis on:

- Promoting a culture of continuous improvement in NHS Scotland
- Devolving power to those best placed to make a difference
- Involving the Scottish people better to promote the right changes for its health care.

The main changes are:

- The abolition of the NHS Trusts
- The creation of Community Health Partnerships
- The integration within NHS Scotland of the health services and the social work services of Local Authorities (by creating Unified Health Boards)
- The creation of a new Scottish Health Council to involve the public in NHS Scotland.

The White Paper also places emphasis on a Health Improvement Challenge which focuses on four groups – children in early years, teenagers, people at work and communities.

WALES

The NHS in Wales was set up in 1948 as part of the NHS for the United Kingdom. The principles on which it was founded remain true today. NHS Wales provides primary, secondary, tertiary and community care to the people of Wales. The Welsh Assembly is responsible for policy direction and for the allocation of funds. Along with its other national counterparts in the UK, NHS Wales has had several reorganisations. In February 2001, *Improving Health in Wales* was launched, with a reform and investment programme to be implemented over the following three years.

The five Health Authorities set up in 1996 to commission health services are being abolished. New arrangements introduced in April 2003 ushered in 22 Local Health Boards co-terminous with Local Authorities. Local Health Boards (LHBs) involve local doctors, nurses and other health professionals, representatives from the local Council, voluntary organisations and the public. As with the PCTs in England, the LHBs assess the needs of the population they serve and ensure that services are there to meet them. In this new system, local government, LHBs and the voluntary sector will work closely so that there is better co-ordination of services between health and social services.

The NHS is the largest employer in Wales, employing around 77,000 staff (over 7% of the Welsh workforce).

There are 15 NHS Trusts, including one all-Wales ambulance trust. Between them, these trusts manage 135 hospitals and around 15,000 beds. There are around 1,900 GPs, 1,000 dentists and some 600 opticians.

The Minister for Health and Social Services in the Welsh Assembly is held politically accountable for policy. The Director of the NHS Wales Department acts as the Chief Executive. Around £3.8 billion was spent in 2003-2004 for a population of 4.2 million.

NORTHERN IRELAND

Northern Ireland is served by four Health and Social Services Boards, each representing a geographical area and its population. The Boards were established under the Health and Social Services (Northern Ireland) Order 1972, as amended by the Health and Personal Social Services (Northern Ireland) Order 1991. Originally the Boards had responsibility for all the health and social services provided within their area, including hospitals, clinics and social services centres. Towards the end of the 1980s central government initiated a series of reforms to the NHS, which affected the way services were provided in the UK.

The Health and Social Services Boards work under government policies and guidelines, overseen by the Department for Health, Social Services and Public Safety (DHSSPS), established by the Departments (NI) Order 1999. The stated mission of the Department is to 'improve people's health and social well-being'. The Department's budget for the financial year 2002/2003 was around £2.5 billion. They employ 1,000 staff directly and there are over 40,000 other staff within the health and social services sector. The Fire Authority employs 2,000. The Department has three main areas of responsibility:

Health and personal social services

Including policy and finance, legislation for hospitals, family practitioner services and community health and personal social services.

Public health

Including policy, legislation and administration action to promote and protect the health and well-being of the population.

Public safety

Including responsibility for policy and legislation for the Fire Services and emergency planning.

Under the DHSSPS are the four Health and Social Services Boards (the Western, Northern, Eastern and Southern Health and Social Services Boards), which act as agents of the Department. The regional boards carry out the bulk of all public expenditure on health in Northern Ireland.

Health Boards purchase health care services from Northern Ireland's Trusts and at the local level from GP centres. There are 19 Trusts of varying sizes, the larger ones covering several major hospitals. GP centres may be large or small practices.

Under the plans announced in the Department's *Corporate Plan 2002/3–2004/5* and under the *Investing for Health Strategy*, Well-being Investment Plans (HWIP) are the new arrangements by which the four HSS Boards will try to secure health and social services for their local populations, improve health and

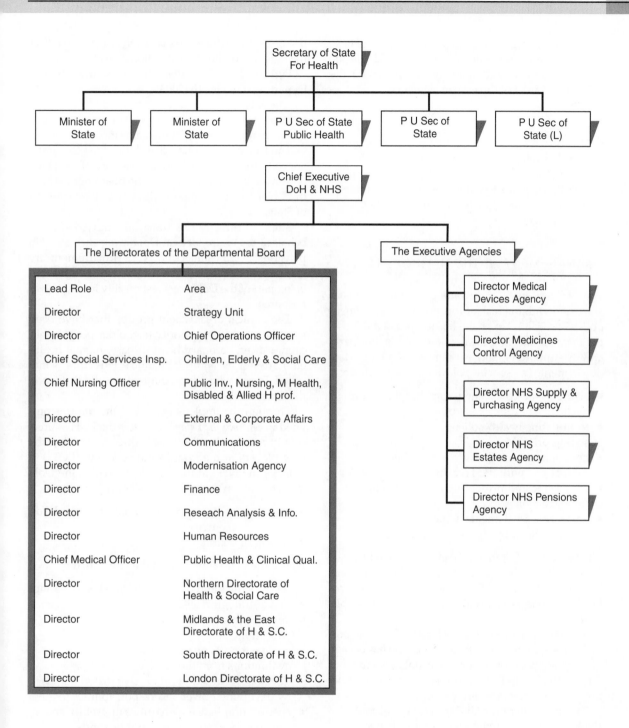

Figure 2.2 The structure of the Department of Health

social well-being and reduce inequalities. These Plans, which became effective in May 2002, are the key planning and accountability documents for the HPSS and consist of three main elements:

- HSS Board plans for commissioning services to their local areas
- HSS Board plans to deliver on the Investing for Health Strategy of the department and reduce inequalities.
- HSS Board plans to deliver on the major under-pinning themes of the Programme for the Government.

MANAGEMENT AT THE NATIONAL LEVEL

The *Secretary of State for Health* is a cabinet minister entrusted with the task of formulating government policy on health. He or she has to operate both as a politician, in meeting the demands of his/her party and its supporters, and as the head of a large state department. The specific role and duties include:

- acting as the government's spokesperson on health
- formulating health policies
- setting priorities
- negotiating annual health service budgets in cabinet and with the Treasury
- overseeing and presenting Bills of Parliament for legislation
- answering parliamentary questions and debating health proposals in Parliament.

The Secretary of State for Health is assisted by two Ministers of Health, and three Parliamentary Undersecretaries of State (one from the House of Lords and one with specific responsibility for public health).

The performance of the Secretary of State is normally assessed on how effective he or she has been in gaining support for government policy inside and outside the Service, and how changes brought under his or her Secretaryship are viewed.

The Parliamentary Undersecretary of State for Public Health has a remit which crosses between various departments in addition to health, including the Environment and Education.

Since April 2002, the posts of NHS Chief Executive and of the Permanent Secretary (as head of the DoH civil service) have been integrated, with the new Chief Executive unifying these two departments. The

rest of the Department has been streamlined to reflect the new role of the DoH at national level.

Figure 2.2 illustrates the structure of the Department of Health (2003).

Students are advised to consult the DoH website (address at the end of the chapter) or an appropriate directory for updates of the organisational structure.

The Departmental Board and the Chief Executive are collectively responsible for the work of the DoH. As the most senior member of the Board of the DoH, the Chief Executive reports directly to the Secretary of State.

Such administrative functions carried out on behalf of the entire NHS at DoH level, such as NHS pensions, NHS estates and NHS procurement are grouped under *Executive Agencies* which whilst still being part of the DoH have responsibility for a set business area.

The clinical areas/client groups that have been identified as having priority (e.g. older people, children, cancer, coronary heart disease, mental health etc.) are led by National Clinical Directors (some called Tzars) who are accountable to the Board via the Chief Medical Officer.

Through the implementation of the reforms outlined in *Shifting the Balance of Power* the DoH's direct role in management will be reduced, allowing the new players in the local health economy (PCTs) to manage the NHS at the local level, whilst the DoH concentrates on doing things that only it can do:

- ensuring the development of national standards
- securing resources
- setting direction.

Hence the main functions of the DoH are to:

- set objectives and direction for the health service
- make strategic decisions
- approve the overall budget and resource allocation
- receive reports on performance and other evaluations from the service
- develop the functions of newly created bodies by devolving power and responsibilities to them
- ensure compliance with duties of probity and transparancy in managing public funds
- ensure that reform is implemented and implementation targets are met.

With the implementation of *The NHS Plan* (2000) being a major priority, the DoH has a *Modernisation Board* which oversees the implementation of the

Plan and publishes an annual report on its progress. The Modernisation Board includes health professionals, patients, citizens and front-line managers.

The *Modernisation Agency* has been set up to help local clinicians and managers in redesigning local services. Its work is closely aligned to achieving NHS Plan targets. The Agency incorporates some of the previous sections of the NHS Executive, including:

- National Patients' Access Team
- National Primary Care Development Team
- National Health Services Collaborative
- National Clinical Governance Support Team
- Changing Workforce Programme
- National Learning Centre
- National Learning NetworkTeam.

The Agency has also taken responsibility for the NHS Leadership Centre, the Beacon programme and the Health and Social Care Awards.

The traditional role of the Department as being the centre that holds the Trusts accountable for their performance is also changing. Other inspection and audit teams, working within a concept of being at 'arm's length' and independent of the DoH will be taking on the monitoring of performance at the local level.

The *Directorates of Health and Social Care* have replaced the eight Regional Offices of the DoH. These are:

- Northern Regional Directorate of Health and Social Care
- Midlands and Eastern Regional Directorate of Health and Social Care
- Southern Regional Directorate of Health and Social Care
- London Regional Directorate of Health and Social Care.

The main role of these four Directorates is to hold the *Strategic Health Authorities* to account for ensuring that there is collaboration and partnership working between the Local Authorities, the NHS Trusts and their partner organisations to deliver improvements in health. Each Regional Directorate in England has between seven and eight Strategic Health Authorities (London however has five).

From April 2002, 28 *Strategic Health Authorities* replaced the previous 95 Health Authorities.

Strategic Health Authorities cover larger populations (around 1.5 million), dividing the country into areas for which each SHA is responsible.

The role of the Strategic Health Authorities is to:

- manage system performance
- drive reform
- ensure delivery of improvement
- ensure that all NHS organisations work together to deliver improvements in health
- create the right strategic framework with stakeholders
- hold PCTs and NHS Trusts to account
- secure performance improvements.

MANAGEMENT AT THE LOCAL LEVEL

PRIMARY CARE

As discussed in Chapter 1 and above, since April 2002, there are new players in the local health economy. The Health Authorities have been replaced by Strategic Health Authorities, and the purchasing/ commissioning role of the now defunct Health Authorities has been devolved to *Primary Care Trusts*.

Primary Care Trusts have evolved out of GP commissioning schemes. They provide a means of involving GPs, community nurses and others in the planning and provision of local health and related services.

PCTs have to assess, plan and secure all health services for the community they serve. The three main responsibilities are to:

- Improve the health of their community by addressing the health neeeds (and inequalities) of the population, promoting its health and working with other organisations to deliver effective and appropriate care
- Develop primary community health care through investment to improve the quality of care and integration of services
- Commission secondary and tertiary care on behalf of the resident population.

Hence PCTs must ensure that there are enough GPs for their population and that they are accessible to patients. They must secure the provision of other primary care health services, i.e. dentists, opticians and pharmacists. Furthermore, apart from setting up contracts with NHS Trust hospitals to provide secondary care, they must provide community care, i.e. health visiting, district nursing, family planning etc. One of the major areas of development will be one-stop health centres, walk-in clinics. They will also develop intermediate care facilities where some procedures along with some facilities currently provided in hospital settings can be provided by the relevant health professional in smaller units in the community. PCTs take the lead on the local Health Improvement and Modernisation Plan (HIMP).

The management structure of the PCTs is centred around the *PCT Board*, and the *Executive* Committee. The PCT Board is made up of:

- The Chairperson
- The Chief Executive
- Officer members
- Non-executive Directors (or members).

The number and type of officer member for each PCT are specified in the PCT's establishment order.

Reflection Point 1

Find out about the SHA for your area. What are its geographical boundaries and where are its offices?

Find out how the country is divided up into all the different SHAs.

The Chief Executive, the Director of Public Health and the Director of Finance are automatically members of the Board. Patients' Forums, when established, will elect a patient non-executive Director to the Board. Additional PCT employees may be appointed to the Board under specification of the establishment order.

The Executive Committee has no more than 15 members. It is made up of the Chief Executive, the Finance Director, up to two members employed by the relevant social services, and Professional Members. Professional members should include:

- at least one public health person
- up to seven medical practitioners
- up to seven nurses
- at least two non-executive members.

Public health members will be Consultants in Public Health medicine or similar and are eligible to be appointed as Chair of the Executive Committee.

By October 2002, there were 304 PCTs in England, the last PCG having ceased.

Care Trusts

The first *Care Trusts* focusing on older people and people with mental health problems were set up in April 2002. By Spring 2003, five Care Trusts had been established. These are Trusts that are able to provide health and social care as integrated care in collaboration between Health and Social Services. They will also be able to deliver and commission health and social care for older people and other clients.

SECONDARY CARE AND TERTIARY CARE

Under the 1990 NHS and Community Care Act, the first wave of 57 Trusts came into existence on 1 April 1991. These covered a range of services, including acute hospitals, community services, mental health, learning difficulties and ambulance services. By April 1994, after the fourth wave, the majority of units (some 400) had opted out of Health Authority management and had become NHS Trusts. The remainder became Trusts by 1996.

The main powers and responsibilities of Trusts are:

- to provide health services through contracts with Health Authorities and GP fundholders
- to manage NHS facilities vested in the Trust
- to generate income through commercial activities and private facilities
- to employ staff as necessary and determine their remunerations and terms of employment
- to provide education and training for NHS staff
- to determine its own management structure without needing approval from the Health Authorities, the NHS Executive or the DoH.

Management of NHS Trusts

Trust Boards comprise a Non-executive Chairman and a Chief Executive together with up to five executive and five non-executive directors.

The executive directors of a Trust hospital include:

- the Chief Executive
- the Director of Finance
- the Medical/Clinical Director
- the Head of Nursing
- one other director (e.g. of Human Resources, Corporate Affairs, or Quality and Customer Services) or these roles can combined with any of the above.

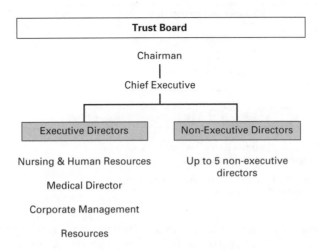

Figure 2.3 The Trust Board. The tasks of the Trust are to determine overall Trust policies, monitor implementation of those policies and maintain the financial viability of the Trust.

The Chairperson, and the non-executive directors, are not full-time employees of the Trust. These are individuals with particular skills and management experience established outside of the Health Service. Two of the non-executive directors have to be local residents. The Chairperson and the non-executive Directors are appointed (following the Nolan Enquiry recommendation), by the NHS Appointments Commission.

In cases where the Trust has responsibilities for medical training, one of the non-executive directors has to be a person from the relevant medical school.

Trusts have a duty to comply with public health and patient health and safety regulations. Thus they are expected to comply with guidance on the notification of defects, of adverse reactions to drugs, and of communicable diseases. They also have to participate in emergency and contingency planning.

Unlike private hospitals, Trusts have to respond to quality standards demanded by the Department of Health (DoH) under such initiatives as quality and performance management. They have to provide statistical information required by the DoH for the purpose of monitoring. Trusts have to allow access to DoH and Home Office Inspectors. All Trusts now have to set up a Patients' Forum, and Patient Advice and Liaison Services (PALS).

Trust management structure

The internal management of NHS Trusts may vary depending on the types of hospitals and services provided. Trusts have full autonomy in deciding on their management structure (Figure 2.4). Most commonly, inpatient services in general hospital Trusts are grouped under specialties which are managed as *directorates*, e.g. medical directorate, child health directorate, etc. These may include one or several wards. Directorates are headed by a Clinical Director, who is assisted by a Senior Nurse and a Business Manager. The Clinical Director is a consultant within that specialty, with management responsibility to ensure that the directorate performs in accordance with plans and objectives agreed by the Chief Executive and the Trust Board. Directorates are given a budget to cover:

- staffing costs
- drugs and appliances
- funds to purchase other clinical support services, e.g. diagnostic and paramedical services
- hotel services including domestic, catering and portering and linen services
- building and maintenance
- administrative costs and supplies.

Other clinical services, e.g. radiography, pathology, physiological measurement, paramedical services, are

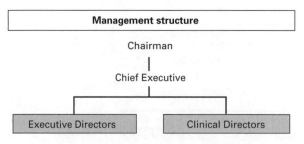

1. Executive Groups – Executive Directors, Clinical Directors and Chief Executive.

2. Operational Group – Executive Directors, General Managers, Service Managers.

Figure 2.4 The management structure of a Trust. This Trust is divided into directorates, each responsible for carrying out a distinct area of service. Each surgical and medical directorate has a clinical director, who is a consultant in the relevant specialty. The support directorates, which provide support services to surgery and medicine, also have directors. In addition, each directorate has a service/business manager, and there are four general managers with overall responsibility for surgery, medicine, theatres and pathology.

grouped under functional lines and set up as business units in their own right, with their own budgets and income from the services they provide to the inpatient directorates and to those outside the Trust.

All non-clinical services are organised along functional lines (e.g. estate services, medical records administration, portering services), with functional heads accountable to a Support Services Manager. Hotel services, such as domestic, linen and catering services (and portering and security more recently), have been subject to a programme of competitive tendering first introduced in 1983. All support services are expected to be managed along commercial lines in order to improve efficiency and cost-effectiveness. Trusts were expected to have more flexibility in introducing commercial and business systems prevalent in the business world.

COMMUNITY NHS TRUSTS

Community NHS Trusts provide such services as health visiting, school medical and nursing services, community chiropody, community dentistry, community nursing, child health, family planning, and well-women and well-men services. These generally have a directorate management structure, but directorates are formed along lines of geographical sectors, and directors may not necessarily be from the ranks of doctors. Community NHS Trusts also exist for mental illness and learning disability services. These have internal management arrangements which combine geographical sectorisation and specialty divisions.

Ambulance services and blood transfusion services were previously managed by Regions for groups of user Districts. Ambulance services have been allowed to set themselves up as NHS Trusts. The Blood Transfusion Service has been re-organised under a new Blood Transfusion Authority.

Reflection Point 2

From your work experience or personal contact, find out what services are offered by different GPs in your area. Try to get an opportunity to ask members of staff how these services have been developed or extended recently. You may come across rural practices that are operating as satellite out-patient departments, working with visiting consultants. Find out about these flexible arrangements.

Reflection Point 3

What other kinds of Trusts have you come across? Try looking in your telephone directory under health services and see how many and what kind of trusts are listed there.

MERGERS OF TRUSTS AND NEW FREEDOMS

Throughout the 1990s Trusts have merged where it has been beneficial to reduce costs through economies of scale. There currently are some 275 NHS Trusts providing Secondary and Tertiary care.

In 2002, the creation of NHS Foundation Trusts was announced. These would be from the ranks of Trusts that were already achieving 3-star ratings under the performance rating system. They are expected to be 'legal entities operating outside of the direction of the Secretary of State for Health'.

Foundation Hospitals will be able to:

- Retain the proceeds from land sales
- Decide their own borrowing requirement for investment in services
- Use new pay systems to modernise the work-force and introduce incentive schemes for staff.

Foundation Trusts can be established as 'public interest companies' operating not for profit.

Instead of direct line management to the DoH, Foundation Trusts will be accountable through performance contracts with PCTs and other commissioners, and through Independent Inspection like the Commission for Audit and Inspection (CHAI).

SPECIAL HEALTH AUTHORITIES

There are a number of Special Health Authorities in the NHS, designated as such because of the roles they play, which do not fit the above pattern of commissioning or planning within Strategic Health Authorities. Some of these were created before 1997 and some since.

The Special Hospitals (i.e. Ashworth, Broadmoor and Rampton) were set up as Special Health Authorities on their transfer from Home Office management to the NHS. Thus Ashworth Hospital Authority is a Special Health Authority which is responsible for the forensic mental health servies provided at Ashworth Hospital.

Other Special Health Authorities are:

- Broadmoor Hospital Authority
- Rampton Hospital Authority
- The Health Development Agency
- The Mental Health Act Commission
- The UK Transplant Authority
- The National Blood Authority
- The National Clinical Assessment Authority

- The Public Health Laboratory Service
- The National Institute for Clinical Excellence
- The NHS Information Authority
- The NHS Litigation Agency
- The NHS Purchasing and Pricing Authority
- The Prescription Pricing Authority.

Reflection Point 4

If you are working in a Trust or have been involved with a Trust as part of your work, try and find out about its management structure. Many Trusts produce brochures explaining their structure. Compare your findings with the roles and functions outlined above.

Try and identify which services have been subject to competitive tendering (e.g. linen services or cleaning). Try and find out whether this has been successful or whether any problems have been experienced.

QUALITY AND PERFORMANCE MANAGEMENT

In the White Paper *A First Class Service* (1998), the government set out its framework for achieving, maintaining and improving quality. The main components of this framework were:

- Setting quality standards with the help of
  - the National Institute for Clinical Excellence
  - the National Service Framework
- Delivering quality standards through
  - clinical governance
  - life-long learning
  - professional regulation
- Assessing and monitoring performance via a National Framework focusing on six key areas:
  - health improvement
  - fair access to services
  - effective delivery of health care
  - efficiency
  - patient and carer experience
  - health outcomes of NHS care.

The National Institute for Clinical Excellence was set up to evaluate new and existing clinical procedures and treatment, assessing their clinical effectiveness and issuing guidance to practitioners and managers in the NHS.

The National Service Framework is a set of guidelines setting out the service framework for particular client groups, e.g. the elderly, cancer sufferers, coronary heart disease sufferers, mental health and children's health etc.

The Commission for Health Improvement (CHI) has now merged with the Social Services Inspectorate to form the Commission for Audit and Inspections (CHAI) undertakes regular inspections of Trust services – four-yearly for those performing well and two-yearly for those rated as Red.

A national survey of patients and user experience will provide annual feedback on the issues that matter most to patients, service users and their carers.

HEALTH IMPROVEMENT AND MODERNISATION PROGRAMMES (HIMPs)

The link between poverty and poor health had been established by research for the Black Report and the Acheson Report. The government Green Paper *Our Healthier Nation* picked up this theme and strongly recommended the need for new partnerships between the NHS, Local Authorities and the private and voluntary sectors in developing programmes to improve health outcomes for the local community.

Since 1999 HIMPs have been set up. *Our Healthier Nation* identified the following three settings in particular for action:

- Healthy schools – focusing on children
- Healthy workplaces – focusing on adults
- Healthy neighbourhoods – focusing on older people.

HIMPs embody the government's aim of building high quality public services, strong communities and establishing a system of integrated health and social care based on partnerships within the NHS and other key local players. Partnership working is now a statutory obligation. The PCTs take the lead in ensuring that these HIMPs are carried out and implemented.

AMBULANCE SERVICES

Ambulance services are required for the transportation of emergency and urgent cases to hospital, and for inter-hospital transportation. They are also required for a large number of non-emergency cases, e.g. non-ambulant patients being discharged, or being transported to and from outpatient and day hospital attendances. There are around 37 ambulance services in England, 5 in Wales, 1 in Northern Ireland and 1 in Scotland. By 1997 all of these had become NHS Trusts or had become part of a larger Trust.

Non-emergency journeys make up around 80% of all journeys. For instance, during the 1995 financial year the ambulance services in England undertook 3,625 million emergency and 14,210 million non-emergency journeys.

Concerns about the ambulance services have in the past been focused on the following:

- status of an emergency service
- operational cost-effectiveness
- response times.

A review of standards in 1996 recommended that more meaningful standards be developed. In the case of the ambulance service the recommendation is that in immediate life-threatening cases response should be within eight minutes, both in urban and in rural areas.

The ambulance services underwent considerable changes in the 1980s and early 1990s. A variety of measures have been introduced to improve efficiency.

- ambulance controls are fully automated
- emergency ambulance vehicles are equipped and manned by specially trained crews with paramedical skills
- volunteer drivers and vehicles are used for non-urgent 'hospital transport'
- a variety of vehicles, e.g. helicopters, high-speed cars and motorcycles are used to improve response time.

Emphasis is on stabilising the patient on arrival and preparing for transportation to the appropriate service.

Requisitioning an ambulance for a patient in contact with the NHS requires authorisation from the doctor and should specify the type of ambulance required (sitting cases, stretcher, escorted or sole traveller, etc.).

The ambulance service is required to respond to all 999 calls made by members of the public. All calls are logged automatically and it is expected that all ambulance controls will be able to prioritise 999 calls.

THE BLOOD TRANSFUSION SERVICE

The national blood transfusion service began in 1946. Currently the service in England is managed by the National Blood Authority (NBA), which was created in 1993 to replace the Central Blood Laboratories Authority and the National Directorate of the National Blood Transfusion Service.

The NBA has become responsible for 15 Regional Transfusion Centres (RTCs) since 1994. The objectives of the NBA are to:

* maintain and promote blood and blood product supply based on a system of voluntary donors
* implement a cost-effective national strategy to ensure adequate supply
* meet national needs
* ensure high standards of safety and quality
* ensure cost-efficient operation of the Blood Centres, the Bio-Products Laboratory and the International Blood Group Reference Laboratory as parts of the national service.

Under plans approved in 1995 to reorganise the blood service, there are now three geographical zones with administration centres in Bristol, Leeds and Colindale (North London). Bulk processing and testing is being consolidated in 10 centres but the 15 centres retain various functions in addition to storing and supplying functions. A national computer system has been introduced to improve organisation of donation, inventory and stock control.

The NHS uses around 5,000 litres of blood a day and demand has been rising by around 4% each year. Only 5% of the population are donors, hence the NBA's struggle is constantly to recruit and retain more donors. Blood has a relatively short shelf-life, and also needs to be compatible with the recipient's own blood group. There are four main blood groups (A, B, O and AB), with either rhesus-positive or rhesus-negative type. Group O negative is a universal type and can be given in an emergency to anyone. In the UK the majority of people are of A and O blood groups.

A major change in blood transfusion therapy has been 'component therapy', enabling patients to be supplied with the specific blood product they require. There are a number of different blood products as follows:

* Red blood cells contain haemoglobin, which carries oxygen around the body. These are used in cases of anaemia and during operations. Red blood cells have a shelf-life of 35 days.
* White cells are essential for fighting infections and are given to patients who for one reason or another have insufficient amounts or who are unable to produce their own.
* Platelets are essential in the clotting process and are used in the treatment of leukemia. Platelets last for 3 to 5 days only.
* Plasma is a liquid with many useful components including Factor VIII, needed for treatment of haemophilia, human albumen used in the treatment of severe burns, immunoglobulins used against infectious diseases like measles and hepatitis.

The Blood Centres are reimbursed by the hospitals for the products ordered and used.

Reflection Point 5

How does the blood service manage when supplies are low? Have you been aware of advertising either locally or nationally for blood? Make sure you know what your blood type is and be aware that it is enormously important that individuals volunteer to give blood.

THE PRIVATE SECTOR

The private sector is a small but important part of health care in the UK. In the 1980s, with the application of tight finance in the NHS and various incentives given by government, the private and voluntary sector received a major boost. By 1990 it was estimated that the private and voluntary sector provided up to 15% of all health care beds in the UK.

The private sector is made up of private hospitals and facilities (which include profit-making and non-profit-making organisations) and private health insurance. It provides an alternative to the NHS for those willing and able to pay. It is intended to offer its patients greater choice, a generally better standard of hotel services and less worry about waiting for operations. In some cases it complements existing NHS services by providing services, at a charge, which the NHS is unwilling or unable to provide (e.g. some types of cosmetic surgery).

Before the 1980s, the major providers of private inpatient services in the UK were the non-profit hospitals (e.g. Nuffield, BUPA); in 1979 these made up 72% of the sector. In the 1980s a number of for-profit companies expanded (e.g. AMI, Human Inc., Charter Medical), increasing the number of private hospital beds to near saturation point by the end of the decade, with reports of companies making losses due to overprovision.

The most dramatic increases of the 1980s were in private nursing and residential home beds. These increases were due to:

- a government squeeze on NHS and Local Authority spending
- a guarantee of social security support for patients discharged to private homes
- pursuit of long-standing policy of transferring care for the mentally ill and those with learning difficulties to the community, creating demand for nursing home places
- implementation of hospital closure programmes.

The NHS Plan (2000) formally announced a concordat between the NHS and the private sector. The desire to make the NHS a truly client-centred service aiming to reduce waiting lists and waiting times has led the government to pledge that where necessary, NHS money will be used to treat NHS patients in private hospitals or even abroad.

Private nursing homes may also be run by voluntary organisations with charitable status.

THE VOLUNTARY SECTOR

The voluntary sector has existed by the side of the NHS in order to provide services and undertake research into particular conditions which the NHS has not been able to provide. The majority of these rely on voluntary donations, and contributions from statutory bodies. The Marie Curie Foundation and the Macmillan Foundation are voluntary

organisations which provide community nursing services for patients with cancer. St Christopher's Hospices provide hospice services for the terminally ill funded by the voluntary sector. These organisations are all run as charities, relying on fundraising to pay for the services they provide.

Considerable criticisms were aimed at the National Lottery when it was first launched, for adversely affecting the voluntary organisations that support health services. The government has since made it possible for lottery money to be used to fund health projects such as developing health advice and fitness centres.

It is also likely that reduced resources within the NHS will mean that the voluntary organisations will be relied upon more and more to fill the gaps.

Reflection Point 6

- Discuss with colleagues what kind of services might be funded via the lottery and why.

- Find out about voluntary services available in your area by consulting the telephone directory. For example, is there a hospice in your area?

ISSUES FACING THE NHS

Box 2.1 Changes in GP contracts

- Introducing charges for certain services
- Applying strong budgetary control
- Implementing cost reduction and efficiency measures
- Introducing an 'enterprise culture'
- Introducing business management
- Introducing an 'internal market' and competition
- Creating incentives for the private and voluntary sector
- Shifting some of the service burden to the voluntary sector
- Creating incentives for private health insurance.

FUNDING

The cost of the NHS has been a major preoccupation for all governments. Box 2.1 lists the measures that governments have taken to try and control the cost to the taxpayer.

The increases in management costs in the new NHS have been justified on the grounds that the NHS had been previously 'undermanaged'. Under the New Labour government, initial commitment has been made to reduce drastically the cost of management bureaucracy within the NHS and to divert these funds to direct patient care. With *The NHS Plan* (2000) the government has pledged to increase funding year on year in real terms in order to reach by 2008 the average of the European Union countries. The government is however looking to see reform go hand in hand with investment in order to make the service truly fit for the 21st century.

PUBLIC HEALTH AND THE PRIMARY CARE-LED NHS

Maintaining a balance between preventative and curative care (a balance between primary, secondary and tertiary care) and between the acute/glamorous/high-tech and the so-called 'Cinderella' services (mental health/care of the elderly) has been a major concern.

There have also been persistent misgivings that the NHS on its own can only be doomed to a curative and rehabilitation role without the assistance of other agencies in enabling and providing possibilities for members of the public to make healthier behaviour and habit changes.

Nowadays, partnership working between Health and Social Services and other agencies involved in housing, schools, leisure, policing and local businesses is relied upon to deliver real improvements in people's health and lifestyle.

 Exercises

- In addition to the further reading suggested below, it is also recommended that you keep up to date with current affairs as they relate to the health service and, if possible, seek further information through one of the health service related journals such as *The Health Service Journal*, which is available from most good newsagents.

- When you are at work or on a practice placement, ask to see any information relating to the management structure and roles, such as the Trust handbook or practice leaflet.

CONCLUSION

This chapter has outlined the present structure of the NHS, and has given some indication of how it is likely to develop in the future. Changes in the way in which local health services are delivered are likely to have a significant impact on the way that GP practices and Trusts work and therefore it is important to keep abreast of developments. Furthermore, an understanding of how services are accountable will help all medical secretaries to appreciate the importance of their role and function in the effective delivery of quality health services.

Further reading

DoH 2000 The NHS Plan – A plan for investment, a plan for reform. HMSO, London

DoH 1998 The new NHS – modern, dependable (White Paper). HMSO, London

DoH 1998 A first class service. HMSO, London

DoH 1988 Our healthier nation (Green Paper). HMSO, London

Drury M, Hobden-Clarke L 1994 The practice manager. Radcliffe Medical Press, Oxford

Ham C 1994 Management and competition in the new NHS. Radcliffe Medical Press, Oxford

Ham C 1990 The new NHS. Radcliffe Medical Press, Oxford

Johnson N 1990 Reconstructing the Welfare State – a decade of change 1980-1990. Harvester Wheatsheaf, London

NHS Confederation. 2002 NHS handbook 2001/2002. JMH Publishing, London

NHSME 1994 Towards a primary care-led NHS. NHS Management Executive www.doh.gov.uk

Chapter **3**

The legislative context of medical secretarial practice

Vincent Leach, Ingrid Anstey

OBJECTIVES

- To describe trespass and negligence
- To explain the laws that are specific to the health services
- To consider how to prevent and manage complaints
- To examine the main aspects of employment law
- To consider how to deal with health and safety in the work place.

INTRODUCTION

All citizens of the state are subject to the law. There are additional rules and regulations for workers in health care. This chapter gives a brief overview of the different types of law and how they affect the health service, your fellow health professionals and your role as a medical secretary. On completion of this chapter you should have some knowledge of the law as it affects health care workers and be aware of some of the legal pitfalls that may be met. If a legal opinion is required the appropriate authority must be consulted.

Before reading this chapter you may find it useful to:

- Look for some pamphlets on health and safety at work
- Obtain any instructions that are available concerning complaints at your place of work

- Obtain copies of the Patient's Charter, your Hospital Trust charter standards, your practice charter, even if not employed in general practice.

THE LAW AND YOU

The advances in modern medicine, and the increased knowledge of medical matters via the media have increased people's expectations of health care. When these expectations are not achieved, there is an increasing tendency to complain and to go to law to claim compensation. Consequently, it is essential that all workers in health care have some knowledge of the legal framework within which they work, and the legal pitfalls they may meet. Although legal matters are primarily the responsibility of the health care professionals, as an essential member of the health care team, the medical secretary has a responsibility to ensure the efficient management of the team, and to look after the interests of colleagues and people using the service.

CIVIL LIBERTIES AND RIGHTS

All laws develop originally from the principles of rights, going back to Magna Carta in England, the declaration of the French Revolution and the declaration of American independence. Essentially these are:

- The right to life
- The right to freedom, including freedom from interference, and freedom of movement
- Freedom of speech and right of assembly
- Equality under the law and the right to a fair trial
- The right to privacy
- The right to health and happiness, including a standard of living to achieve health and well-being
- The right to own property.

These have been incorporated in the United Nations Declaration of Universal Human Rights. They might be called the fundamental human rights, but there are additional civil rights, which might vary in different countries. In the United Kingdom we have civil rights such as:

- The right to free health care
- The right to free education
- The right to have clean air and water.

From these rights laws have been enacted and breaking these laws may bring about penalties. It should be noted that the European Convention on Human Rights has now been incorporated into English law. The full impact of accepting the European Convention has yet to be realised. As a member of the European Union, we are subject to the Treaty of Rome and to the European Court of Justice.

It must be remembered that if a right is demanded then someone has to fulfill that right. With rights go responsibilities. In order for you to demand a right then you must observe others' rights. If others demand the right of free education you have to pay taxes.

STATUTE LAW AND COMMON LAW

There are two sources of law which will both divide into criminal law and civil law. *Statute law* relates to laws as laid down in Acts of Parliament. *Common law* relates to how these laws are modified in the court of law and how they evolve. This is by cases that have been sent to court and interpretations made of statute law and previous cases. This applies especially where a case has gone to the Court of Appeal and the House of Lords. The House of Lords in its judicial capacity is the highest court in the country. The House of Lords will give a judgment where there is a significant point of law at stake. Tony Bland was severely brain-damaged in the Hillsborough disaster. He was in a persistent vegetative state (PVS). The House of Lords decided that his life was of no value to him and that hydration and nutrition could be withheld. This ruling was necessary to prevent his doctors being charged with murder because they caused his 'death' by starvation. Certain cases may also go to the European Court of Justice. Statute law will override common law in any conflict between the two.

CRIMINAL LAW

Criminal law is punitive law initiated by the state against an individual. Some examples of the matters covered by criminal law include:

- To protect persons and animals from violence and cruelty
- To protect vulnerable members of society against abuse of person and property

- To prevent offence to others, for example public nuisances
- To protect property, for example against theft and damage.

Criminal acts include driving offences, burglary, assault, manslaughter and murder.

A health care worker is just as liable to prosecution for theft as a burglar entering your home. Intentions may be critical in deciding whether or not there is legal culpability. For example, in the terminally ill cancer patient the only way of controlling the pain might be with a very high dose of morphine that could prove to be fatal. In this case, the intention is clearly to control pain and not to kill and death is the unintended, possibly unfortunate, side effect. This is the so-called double effect.

Taking a person's property and putting it in a safe for safe keeping might be acceptable, if the person could not give consent. But, putting the property in your locker for safe keeping could easily be open to several interpretations. If the property were to be found in your home, your good intentions would be very difficult to prove. So the facts of a case may be used to infer intentions even if the act was intended innocently.

Reflection Point 1

From your experience, think of examples where actions may be misconstrued or where, if things go wrong, there may be a criminal offence.

Consider the following example: You are working as a ward clerk. It is a busy day with new patients arriving for admission and other patients being discharged. You notice that lockers are not being checked because of the speed of turnover – what might the consequences be? What if you notice a nurse taking a watch and some money from an elderly patient's locker? In what ways could you interpret this act? What sort of procedure should be carried out here?

CIVIL LAW

Civil law covers situations where individuals seek recompense for a harm that has been done to them. Civil law defines the rights and duties of individuals to one another and provides a system of remedies such as actions to award damages to compensate the wronged individual. Civil courts do not punish the wrongdoer; they only assess the level of damage and the compensation that must be paid. If a wrong act is committed under civil law it is known as a tort, as opposed to a crime, which is a wrongdoing committed under criminal law.

These torts include the following categories of special interest in health care:

- trespass
- negligence.

TRESPASS TO THE PERSON

It is a matter of law that every individual has the unalienable right to personal freedom and in the law of torts this amounts to the actionable wrong doing of trespass. Trespass to the person is commonly known as a battery which can also amount to a criminal offence as well as a civil wrong.

Definition: The intention and direct application of unjustifiable physical force to another person in a way known to be objectionable.

Intentional: There must be what has been described as 'wilful interference'; there is no trespass if the contact is accidental. The intention is to the contact itself and is therefore actionable *per se*. This means that there is no need to prove actual harm.

Direct: The contact between the wrong-doer and the victim must be direct. It will still be considered physical even when applied by an instrument. 'Force' has been widely interpreted to cover all forms of physical contact.

Objectionable: Originally the contact had to be 'hostile', meaning 'in anger'. Nowadays this includes any contact considered by the victim to be aggressive, invasive or offensive.

- Not all touching is trespass, but if physical contact is deemed to be offensive, aggressive or invasive it could be considered to be trespass.
- Trespass does not have to result in actual physical harm in order to be battery. Just touching somebody could be considered trespass if it were done in an offensive or aggressive way.
- If consent to be touched is granted then there is

no claim for trespass or battery. Consent is discussed in detail below, but it should be noted that it could be either expressed or implied, and oral or written.

- Trespass to the person also includes assault and false imprisonment.

There are exceptions in the law, for example in cases where people may need to be restrained in order to avoid being a danger to themselves or to others. No battery is committed where such acts are based on lawful authority.

The medical context

All forms of physical examination and treatment require the patient's consent. Consent is a subject that presents legal and ethical problems. Essentially it is a legal matter first and foremost. Medical treatment may be considered battery without this consent. In order for what otherwise might be a trespass, the defendant must show that the claimant consented to the act. 'Real' consent must be a voluntary, informed and competent agreement to specific contact, either expressly given or implied, orally or in written form.

- The patient must be willing. Their consent must be voluntary and is not valid if it has been coerced or induced by mistake.
- The patient must be informed, i.e. they must be given an explanation by the medical practitioner as to the general nature and purpose of the proposed treatment.

Chatterton v Geerson 1981 3 WLR 1003

A patient underwent a particular operation to relieve her of acute pain. Unfortunately the treatment was not only unsuccessful, but left her numb in one leg and foot, seriously affecting her ability to walk. She claimed that as the doctor had failed to explain that this operation might result in this side effect, she had not given the appropriate informed consent and sued in trespass. The court concluded that while the doctor may have been NEGLIGENT in failing to disclose the risks involved, the fact that she understood the nature and the purpose of the operation meant her consent was real enough for her action in TRESPASS to fail.

- The patient must be competent i.e. they must be capable of understanding what is being proposed.

This raises important concerns. If a person has a learning handicap or is mentally ill, are they capable of understanding the nature and purpose of treatment? In the case of children, at what age may they be considered competent to make a decision? Parental consent is commonly required, but legal principles allow that young people can agree to medical treatment, providing they can understand the nature and the consequences of the treatment and the consequences of not having treatment. This principle was established in the classic case of Gillick.

The Gillick case

Mrs Gillick objected when her sixteen-year-old daughter was prescribed the pill without her mother's consent. The case went as far as the House of Lords and established that a young person with sufficient understanding and intelligence to understand what is proposed may give consent. This is known as 'Gillick competence'. A more difficult situation is where a young or incompetent person refuses life-saving treatment. They may be judged not to understand the consequences of their decisions and others are obliged to make those decisions for them. Sometimes only a court of law may make the decision, but in general the young person's consent to consulting their parent should be sought wherever possible.

In the case of the unconscious patient unable to give consent, treatment can proceed provided it is justified on the basis of necessity.

There can be implied consent; holding out one's arm for a blood sample to be taken may be construed as consent.

One other lawful excuse linked to consent occurs in what the courts describe as 'ordinary conduct of everyday life'. It would be impossible to regulate for every occasion when uninvited physical contact arise, particularly in public places such as supermarkets and streets.

Consent can be implied by conduct or expressly given. Clearly it is more sensible to ensure the consent, particularly to medical treatment, is written, but oral consent is still sufficient.

Note: All those who are incompetent to consent to treatment may still receive treatment if it is in their best interests.

Reflection Point 2

You are working in a GP practice where minor surgery is carried out regularly under local anaesthetic. Is it necessary to have written consent?

While you are in work placements, check the procedures for obtaining patient consent and which members of staff are involved. How old must you be to sign your own consent?

Relevance to the medical secretary's role

As a secretary, you may be involved in ensuring that consent has been given before a procedure is performed.

As you will have seen from the examples and reflection points, consent is a very important concept to understand.

Chaperone duties. You may be required to 'sit in' while the doctor or nurse treats or examines a patient, to witness the examination and what has taken place. Medical practitioners are presented with a particular problem where a patient's competence may be in question, for example:

- Young people unaccompanied by their parents
- Patient with mental disorders
- Senile patients
- People with deafness or other sensory loss
- Female patient being examined by a male doctor in the event of a trespass or battery allegation, you may therefore be required to give evidence.

Consent forms. Patients are required to complete consent forms before operations. A sample consent form is illustrated. You may be asked to get the form signed. This is a very important task, and you must be careful that the consent given is valid. If in doubt, or if the patient is in doubt, you must refer back to the relevant medical staff. The consultant may need to discuss the proposed operation with the patient again. It is not your role to discuss the patient's concerns with him or her. Relevant clinical professionals must make all decisions on matters of consent, as they are ultimately accountable for decisions of this kind. If asked to obtain a patient's consent you, perhaps, should

ensure that it is within your role to do that. A health care professional should obtain consent.

NEGLIGENCE

Negligence is perhaps the most common tort or wrongdoing that confronts the individual working in a health care setting.

The law

In law, negligence means failing to take reasonable care to avoid acts or omissions that you can reasonably foresee would be likely to injure another person. In order to show that the wrong-doer was negligent the claimant must prove that three key factors are present:

- Duty of care: Where harm is foreseeable a duty to take reasonable care is owed by the wrong-doer towards that person
- Breach of duty: The wrong doer has acted NEGLIGENTLY in that they have failed to meet the standard of care owed
- Damage: Failing to meet the standard of care has CAUSED the harm done.

The medical context

All health care professionals owe a duty of care towards the patient they treat. The standard of the care expected follows the decision in Bolam v Friern Hospital Management Committee 1957 1 WLR 582. A patient receiving electro-convulsive therapy was given neither relaxant drugs nor physical restraints to prevent injury during treatment and suffered harm as a result. The doctor was found to have administered the therapy competently because he had acted 'in accordance with a practice accepted as proper by a responsible body of men skilled in that particular art'. Accepted practice means that CURRENTLY recognised by the medical profession as whole. Health care professionals are NOT required to provide innovative treatment. A health care professional is therefore negligent if they:

- Perform an operation or administer a treatment below the expected standard of competence, or
- Fail to disclose KNOWN risks linked to the operation or treatment proposed that any other competent medical advisor would have disclosed.

SAMPLE CONSENT FORM

For medical or dental investigation, treatment or operation

DOCTORS OR DENTISTS (This part to be completed by doctor or dentist.)

See notes on the reverse

Type of operation, investigation or treatment for which written evidence of consent is considered appropriate

I confirm that I have explained the operation, investigation or treatment, and such appropriate options as are available and the type of anaesthetic, if any (general/local/sedation) proposed, to the patient in terms that in my judgment are suited to the understanding of the patient and/or to one of the parents or guardians of the patient.

Signature .... Date ....

Name of doctor or dentist ....

PATIENT/PARENT/GUARDIAN

1. Please read this form and the notes overleaf very carefully.

2. If there is anything that you don't understand about the explanation, or if you want more information, you should ask the doctor or dentist.

3. Please check that all the information on the form is correct. If it is, and you understand the explanation, then sign the form.

I am the patient/parent/guardian (delete as necessary).

I agree	• to what is proposed which has been explained to me by the doctor/dentist named on this form.
	• The use of the type of anaesthetic that I have been told about.
I understand	• that the procedure may not be done by the doctor/dentist who has been treating me so far.
	• That any procedure in addition to the investigation or treatment described on this form will only be carried out if it is necessary and in my best interests and can be justified for medical reasons.
I have told	• the doctor or dentist about the procedures listed below I would not wish to be carried out straightaway without my having the opportunity to consider them first.

Figure 3.1 A sample consent form

N.B. In the interests of advancing medical knowledge, a health care professional is not necessarily negligent if they can justify a treatment not commonly considered to be accepted practice.

Vicarious liability

It is a matter of law that the GP and, in the hospital, the Trust are legally responsible for the conduct of all their employees, who may also, where appropriate, share this responsibility This is known as vicarious liability and it means that the Trusts or GP are liable for any negligent acts of other professionals working for them. However, all team members have a requirement to fulfill their individual duties adequately and the conduct generally of health care professionals towards those they treat is regulated both by Legislation and Common Law.

Under the Occupiers Liability Act 1957, both GPs and Health Authorities have a duty of care towards visitors to ensure their safety whilst on their premises. Note that there is a higher duty of care towards children, and special care must be taken to ensure that they come to no harm. As a medical secretary, you may be responsible for ensuring that equipment and drugs are well out of reach, and that the premises that you work on are kept safe and clean. (See also Chapters 10, 15 and 17 on general practice and safety in the clinical environment.)

Relevance to the medical secretary's role

You may feel that the question of negligence is a matter for health care professionals and outside the role of the medical secretary. It must be emphasised again that the secretary is an essential member of the health care team.

Legal responsibility for the patient does not begin or end with the medical treatment required. All staff have a duty to ensure that all aspects of patient care are competently handled, and this includes the relevant paperwork and all communications with patients. A misspelling in a discharge letter may mean the GP prescribes the wrong medication. Omitting to send a referral letter may mean a person needing urgent treatment suffers unduly or even dies. An X-ray is useless unless the clinician receives the result at the right time. The clinical notes are essential to ensure the clinician has all the relevant facts of a case.

Legally, medical secretaries also have a requirement to fulfill their individual duties adequately.

Surgeries and hospitals may list administrative tasks that staff can refer to when necessary. An agreed standard policy will exist for many of these duties.

As a medical secretary you have a crucial role in many of these tasks.

There is only one golden rule – if in any doubt consult your employer or superior.

LAWS SPECIFIC TO HEALTH SERVICE PROCEDURES

There is a whole range of laws and regulations covering health care. The following sections deal with some of the more important points for you to know about as a medical secretary, and your role in ensuring that the proper procedures are observed.

PREGNANCY

The law

In pregnancy, the woman's doctor owes her a duty, not only to safeguard her own well-being, but also to ensure the healthy development of the baby. In the event, however, that there is a conflict between the well-being of the mother and that of the child precedence must be given to the health of the mother. However, the doctor risks prosecution for gross negligence or even manslaughter if the baby subsequently dies. The doctor's primary consideration must be for the mother, but he or she is expected to minimise the risks of harm to the fetus as well.

It is a criminal offence for anyone other than a registered practitioner or midwife to assist at a birth except in an emergency. Although the mother is lawfully entitled to give birth alone, she risks prosecution for gross negligence or manslaughter if the baby dies.

- Doctors or nurses can be prosecuted for negligence where incompetence harms either the mother or the child.
- Consent must be obtained from the woman for any invasive antenatal treatments. Consent may be implied, however, for any treatment that takes place during the birth itself. However, verbal consent is usually possible.
- Any refusal of treatment must be respected, except in an emergency; to save lives doctors must risk committing battery. The doctor's

defence would be that it was a necessity, or that the woman was deemed incompetent to refuse. For conscientious or other reasons a doctor may ignore the contents of a living will. In those cases the doctor's action may have to be defended in a court of law.

The medical secretary's role

GP surgeries commonly have an antenatal programme consisting of a series of check-ups, tests and examinations. The relevant forms generally include

1: A maternity care sheet
2: A maternity care pack.

The two main administrative duties are:

- Ensuring the forms are correctly completed, particularly information relating to midwifery services, and sections of the forms relating to patient details for blood tests, other clinical tests and screening
- Making sure appointments are made and are being kept. This is particularly relevant to midwife bookings. Failure to attend for antenatal examinations could mean serious risk to mother and baby.

On hospital admission, it is important to check:

- That medical records contained in the pregnancy pack are present
- That the patient has been informed of the hospital facilities
- That all admission forms are complete and correct
- That medical staff have received all clinical and personal data.

If on admission a patient informs you that she objects to certain medical procedures being used (for example, the use of particular drugs during delivery), you must ensure that the medical staff know of this so that they can discuss it further with the patient if necessary.

TERMINATION OF PREGNANCY

The law

The Abortion Act of 1967 introduced lawful termination, but it contains strict provisions as to when such a termination can be performed, and by whom.

The key points to note are:

- Special rules apply in emergency cases
- Fathers have no legal rights to prevent termination
- Health care staff can be exempt from participating in a termination if they have expressed their conscientious objection to such procedures
- The termination must be carried out in a place specified by the law, i.e. a registered clinic or hospital.

The medical issues

The Abortion Act states that a termination is lawful when two registered medical practitioners are of the opinion that the particular case meets at least one of the following criteria:

- There is a risk to the woman of physical or mental injury (before 24 weeks)
- There is a risk of grave permanent damage to her physical or mental health
- The risk of loss of life is greater if the pregnancy is continued than if it is terminated
- There is a substantial risk that the child born would suffer from such physical or mental abnormalities as to be seriously handicapped (this judgment may not be based purely on the medical assessment).

Other adverse risks can be considered if the pregnancy continues, for example, the mother's ability to cope with, and adequately care for, existing children, especially if a severely handicapped child is born.

Termination of pregnancy is not to be carried out for social reasons. A termination should not be carried out because the pregnancy would interfere with a career unless it can be shown that the birth of a child would have a serious psychological effect.

The medical secretary's role

Once more, it is essential that the administrative duties around termination are carried out competently and accurately. This includes:

- Ensuring appointments are correctly made. This is particularly important when the length of pregnancy is an issue, and where the patient may require counselling

- Checking consent forms are accurately completed and signed.

PROCEDURES ON THE DEATH OF A PATIENT

The law

> **Box 3.1 Conditions for reporting a death to the coroner**
>
> 1. Deceased not attended by doctor in last illness
> 2. Deceased not attended by doctor in last 14 days of illness
> 3. Cause unknown
> 4. Death unexpectedly sudden
> 5. Death due to industrial disease
> 6. Unnatural causes, including rare diseases
> 7. Cases of violence and accidents
> 8. Neglect
> 9. Abortion
> 10. Any suspicious circumstances
> 11. Death in police custody or prison
>
> In some areas a coroner asks for all deaths within 24 hours of admission to hospital to be reported.
>
> Following the enquiry into the activities of the multiple murderer Harold Shipman, there will probably be changes in the procedure for certification and registration of deaths.

In law there is a distinction made between natural death in ordinary circumstances and exceptional death, where death has occurred through unnatural causes or in exceptional circumstances or both. Procedures regulating a normal death are contained in the Births and Deaths Registration Act 1953. Procedures regulating exceptional deaths are contained in both the 1953 legislation and the Coroners' Act 1988. Box 3.1 lists the deaths that are reportable to the coroner.

Note also the Human Tissue Act 1961. This regulates organ donation, post-mortem procedures and bodies donated for teaching purposes.

The medical context

There is a standard procedure in the event of a normal death. The doctor issues a death certificate that is sent to the registrar and the doctor retains a counterfoil certificate. The informant (normally a relative or hospital secretary) notifies the registrar of the deceased's details.

The registrar issues a certificate for disposal of the body.

Documents required for cremation include an application obtained from the funeral director/undertaker. The form confirms the deceased's wishes and that death is due to natural causes. Other forms that are required include:

- Medical certificate from deceased's GP, disclosing any interest in the deceased (e.g. the deceased's estate). The doctor issuing the death certificate usually completes this certificate
- Medical certificate issued by an independent senior practitioner, or pathologist in the event of a post-mortem. This second doctor has to consult with the doctor issuing the death certificate and examine the body of the deceased.
- A third doctor, the referee on behalf of the crematorium, signs the third part of the certificate to sanction the cremation.

The procedure in the event of an exceptional death is as follows. The doctor issues the death certificate, initialing Box A that he is reporting to the coroner and sends this to the registrar. The doctor may notify the coroner direct. The coroner receives the GP's or hospital doctor's report by phone. The registrar may not be satisfied as to the cause of death or other irregularities and notify the coroner. The coroner may:

- Take no further action and report to the registrar, who will then register the death and issue a disposal certificate
- Order a post-mortem and take no further action – again reporting back to the registrar
- Order an inquest.

The inquest is an investigative process aimed at establishing (usually publicly) the cause of death. The verdict can include death by misadventure, unlawful killing and natural causes. The coroner reports back to the registrar who enters death in the register and issues a disposal certificate. If there is to be investigation of a possible criminal act the coroner will adjourn the hearing until the investigations are complete. In those circumstances he will often not give permission for burial to take place.

The medical secretary's role

Generally speaking, there are few administrative duties required. However, in the event of the deceased having no one else to act as official informant to register the death, you should refer to the instructions on the right hand side of the medical certificate, ensuring that you supply the registrar with all the details of the deceased that are required. This includes, if possible, the deceased's medical card. Alternatively, you may be asked by the bereaved and possibly bewildered relatives to assist in collating and completing the required paperwork.

Finally, the GP or hospital may, in the event of a coroner's inquest, be asked to give medical evidence. You must ensure that all the deceased's medical records are available and up to date. You should also be aware that if the doctor decides in the circumstances of a normal death to arrange a post-mortem by a pathologist you may be required to record the relatives' consent, and prepare the post-mortem report.

For hundreds of years it has been the usual practice to preserve and store specimens removed at operation or at post-mortem. These specimens are vital for teaching and research. In addition, organs are needed for transplantation. At Alder Hey Hospital in Liverpool some parents realised that their dead children had been buried with large numbers of organs removed. Now there is great controversy as to what may be retained after operation or post-mortem. What constitutes a sample or specimen? After operation permission must be sought for preservation of samples and organs. Consent is the key.

Medical secretaries must be prepared to keep up to date as opinions, laws, and policies change.

SICKNESS CERTIFICATES

The law

Provision has now been made for patients to complete their own medical certificates, along with the continued practice of using a GP's certificate when required.

The medical issues

For the first 7 days of illness the patient completes a sickness certificate obtainable from the employer.

For any illness that does continue, or is likely to continue, after the seventh day, the GP is required to complete the relevant certificate if in his opinion the patient is unfit for work. Certificates can cover illness lasting up to 2 weeks, or illness lasting up to 6 months. There is a special certificate for hospital in-patients. There is also a special certificate (Med 5) for use when the patient has not been able to obtain the certificate within the time limit.

The medical secretary's role

As these certificates are available from surgeries, staff will be required to issue patients' forms for them to complete. Ensure that patients know that the completed certificate must be sent to their local Department of Work and Pensions. You may also be required to assist the doctor in issuing other reports for various purposes including insurance policies. It is important to realise that a medical secretary may not sign the form.

THE MENTAL HEALTH ACT 1983

Under the Mental Health Act, Section 1(2) provides for the definition for mental disorder, broadly defined as 'mental illness, arrested or incomplete development of mind, psychopathic disorder or any other disorder or disability of mind'. This is further classified into four distinct legal (as opposed to clinical) forms of disorder. These are:

Mental Illness – this is not defined, which is strange in a mental health act, especially since this is the most common form of mental disorder for which people are dealt with under the Act. While no legal definition exists, mental illness is considered to include clinical conditions such as severe depression, where there is a risk of suicide, and some cases of schizophrenia.

Severe Mental Impairment – this is a state of arrested or incomplete development of mind that includes severe impairment of intelligence and social functioning and is linked to aggressive or seriously irresponsible behaviour.

Mental Impairment – this is considered to be significant rather than severe.

Psychopathic Disorder – this is a persistent disorder or disability which results in abnormally aggressive or seriously irresponsible behaviour.

The Act excludes promiscuous or immoral behaviour, deviancy, drug dependency or abuse.

The Act makes a crucial distinction between *informal voluntary* patients and those *compulsorily* admitted, in two key respects:

- Voluntary patients have the right to discharge themselves
- Voluntary patients have the right to refuse any treatment

Informal admission of voluntary patients is the same procedure as normal admission to hospital for physical treatment. It requires:

- Consultation with GP
- Assessment of condition on admission.

Section 2 of the Act covers *compulsory admission* of *involuntary* patients. 'Involuntary' does not necessarily mean that the patient refuses to go – it means that they *must* go, whether they consent or not. This is because their mental disorder is considered clinically too serious for self-help. The grounds for assessment are:

- The patient is suffering from a mental disorder which justifies assessment
- There is a risk to personal or public health and safety.

The period for assessment is up to 28 days

Section 3 of the Act covers *compulsory admission for treatment*. It depends upon:

- Whether the patient is suffering from the type of mental disorder which justifies hospital treatment, and, in psychopathic disorder and mental impairment, whether the disorder can be alleviated or deterioration prevented
- Whether treatment is necessary for personal and public health and safety.

The period for treatment is initially up to 6 months, subject to a further 6 months, and then at yearly intervals.

Under Section 3, a patient whose mental condition is serious enough to justify compulsory admission but is still classified as a 'minor disorder' must be capable of being treated.

There is no such treatability requirement for those suffering from 'mental illness' or 'severe mental impairment'. This is only qualified by the treatability requirement on applications to renew detention (except in cases where the patient is unable to care for themselves and should not be discharged).

Procedure for compulsory admission is the same for both assessment and/or treatment:

- A recommendation must be made by two registered practitioners, one of whom must be an approved specialist
- An application must be made by an Approved Social Worker (ASW) or the nearest relative. The social worker must consult with (or have tried to consult with) the nearest relative. If the relative objects, the ASW must apply to the County Court on the basis that the objection is unreasonable.
- Applications and recommendations must be received and agreed by the hospital manager who is responsible under the MHA for detaining patients compulsorily.

General points

If, following criminal proceedings, or following a hospital order made by the courts on conviction, informal *voluntary* in-patients are remanded in hospital, they can be compulsorily detained for up to 72 hours if the doctor in charge of treatment considers this appropriate and if the hospital manager approves the recommendation.

Under Section 4, patients may be admitted as emergencies for assessment for up to 72 hours, initially, as an 'urgent necessity'. On a doctor's recommendation this may lead to Section 2 being implemented.

Vagrants and those generally 'at risk' can be compulsorily removed to a psychiatric unit for 72 hours as an appropriate place of safety.

Mentally handicapped patients are regarded as generally outside the provisions of the MHA in that a permanent mental disorder of this type is not contemplated in the Act's definition. Nevertheless, should such a person be regarded as a threat to health and safety, they could still be admitted under the MHA provision.

Consent to treatment

The essential distinction between informal and compulsorily admitted patients is that

- Voluntary patients must consent to treatment
- Compulsorily detained patients can be given routine psychiatric treatment without their consent, but they must give their consent to any physical treatment proposed.

N.B. The usual rules apply to those deemed incompetent to consent. However, a mental illness does not automatically render a patient incompetent to refuse or consent to treatment.

The Mental Health Tribunal is an independent body that hears applications to consider whether the detention of a patient under Section 2 should be renewed at each point of detention. It was set up to provide patients with the means to object to any compulsory procedure they consider should not have been followed. It is not a forum for patients' complaints.

The Court of Protection is an official department of the High Court under the MHA. Its purpose is to regulate the affairs of those with mental incapacity. If a person is sufficiently competent to appoint a Power of Attorney, that person can then act on the patient's behalf once they become incapable. This power must be registered with the Court, which ensures that the power cannot be revoked with judicial consent. The Court retains supervisory powers to cancel power if the donor remains incapable, the registration expires, it was obtained by fraud or under undue pressure or the attorney is deemed unsuitable, and then the Court assumes responsibility. Where no attorney is appointed, the patient's affairs must be placed with the Court, accompanied by a medical certificate confirming incapacity.

Discharge procedures for compulsorily detained patients

The Act gives the following people authority to discharge patients who have been detained compulsorily:

- Registered medical officer
- Hospital manager
- Nearest relative
- Mental Health Review Tribunal (MHRT).

The MHRT directs that a person detained under Section 2 is discharged if, at the time the MHRT considers the case, the person concerned does not have a mental disorder of a nature or degree which warrants detention in hospital for assessment, or assessment followed by treatment, or detention is not justified in the interests of the person's own health and safety, or with a view to the protection of others.

If the above criteria are not met, the Act requires the MHRT to take into account the following matters, in considering whether to use its general discretion to end a Section 2 admission:

- The likelihood of medical treatment alleviating or preventing a deterioration of the person's condition
- In the case of mental illness or severe mental impairment, the likelihood of the person, if discharged from hospital, being able to care for him/herself or obtain the care needed, or the likelihood of the person being able to avoid being seriously exploited.

In the case of people who have been transferred from prison to hospital, and who are subject to a Restriction Direction, the MHRT cannot discharge without the agreement of the Home Office. These will mainly be the cases in the Special Hospitals such as Rampton.

The medical secretary's role

It may be the duty of a medical secretary to fill in relevant documentation for any of these procedures. As always, accuracy is essential. You may also be asked to act as a chaperone in some of the situations described above.

THE GOVERNING BODIES

In addition to the laws of the land, doctors, nurses and other health care professionals are also regulated by their governing bodies, which have statutory power to regulate these professions and to ensure that practitioners who are in breach of their rules are not able to practise. They have a very significant role in protecting the public.

GENERAL MEDICAL COUNCIL (GMC)

To function as a medical practitioner, of whatever type, it is necessary to obtain registration by the GMC – hence the phrase 'Registered Medical Practitioner'. The GMC has a mixture of medical and lay members, was set up by Act of Parliament and is concerned with the standards of medical education, and the ethical and professional standards of practising doctors. Doctors thought to be negligent will be subject to investigation by the GMC. Whistle blowing by colleagues, in the past thought to be unprofessional, is now acceptable providing the correct procedures are followed. The GMC will decide on appropriate action and has brought in systems of regular appraisal and audit to try to raise standards. Doctors who act in an unprofessional way due to ill health may be suspended until they have been adequately treated. If the offence has been a criminal or other serious unprofessional offence, suspension from the medical register may be permanent.

THE NURSING AND MIDWIFERY COUNCIL (NMC)

For nurses, midwives and health visitors the governing body is the Nursing and Midwifery Council (NMC). The NMC has a similar statutory regulatory role to that of the GMC. It is responsible for maintaining the register of professionals who are permitted to practise as nurses and regulates the boundaries of nursing practice. It also provides guidance on ethical issues.

AMSPAR is the comparable organisation for medical secretaries (the Association of Medical Secretaries, Practice Administrators and Receptionists), although it does not have statutory powers over its membership.

Although the issues covered by the NMC and the GMC may not be directly applicable to the work of a medical secretary, nevertheless all workers in health care have to work in the environment set by the law and the statutory bodies.

CHARTERS AND COMPLAINTS

Laws are just one aspect of the rules and regulations that protect patients and govern professionals' behaviour in the health service. Patients and other users of the health service have certain rights, such as those covered by the Patient's Charter. This next section looks at these rights, and, more importantly, at how to deal with the complaints that may emerge if patients do not feel they have received the respect or treatment to which they are entitled. Whenever there is a complaint, people are liable to feel aggrieved, hurt and that their professional position has been challenged or undermined. However, dealt with in the right way, complaints should help to preserve professional standards and improve the standards of health care.

THE PATIENT'S CHARTER

The Patient's Charter, which was introduced in 1992, sets standards and encourages people to complain if those standards are not reached. It lays down guidelines for acceptable standards of care to be delivered to patients and their families in all areas of the NHS. It covers waiting times in open waiting areas, acceptable waiting times for surgery or first appointments, the right to emergency treatment and the right to referral for a second opinion in consultation with a patient's GP. The Charter also gives information about community services, ambulance, dentistry and pharmaceutical services, and has a separate section on the rights and standards that patients should expect from maternity services. The aim is to promote high standards of health care in the UK and the Charter underlines the fundamental values of the NHS, alongside the rights of the patient.

The Department of Health sets guidelines and standards through initiatives and circulars. Hospitals and GP practices are expected to publish their own charters. In general practice there may be an undertaking to offer emergency appointments immediately, or at least on the same day, depending on the degree of urgency. A practice may also offer an undertaking that no appointment is delayed more than 48 hours. Such standards may go to make up the mission statement of the practice or hospital trust. Many organisations publish their mission statements.

Reflection Point 3

The Labour government has reviewed the Patient's Charter in order that it should reflect not only patient's rights but also their responsibilities. Look at a copy of the Patient's Charter. Have you seen (1) your own GP's practice charter (2) your local hospital's charter ? Do they inform the public of their rights and responsibilities? Have they improved services and made providers more accountable? Discuss this with colleagues when you are on placement.

COPING WITH COMPLAINTS

In the past few years, physical aggression against NHS staff has increased enormously. All staff should have training in aggression management. Very often a complainant is merely seeking information as to the reason for a delay or why something appeared to go wrong. Similarly, a person who behaves aggressively may in fact be very frightened or worried. Responding with aggression, sarcasm or belittling the complainant will make the situation worse, and verbal abuse may develop into physical abuse. An inappropriate response may convert a simple inquiry or an expression of anxiety into a formal complaint. Keeping calm and being prepared to understand the other person's point of view or problem will take the heat out of most situations. Make sure that the complainant understands that their complaint will go to the appropriate authority and that it will not be ignored.

Reflection Point 4

Many Trusts have a 'complaints, suggestions or compliments' brochure – what are they trying to suggest here? Try to obtain a copy and find out who is involved in any procedures – which of the above three are going to require procedures? Find out about PALS and Patient Liaison.

COMPLAINTS IN HOSPITAL

In hospital practice there will be procedures for dealing with complaints and a 'Consumer Relations Officer' who will have the authority, the knowledge and the expertise to handle the problem. A sample complaints form is illustrated.

A complaint may be referred to the consultant concerned, so that the complainant may be offered an explanation or, possibly, an apology. A complaint about administration, for example delay in waiting rooms, may be referred to the manager of the unit. A complaint concerning clinical competence will usually be referred to a panel of doctors and laypersons. Many complaints will go straight to hospital man-

agement from the person involved. Complaints may come from a solicitor or from the local Patient Advice Liason Service (PALS) or Public Involvement Forum (PPI). There will normally be an internal mechanism for handling complaints. This mechanism varies from hospital to hospital.

GENERAL PRACTICE COMPLAINTS

In general practice there should be a procedure for handling complaints – this has been obligatory since 1 April 1996. Someone should be appointed to handle complaints. If it is a complaint over appointments or obtaining repeat prescriptions, the appropriate person to handle the complaint may be the practice manager. On clinical matters, the medical partners should handle the complaint. The ultimate responsibility lies with the medical partnership and the involvement of a partner is often essential.

- If the complaint cannot be satisfactorily dealt with at practice level then the complainant, who may not be the patient, may take the complaint to the Public Involvement Forum (PPI) or Primary Care Trust (PCT).
- The complaint may be verbal or in writing.
- Anyone may access the NHS complaints procedure, including relatives or carers and clients.
- Anyone may complain on behalf of another person with written permission.
- The complaint should be made as soon as possible after the event, normally not more than 6 months after the event or 6 months after the injury became apparent.
- A convener will examine the facts after contacting the practice. The convener may suggest changes in the practice or even obtain an apology from the practice.
- If the complainant is not satisfied, an Independent Review Panel may be requested.
- The convener may decide the complaint is sufficiently serious to refer to an Independent Review Panel, and will prepare a report setting out the results of the investigations and making recommendations.
- If the complainant is still not satisfied, there is still the right to refer the case to the NHS Ombudsman.

In all these proceedings, support, information and advice may be obtained from Patient Advice Liason Services.

HELP US TO HELP YOU

HOW TO 'COMPLAIN, MAKE SUGGESTIONS OR COMPLIMENT US'

The Newtown Health Care NHS Trust is committed to looking at ways to improve our service to you. You can help us by telling us what you think of the services we provide, good or bad.

- If you have any suggestions, comments or complaints to make about the services we provide, and the way we provide them, we would be happy to hear from you. We value your comments and can use them when making changes to our services.

- You can use this form to write your comments or complaints on.

- If you need any help or advice to fill in this form, the ward or department staff would be pleased to help you.

- You may wish to contact the Patient Advice Liason Service for free Independent Advice.

YOU CAN MAKE YOUR COMPLAINT BY FOLLOWING THESE GUIDELINES:

- If something happens which causes you concern, we would like to try and put it right straight away. Our staff will make every effort to address your concerns and sort out your problems. If they cannot help, they will arrange for you to speak to someone who can.

- If your complaint is not resolved at that stage you may wish to see your Consultant or the Senior Manager for the area concerned.

- If you are still dissatisfied and wish to make a formal complaint you should contact The Customer Services Manager, Newtown Health Care NHS Trust. Telephone:

OUR STANDARDS FOR DEALING WITH FORMAL COMPLAINTS ARE:

- You can expect us to write to you within 2 days to tell you we have received your letter or call.

- You can expect us to send you a full written response within 28 days.

- If for any reason we are unable to complete the investigation within 28 days, we shall write to you and offer an explanation for the delay.

You may receive a call from someone at the Trust at a later date asking if you were happy with the way in which your complaint was dealt with. You are not obliged to comment on this if you do not wish to.

DATE OF EVENT ....
Suggestion ☐   Comment ☐   Complaint ☐   *(Please tick)*

Similar forms are used by the PCTs.

Figure 3.2 A sample complaints from from a hospital trust

THE HEALTH SERVICE COMMISSIONER (THE OMBUDSMAN)

Essentially, the ombudsman is the final appeal when other mechanisms have failed to produce a satisfactory result for a complainant. All other mechanisms for complaining, outside the law, must have been used. The ombudsman has powers similar to a High Court and can require documents and persons to assist his investigations, but his investigations are carried out in private. In general, he will not investigate if there are ongoing legal or disciplinary investigations.

Originally the ombudsman was only concerned with maladministration within the NHS, but the remit has now been extended to cover clinical matters. Examples of maladministration are:

- Bias, neglect, delay, inattention, ineptitude, perversity, turpitude, arbitrariness, rudeness
- Unwillingness to treat the person as a person with rights
- Failure to answer reasonable questions
- Showing bias because of colour, sex, or any other grounds.

The ombudsman has the power to investigate complaints of a clinical nature once other disciplinary or legal investigations are complete.

It must be remembered there are other mechanisms for complaint. The GMC has been mentioned, with the example of a case of fitness to practise due to ill health or incompetence or unprofessional conduct. A civil action may be instigated to obtain compensation. In some instances the police may bring an action if there is suspicion of criminal neglect.

The medical secretary's role

The primary reason for complaints and resultant lawsuits is often not medical injury itself, but the failure of communication. Medical secretaries are an essential and vital link in that chain of communication. The handling of a complaint, and the handling of a difficult or aggressive person may make a great difference to the outcome of the complaint, reducing stress upon the health care team and also on the complainant. Going through a complaints procedure is just as stressful to the complainant as to the doctor. The best prevention against complaints is to show that you are treating the other person with respect and understanding and, above all, that you care.

EMPLOYMENT LAW

There are also laws that you need to be aware of in your role as an employee within the health service. Employment laws cover the duties and rights of both employers and employees, and are derived through common law and statutory provision, i.e. have been passed by Parliament. The principal legislation regulating employment is the Employment Rights Act 1996. An employment contract is an agreement between employer and employee which contains general terms and conditions, namely:

- Conditions of pay, including holiday benefits and sick pay
- Hours of work.

THE LAW

Within two months of starting work, a statement of particular terms must be sent to the employee, including:

- Job description
- Notice requirements
- Disciplinary procedures (and grievances)
- Length of contract
- Holiday entitlement.

Certain rights and responsibilities affecting both employer and employee have either been incorporated, or implied, by law into all usual employment contracts. Employees' rights include:

- Receiving notice
- Redundancy pay
- Maternity leave
- Protection from discrimination or unfair dismissal
- Conditions of pay including pension schemes and authorised deductions (National Insurance and PAYE)
- Protection from discrimination under the Equal Pay Act 1971, the Sex Discrimination Act 1975, the Treaty of Rome article 119 and the EU equal pay directive and equal treatment directive
- Conditions of employment under the EU Working Hours Directive

Duties to be met by either employer or employee include:

- Conduct which ensures mutual trust and confidence

- Confidentiality (not disclosing employers' confidential information elsewhere)
- Obeying employers' responsible and lawful orders
- Using reasonable care and skill in carrying out employment
- Providing, as an employer, a safe and healthy working environment for staff; this duty is regulated by the Health and Safety at Work Act 1974 and by later supplementary regulations.

Relevance to the medical secretary's role

When taking up employment as a medical secretary, you need to check that you receive your initial contract or letter of appointment, and the statement of particular terms applicable to your role, within two months of starting work. You should note all the terms carefully, particularly the job description. If this includes any duties you are not prepared to undertake, you need to make this clear immediately. An employee who refuses to fulfill all *contractual* obligations may not be able to claim unfair dismissal.

Employees' rights are incorporated by law into the contract and cannot be excluded. Note, however, that these rights can only be exercised after a period of continuous employment. Check this with your practice or hospital manager or official trades union representative. Note that you are legally entitled to join a trades union, or to refuse to do so, if you wish. You are by law protected from verbal and physical harassment during your work. If such an event occurs, it must be reported immediately to your employer or trades union official.

HEALTH AND SAFETY AT WORK ACT 1974

The 1974 Health and Safety at Work Act does not only apply to shops and factories. It lays down an approach to occupational health, safety and welfare and it applies to many premises that are not covered by previous legislation, including laboratories, hospitals and general practice surgeries. Although the occupiers of these premises already owed their visitors the common duty of care, as laid down in the 1957 Occupier's Liability Act, this duty only required reasonable precautions to be taken for their well-being.

The 1974 Act lays down duties on employers (including the self-employed) to provide and maintain a safe place of work. Its aim is to make all employers and employees aware of the need for safety at the place of work. The main requirements are that:

- All facilities are suitable, clean and safe
- Equipment used is safe, with adequate protection provided where necessary
- Hazardous substances are controlled and safely handled
- Refreshment breaks are allowed where rest periods are essential in the operation of certain equipment
- There must be adequate lighting and heating
- There must be provision to prevent industrial diseases such as deafness
- Prevention of Repetitive Stress Injury
- Prevention of eye strain from use of VDUs.

The medical context

The Health and Safety at Work Act is very important in terms of working conditions within the health service. Further regulations of relevance in hospitals and surgery premises are the Control of Substances Hazardous to Health Regulations (COSHH), introduced in 1988, and the regulations introduced by the EC in 1993 (see also Chapter 17). In addition, there is a responsibility to ensure that people visiting the hospital or practice are not put at risk. Public liability insurance is necessary and the certificate must be on public view.

In general practice, it is the practitioner who employs the staff; in the hospital, the Trust employs the staff. Particular areas of concern exist in a surgery or hospital regarding health and safety. These include:

- Handling hazardous substances, including medications, patients' samples, instruments
- Use of X-ray equipment and other potentially dangerous equipment
- Use of VDU screens and X-ray equipment
- Handling difficult or dangerous patients
- Maintaining a particularly thorough standard of hygiene
- Increasing attention is being given to the avoidance of Repetitive Stress Injury (RSI)
- Stress in the work place is now considered a major cause of illness.

Your employer is obliged by law to provide a healthy and safe environment. You should check the surgery's or hospital's standard policy on this, especially as regards handling potentially dangerous equipment or substances (see also Chapter 17). Most noticeably, there should be a policy about the handling of needles and sharps that covers methods of handling them and action in the event of injury. There should be a written policy statement to provide working conditions that are as safe and healthy as possible and to enlist the support of employees to achieve this objective. In addition, employees have a duty to take reasonable care to avoid injury and harm to themselves and their colleagues, and not to misuse equipment and clothing provided for their safety. Employers should offer hepatitis B and other immunisations where appropriate.

It should be noted that employers are only responsible for injuries that occur in the course of an employee's contractual duties. They are not responsible for any activities on your part that result in injury that are not part of your contractual duties. All accidents, no matter how trivial, to patients, staff and visitors must be recorded in an accident book. The book must be kept in a prominent place. The subject is considered elsewhere but it is worth repeating that all specimens, needles and instruments should be considered to be infected. There is no way of knowing which patient has HIV or hepatitis. The hospital infection MRSA is also becoming more prevalent.

The medical secretary is often in a good position to spot possible dangers and hazards, such as a cable crossing the floor, or a place where water has been spilt. If you notice a potential hazard and you cannot deal with it yourself then you should report it to the appropriate person.

THE WHITLEY COUNCIL

The Whitley Council has been involved in setting pay scales within the NHS since 1947. Its remit includes:

- 'To secure the greatest possible measure of cooperation between management and staff of the NHS with a view to increasing efficiency and ensuring the well-being of those employed in the services'
- 'To provide machinery for the negotiations of pay and conditions of service' (General Whitley Council).

The Council has several functional committees covering many professional, administrative and clerical grades of staff. The Whitley Council also has the very important function of hearing appeals if employees are aggrieved by a disciplinary action

taken by an employer. However, Trust hospitals and GPs are not obliged to pay Whitley scales, and whilst there are some advantages in having an independent system of arbitration to settle disputes, and a national standard does reduce the risk of exploitation, the effect of the Whitley Council is gradually diminishing.

DISCRIMINATION AND HARASSMENT

Employment law also links to acts that cover racial and sexual discrimination. These acts prevent an employer discriminating against an employee and ensure equal pay. An employer may not discriminate against an employee on the grounds of gender (including marital status), race, colour, religion, nationality, ethnic group or disability.

SEXUAL HARASSMENT

The Sex Discrimination Act does not specifically mention sexual harassment, but it has been interpreted in common law that an employer discriminates against a woman on the grounds of sex if he treats her less favourably than he treats or would treat a man and the woman suffers a detriment. Significant awards have been made in the courts. In addition, such actions may be construed as constructive dismissal by an industrial tribunal.

Examples of some actions that may constitute sexual harassment include:

- Unwanted and unnecessary physical contact
- Demands for sexual favours with a prospect of promotion or other favours
- Suggestive, lewd, gender-related remarks and innuendoes which are derogatory and offensive
- Sexual assault.

It is possible for men to suffer from sexual discrimination and harassment in the same way as women.

THE DISABILITY DISCRIMINATION ACT 1995

The law

Disability is defined as 'a physical or mental impairment that has a substantial and long term adverse effect on a person's ability to carry out normal day-to-day activities'. The Act makes it illegal for providers of goods, facilities or services to discriminate against people with disabilities. It is also unlawful for an employer of more than 20 people to discriminate against a person with disability, because of their disability. Employers have to make reasonable arrangements to enable people with disabilities to be employed.

The medical context

Hospitals, Health Authorities and possibly some larger practices may have to, for example:

- Alter premises
- Modify procedures
- Supply additional training and training manuals, say, in dealing with deaf or visually handicapped people
- Provide a reader or interpreter.

Health care is a service, and a person with a disability must be offered the same services as anyone else. Services required might include:

- Wheel chair access, and the provision of lifts and hand rails
- Facilities for interpreters for the hard of hearing
- Sighted persons available for reading forms and documents
- Access for guide dogs for a blind person.

The Act means that if someone is disfigured it would be wrong to insist that they sit in a room by themselves whilst waiting for attention. If they prefer to sit by themselves that would be a different matter.

A deaf person may be holding up a queue; it is wrong to ask them to step aside to let other people come first. However, if a person is jeopardising the service for others then the provider would be justified in not providing the same service. Examples could be a person with a disability endangering themselves or others, or disrupting the service for others by unruly behaviour.

Relevance to the medical secretary's role

As a secretary, you cannot be expected to know all the regulations concerning employment. It is, however, important that you know they exist for your protection and the protection of others. If you are unsure, or if you think something is unfair or dangerous, seek advice from your manager, union official or employer. If your employers do not recognise trades unions, the Citizen's Advice Bureau or a solicitor may be your only way of getting advice. For members of AMSPAR there is a legal help line.

CONCLUSION

This chapter has provided an outline of the principles of the laws that affect the health service and also some details about the particular laws you need to be aware of as a medical secretary. These include:

- The legal responsibilities of other members of the health care team
- Your responsibility as part of the health care team to ensure that patients' rights are protected
- Your responsibility as a member of the clinical team to ensure its smooth running and reduce the risk of errors
- Your role as a medical secretary in ensuring that the proper procedures are observed when dealing with legal duties
- The importance of dealing with complaints appropriately when patients believe their rights have been breached
- Your rights as an employee within the health service.

The chapter has demonstrated some of the problems and difficulties of working in health care and how, unwittingly, it is possible to fall foul of the law. Fortunately, there are many sources of advice, including AMSPAR, the Local Medical Committee, and hospitals and Trusts with in-house expertise. There is also one golden rule for all workers in health care: if in any doubt, consult the appropriate authority.

Exercises

Obtain a recent copy of Medeconomics, which goes to every general practice and gives the current Whitley scales with a brief outline of the responsibilities of each grade.

During placements, try to find an opportunity to discuss legal problems with a practice manager or GP. What do they think are the key issues for medical secretaries?

Further reading

BMA 1992 Rights and responsibilities of doctors. BMJ, London

BMA 2001 Injury prevention. BMJ, London

References

BMA 2004 Medical ethics today. BMJ, London

Brazier 1992 Medicine, patients and the law. Penguin, Harmondsworth

DoH 2001 Code of practice for NHS employers

DoH website is a great source of information on such topics as Data Protection Acts, Whitley Council and so on. At www.doh.gov.uk

Dyer C (ed) 1992 Doctors, patients and the law. Blackwell Scientific Publications, London

GMC 2001 Good medical practice. GMC, London

GMC 1998 Seeking patients' consent: the ethical considerations. GMC, London

GMC 1998 Maintaining good medical practice. GMC, London

GMC-uk.org Contains much information on ethics and the fitness to practice

Gostin L 1983 A practical guide to mental health law. MIND Publications, London

Health and Safety Commission Guidance on the recording of accidents and incidents in the health services

Health and Safety Executive Essentials of health and safety at work

Kennedy I, Grubb A 1994 Medical law, 2nd edn. Butterworth Heinemann, Oxford

Knight B 1992 Legal aspects of medical practice, 5th edn. Churchill Livingstone, Edinburgh

McLean SAM 1989 A patient's right to know. Dartmouth, England

Nigel Turner's Hyperguide to the Mental Health Act at www.hyperguide.co.uk/mha. This is a very full account of the Mental Health Act and much more readable then the actual acts. The extracts on the mental health acts are modified from that site.

Chapter 4

Ethics and etiquette

Vincent Leach

OBJECTIVES

- To consider the relationship between law and ethics

- To outline some important codes of ethics

- To describe the main ethical principles

- To examine some aspects of ethics in the medical secretarial role

- To consider some aspects of etiquette in the medical context.

INTRODUCTION

Law tells us what we must do.
Ethics tells us what we ought to do.
Etiquette tells us what we should do.

We have seen in Chapter 3 that many problems in law have an ethical basis or content. Ideally, laws should reflect the moral and ethical standards of the age. Sometimes law is ahead and sometimes it is behind the ethical and moral standards of the country or generation concerned.

At the end of this chapter you should have a basic understanding of medical ethics, and of some of the problems brought about by modern technological medicine and resource allocation and limitation. It is essential that all workers in health care have a general idea of the ethical framework in which doctors and nurses operate.

In addition, there is a discussion of etiquette and how we should treat colleagues and the users of the health services. Professional etiquette is a complex issue for health care professionals, and in this chapter we will be looking at how medical secretaries must be aware of both medical etiquette and their own professional code of conduct set down by AMSPAR (Association of Medical Secretaries, Practice Managers, Administrators and Receptionists).

LAW AND ETHICS

The rapid advance in medical technology can create ethical problems ahead of legal directives. For example, advances in genetic screening may mean that in the future, problems such as heart disease or cancer can be predictable before there is clinical disease. This could mean that getting insurance or a mortgage becomes more difficult or more expensive. You may be aware of debates over *in vitro* fertilisation, surrogacy and the prolongation of the lives of severely malformed babies. The management of patients in persistent vegetative state (PVS) has become a major topic since the death of Tony Bland following the Hillsborough disaster. Euthanasia is a subject that is often discussed in the media.

As a medical secretary you may feel these issues are not of direct interest to you. However, they are becoming matters for great public debate in the media and elsewhere, and everyone should take an interest in these topics in a democratic society. Many secretaries now work in accident and emergency departments, intensive care units, special care baby units, and even on general wards, where these problems arise almost daily. It is important that as a key member of the health care team you are aware of the ethical dilemmas of modern medicine, and have some understanding of the difficulties of working as a health care professional. It is also important that you realise that the actions of a secretary may ease or worsen the problems of patients and their relatives.

As in legal matters, it is essential that you have some knowledge of medical ethics and the framework of modern medicine. People will ask you questions, so being aware of ethical problems and dilemmas will help you to avoid possible errors and pitfalls. As always, if in doubt ask the appropriate authority.

ETHICAL CODES

You will understand that doing the right thing is not always a case of not acting illegally. Ethics is

the word used to describe the philosophical study of right and wrong. Later in this chapter, we will be looking at some of the frameworks and principles of ethics. Firstly, it is helpful to look at an example of an ethical code in medical practice. The most well known example of this is the Hippocratic oath, which provides guidance to help doctors know how they should behave, and reassures their patients that they will be treated as well as possible.

> ### Box 4.1 The modern Hippocratic Oath: the Declaration of Geneva
>
> I solemnly pledge myself to consecrate my life to the service of humanity.
> - I will give to my teachers the respect and gratitude that is their due.
> - I will practice my profession with conscience and dignity.
> - The health of my patient will be my first consideration.
> - I will respect the secrets which are confided in me, even after my patient has died.
> - I will maintain, by all means in my power, the honour and the noble tradition of the medical profession.
> - My colleagues will be my brothers.
> - I will not permit considerations of religion, nationality, race, party politics or social standing to intervene between my duty and my patient.
> - I will maintain the utmost respect for human life from its beginning, even under threat, and I will not use my medical knowledge contrary to the laws of humanity.

THE HIPPOCRATIC OATH

The Hippocratic oath, probably written in the 5th century BC, is the most famous ethical code and is still taken by some, but by no means all, medical students today. The oath has been updated to form the Declaration of Geneva. The texts are written at the end of this chapter.

It is difficult, if not impossible, to establish hard and fast rules to cover all eventualities and situations in modern medicine. Modern medical ethics reflects the influence of many different religions and beliefs. Ethics also tries to establish principles in societies

Reflection Point 1

Some ethical codes are detailed in this chapter. Read them carefully, and think about how they affect your role as a medical secretary working alongside medical professionals.

- Are these principles being adhered to worldwide? Look out for examples of debates on medical problems and developments in the media and discuss them with your colleagues or other students.

- The World Medical Association is an organisation, which debates ethical dilemmas in medical developments. Try to find out more about its impact on ethical thinking.

Reflection Point 2

Compare the AMSPAR Code to the Declaration of Geneva. What similarities and differences can you see?

where many individuals have rejected religious beliefs. Often, ethics comes down to individual conscience and beliefs. Laws are not necessarily the basis of medical ethics, but laws should reflect current feelings and opinions. Medical ethics are often based on principles rather than fixed rules and laws.

In studying this chapter it might be of value to consider each topic in relation to the AMSPAR Ethics Code for medical secretaries. This Code reflects the Declaration of Geneva but is particularly applicable to the secretarial role within the medical team.

ETHICAL PRINCIPLES

THE PRINCIPLE OF DUTY

The technical word for this is deontology. 'Duty' implies that there are certain inviolable rules that should be adhered to. The traditional rules are religious laws. The Ten Commandments from the Old Testament, and part of the background of Judaism, Christianity and the Muslim religions, are a good example; you shall not kill, commit adultery, steal, and you shall respect your parents, and so on. Buddhism has the Noble Truths that are similar rules. Rules such as these imply there is an inherent right and wrong of which we are all conscious.

Box 4.2 The AMSPAR ethics code

AMSPAR members are bound by the following code of conduct:
1. Members will strictly observe and uphold the principles of confidentiality. Anything learned from a patient, a medical practitioner, patients' records or correspondence must never be disclosed to any unauthorised person.
2. Members will establish and maintain professional relationships within the workplace, treating colleagues and employers with respect, refraining from gossip or public criticism of any person. In the event that members have reason to be concerned about the conduct of any colleague or employer (clinical or non-clinical), duty to society at large must outweigh all other considerations and members must report their concerns to the appropriate authorities immediately.
3. Members will strive to foster effective team working with all members of the health care team, placing the needs of patients at the centre of all workplace activities.
4. Members will act within the defined parameters of their personal job role, never taking responsibility for assessing a patient's clinical condition, or initiating prescriptions, and always complying with documented workplace procedures and policies.
5. Members will behave in a manner calculated to maintain the respect and confidence of patients, demonstrating a high standard of professional conduct.
6. Members will make a personal commitment to the principles of continuous professional development and lifelong learning, using all available opportunities to enhance their personal progress and increase their knowledge and understanding.

Reflection Point 3

- Consider 'you shall not kill'. Are there any circumstances in which it would not be unethical to kill another person?

- Are there occasions when to steal might be ethically acceptable?

- Is it always ethically correct to tell the truth?

The difficulty with hard and fast rules is that there are always worthy exceptions. Obviously it would be considered appropriate to kill in self-defence. Unless a pacifist, it would be correct to kill in wartime in defence of one's country. A vegetarian might extend the principle to animal life. It is possible to do great harm if we always tell the truth without considering consequences. An example is how and when we give bad news to a person who has cancer.

Reflection Point 4

Nowadays, it seems straightforward to assume that modern medicine always does 'no harm', but consider the following issues:

- Mr Black is having treatment for raised blood pressure. The treatment makes him lethargic and impotent. Is this doing harm?

- Some inoculations have been linked to cases of brain damage in children. How many cases of brain damage are acceptable to prevent the mass of children getting whooping cough?

- There is a continuing debate about the MMR vaccine.

- Every year there are a considerable number of suicides from paracetamol overdose. Should paracetamol be banned?

Box 4.3 The duties of a doctor registered with the General Medical Council

Patients must be able to trust doctors with their lives and well-being. To justify that trust, we as a profession have a duty to maintain a good standard of practice and care and to show respect for human life. In particular as a doctor you must:

- make the care of your patient your first concern
- treat every patient politely and considerately
- respect patients' dignity and privacy
- listen to patients and respect their views
- give patients information in a way they can understand
- respect the rights of patients to be fully involved in decisions about their care
- keep your professional knowledge and skills up to date
- recognise the limits of your professional competence
- be honest and trustworthy
- avoid abusing your position as a doctor
- work with colleagues in the ways that best serve patients' interests.

In all these matters you must never discriminate unfairly against your patients or colleagues. And you must always be prepared to:

- justify your actions to them
- respect and protect confidential information
- make sure that your personal beliefs do not prejudice your patients' care
- act quickly to protect patients from risk if you have good reason to believe that you or a colleague may not be fit to practice.

THE PRINCIPLE OF CONSEQUENCES

In considering whether or not an act is ethical it may be judged by its outcome, and the technical word for this is consequentialism or utilitarianism. Is the consequence of an act good or bad? Is the action in the person's best interests? Does the action increase the happiness of the person? Does the action benefit society as a whole? Does the action increase the happiness of society as a whole?

Considering consequences alone may lead to further ethical dilemmas and conflicts. A Jehovah's Witness would not accept a blood transfusion, even at

---

Box 4.4 The Tavistock Principles

These principles are for the benefit of all health care workers, not just medical and nursing staff.

Ethical principles

Five major principles should govern health care systems:

1 Health care is a human right.
2 The care of individuals is at the centre of health care delivery but must be viewed and practised within the overall context of continuing work to generate the greatest possible health gains for groups and populations.
3 The responsibilities of the health care delivery system include the prevention of illness and the alleviation of disability.
4 Cooperation with each other and those served is imperative for those working within the health care delivery system.
5 All individuals and groups involved in health care, whether providing access or services, have the continuing responsibility to help improve its quality.

Box 4.5 Advanced directive (living will)

If I should:

- suffer from advanced brain disease such as Alzheimer's Disease
- suffer serious brain damage due to an accident or disease
- be in an advanced or terminal stage of a malignant disease
- be severely incapacitated due to progressive neuro-muscular disease
- be in a condition that is irreversible

I do not wish to be resuscitated, I do not wish a chest infection to be treated, I do not wish to be rehydrated except to relieve obvious suffering.

This is not a comprehensive document but merely indicates some of the features that would be included. The document should be drawn up with medical and or legal advice.

---

the risk of death. Many people believe that life must be prolonged at almost any cost, even at the cost of prolonged suffering. Many believe that life must be prolonged in persistent coma (PVS), or severe dementia, even at great cost to the resources of the health services.

In an attempt to reconcile such cultural differences, a new set of principles has been devised.

Do no harm

The technical phrase is 'non-maleficence'. There is a long tradition, dating from the Hippocratic age, when the saying was 'Above all, do no harm'. (In former times, procedures such as bleeding and purging may have done far more harm than good.)

In modern times it remains difficult to practice medicine without the risk of doing harm. If drugs did not have side effects, if every operation was successful, if risk could be entirely removed, then the principle could be universally applied. However, one can only balance the risks against the possible benefits. A doctor should always try to act in the best interests of the patient. The difficulty is often in deciding what constitutes 'best interests'. Is it in the best interests of the person to be revived from a heart attack and end

up with severe brain damage? A secondary consideration is the best interests of society; for example, whether people suffering from epilepsy should be allowed to drive.

The medical secretary's role

The medical secretary can do harm. Cases of doing harm may legally be cases of negligence. For example, a wrong prescription may do great harm, but the reason for the wrong prescription may be delivery of a wrong message, such as a typing error, by the secretary. Accidents in the operating theatre may arise because of administrative and clerical errors. The wrong kidney may be removed if the notes and X-ray reports are not accurate.

Whilst errors in diagnosis and treatment are obvious instances of harm being done, a much more subtle but no less serious form of harm may arise out of poor communications.

Giving a person bad news requires great skill and understanding. It must be admitted that not all health care professionals have the appropriate skills. As a medical secretary you must not give clinical information without being absolutely certain that you have

Reflection Point 5

Consider what you should do in the following situation. Discussing this scenario with colleagues may be useful.

Mrs White rings up for the result of her cervical smear. What would you say if
(a) if the smear is negative,
(b) if the smear shows abnormal cells?

It may well be that arrangements have been made in a particular department, and with particular patients, that negative results may be given by the secretary. The fact that the secretary will not give the result, but hedges, may in itself cause alarm and panic. For a woman to be told she has abnormal cells in her smear immediately makes her think she will die with cancer of the cervix. Abnormal cells may be due to infection and not all significant abnormalities develop into true malignancy.

the authority to do so. There is great danger in, innocently, giving the results of tests or examinations to patients without first consulting the health care professional concerned. Imagine how much harm may be done if, even with the best of intentions, a secretary makes a comment such as 'Don't worry, this doctor is very good at treating cancer'.

The most important point to remember is that you must consult relevant health professionals regarding the correct procedure in situations like this. Most general practices have a policy to help staff cope with these kinds of problems. Always check with a senior member of the administrative staff on their protocols when you start a work placement or a job.

Do good

'Beneficence' is the technical word; to do good is perhaps the paramount purpose of medicine. It has been said that the motto of the NHS is 'To give years to life, and life to years'. Examples of beneficence in this context include:

- preserving and prolonging life
- recognising and curing disease
- preventing disease

- easing symptoms, including the symptoms associated with dying
- helping people to live as full a life as possible despite the presence of disease or handicap.

Respect for the individual

Respect for 'autonomy of the individual' is the technical phrase. Autonomy means self rule.
Autonomy implies:

- autonomy of thought – the ability to think for oneself, to have likes and dislikes, to have beliefs and the ability to make judgments

Reflection Point 6

Consider the following cases:

- If a patient were suffering from terminal cancer, would it be of benefit to resuscitate him after he has taken an overdose?

- A patient has had a severe stroke, is paralysed, cannot speak, and is distressed by a catheter. Because he cannot swallow he is fed through a gastrostomy (an artificial opening through the abdominal wall). The GP has been called because the patient has developed pneumonia. Should the GP treat the pneumonia?

- When should a foetus be given the status of a human being?

- What serious conditions would justify a termination of pregnancy? Would the presence of cleft palate and hare lip be a justification for termination?

- Is the principle of 'double effect' a fudge to allow doctors to end the life of some patients?

- It is considered to be ethical to withhold treatment if this means prolonging suffering, or if treatment would be futile. Is there a difference between withholding treatment and discontinuing treatment?

- In IVF, should an embryo be selected to be able to benefit a sibling?

- autonomy of will – the ability to make decisions for oneself
- autonomy of action – the ability to perform acts voluntarily.

Respect for individuals is very important and is epitomised by informed consent. We discussed consent in Chapter 3 in its legal context, and identified that fact that treatment without consent may be considered in law to be an assault.

It frequently happens that a person is not autonomous, is not capable of giving consent. For example, a person may be unconscious or otherwise severely ill. In such circumstances the doctor has to act in what is considered to be the patient's best interest.

It can be a great help if there is a written statement from the person stating under what circumstances they would not wish to be resuscitated. A document of this kind is called an Advanced Directive or Living Will. It does carry the weight of law, and to disobey the instructions may give rise to legal penalties. A sample Advanced Directive is given in Box 4.5. If there is an Advanced Directive, the secretary must ensure that it is included in the medical notes and that health care professionals are aware of that fact.

Paternalism

The opposite of respect for autonomy is paternalism. The traditional medical model is paternalistic. Having made a diagnosis, a doctor has in the past been expected to give instructions as to what the patient should do to cure the disease: 'Doctor knows best'. This attitude was acceptable when the doctor was much more highly educated than most of his patients. With increasing education gained from the television and Internet, people now have greater knowledge of medical facts. Increasingly, patients want to know more about their condition, proposed treatments and the consequences of different treatments or of no treatment. Acting in the best interests of the patient, it might be necessary for a doctor *not* to give all the relevant information, and to make the decision for the patient, because the patient is incapacitated by confusion or extreme pain. It may be that some people cannot make decisions for themselves.

Deciding if a person is capable of making decisions and therefore autonomous can present great difficulties. A person of sound mind may refuse any treatment even if this leads to death. There have been

Reflection Point 7

- A simple example is building a by-pass. This may improve the lifestyle of the inhabitants of a village as whole. But if you run a village shop, would you be so keen if you might lose trade?

- A more complex example is using animals for drug testing. Do you think that the benefits to individuals or to society as a whole justify experiments of this kind? You may feel differently depending on whether the tests are aimed at finding a cure for cancer, or just another type of cosmetic.

- Should a girl under the age of 16 be prescribed the pill? This may be considered purely from the deontological point of view. Is it right or wrong? By prescribing the pill are you encouraging an illegal act. From the consequential point of view, is it better that she does not have an unwanted child?

- Should a wife be told her husband has an alcohol problem? Is telling in the patient's best interests? His wife will need to support him and needs appropriate advice and support. Which principle over-rides another? Does confidentiality over-ride benefit?

- What should be done in the case of a 16-year-old who requests a termination of pregnancy, and insists her mother is not informed?

Many of these problems are almost daily occurrences in modern medical practice.

cases of anorexia nervosa (also known as 'slimmer's disease') where individuals have refused treatment and died. Life-saving surgery is sometimes refused. It is especially difficult to decide whether a child can be considered autonomous and free to make decisions about their health care (see discussion of the Gillick case in Chapter 3).

Reflection Point 8

Imagine there is one kidney available for donation. In the ward are the following individuals:

- A child
- A child with severe learning disabilities
- A mother with two children
- A man of 70.

To whom would you give the kidney? Would it make any difference if the normal child is an orphan? Would it make any difference if the mother is an alcoholic who has neglected her children? Would it make any difference if the man is a famous scientist who is close to finding a cure for cancer? Consider the resource constraints within the NHS. Should they have any influence on how decisions are made?

The case of Miss B

Miss B was paralysed from the neck downwards. She was completely helpless and kept alive on a respirator. She was completely rational and decided her life was not worth living. She requested that her respirator be turned off. Her doctors refused this request. An appeal to the courts of law gave permission for the respirator to be turned off.

- Were her doctors acting paternalistically and not respecting her autonomy in refusing to turn off the respirator?
- Was this an act of suicide? Suicide is not illegal, but helping someone to commit suicide is illegal.

Everyone has the right to refuse treatment, even if this refusal leads to their death. In the case of Miss B, she was transferred to another hospital where the respirator was turned off. In the first hospital, it was against the doctors' principles to turn off the respirator. There was respect for the doctors' principles and respect for their autonomy. No doctor can be compelled to act against his/her ethical principles.

Conditions such as termination of pregnancy and prescribing contraception are cases in point. If there is a conflict of conscience the doctor must withdraw from the case. In those circumstances the doctor must refer the patient to another doctor.

The Diane Pretty case

Diane Pretty was suffering from Motor Neurone disease and completely helpless. She could not even feed herself, and was faced with the prospect of death by drowning in her own saliva. She applied to the courts for permission for her husband to help her commit suicide. Permission was not granted. To deliberately kill is murder or assisting suicide, and both these acts are illegal in this country.

When Miss B refused to give permission for her treatment to continue, this was an autonomous act. Diane Pretty's case was considered as an application to sanction a deliberate killing, even though it might be considered just as humane.

Consider the position of a doctor is who treating a person with terminal cancer. The patient is in considerable pain. A dose of morphine, sufficient to control the pain, stops the patient breathing. Is this manslaughter, murder or negligence? The intention was to control pain and the death was a side effect. This is the so-called double effect. (The same principle is used to justify civilian casualties in a bombing raid. The intentions were to damage a military target not the civilians.) In the case of the patient receiving the dose of morphine, if the patient *requested* the high dose of morphine, the doctor's compliance could be considered to be physician-assisted suicide and therefore illegal.

Justice and fairness

A very important ethical principle is that of justice. In an ideal world, 'to each according to his need' would be the universal principle. In all health care systems there are constraints due to limitation of resources. Even if there were no financial limits, there would still be limits on, say, the number of hearts or kidneys available for transplantation.

Reflection Point 9

Is it unfair, in high profile conditions, if publicity in the press and media means that those cases get more resources than other low profile conditions? What difference is it likely to make if a famous person supports a particular cause such as AIDS? Other causes might not attract so much media interest – do they suffer as a result?

Reflection Point 10

- Consider how you would feel if the next time you went to your doctor, you discovered that your next-door neighbour was the new secretary at the practice. How might someone who was HIV positive feel in the same circumstances?

- Look around your office or surgery; can you see areas where confidentiality might be breached?

One school of thought states that all human beings are of equal value. Any decision should be made on the basis that all lives are of equal value. The following quotation is from the Talmud, a Jewish legal text.

> *He who destroys a single life is charged as if he destroyed a whole world and whoever rescues a single life is credited as if he saved the whole world.*

For decisions to be just and fair, all people must have an equal consideration and assessment of their wants and needs. Having assessed the problems, decisions must be made as to what options are possible on the basis of potential benefits. What should be done, and what is best for the patient, considering the patient's priorities? Decisions must be made according to what is available within a particular health care system.

Consider the following case. A mother brings her child to hospital. The child has multiple severe deformities and has not long to live. It may be said that the child has a very poor quality of life. The child is in kidney failure and the mother insists the child has dialysis and, ideally, a kidney transplant.

- Is this the correct use of resources?
- Can a patient demand every possible treatment under the NHS?
- Should one individual demand resources at the expense of other?
- Should a smoker be offered cardiac by-pass surgery?
- Should an alcoholic be offered a liver transplant?

These cases demonstrate the problems in allocating resources between paediatrics, care of the mentally ill, and care of the elderly, as examples. Whether the problem is infertility or serious life-threatening disease, every sufferer wants the maximum resources for their condition.

It is not the responsibility or role of the secretary to make judgments or even to make comments about these matters. If there appears to be an injustice then the person should be referred to the appropriate authority for consideration of his or her case. A citizen has the right to expose injustice and illegal practices to the legal authorities and to the press and media. If injustice is apparent then a secretary's employers should be consulted first. If satisfaction is not received then the secretary perhaps has a moral right to publicise this injustice – whistleblowing – but this will be at some personal risk (see the AMSPAR code of conduct).

ETHICAL ISSUES IN THE MEDICAL SECRETARIAL ROLE

Chapter 5 is devoted to the ideal qualities of the medical secretary. In this chapter, we will discuss the practical considerations of how we promote ethical behaviour, looking at the important principles of confidentiality and discrimination.

Confidentiality

We have discussed the principle of non-maleficence, of not doing harm. The medical secretary is in a position to do great harm by breaching confidentiality. The breach may be innocent, but it may be damaging nonetheless.

Confidentiality of patient information means that only the person concerned has the authority to give permission for any information to be given to a third party.

Some requests for information may appear to be reasonable and innocent. They may appear to be in the best interests of the person concerned. There may be strong and cogent reasons why a wife may not wish her husband to know she is attending her doctor: maybe she has gone to discuss her husband's mental state or drinking habits, or her own personal problems, and does not wish her husband to know. The reasons for an action are a matter of confidence between the person and his or her health care professional and are nothing to do with anyone else. Even the name and address of a person may be of great significance. It is not uncommon for a woman to be frightened that her estranged husband should find out where she is living.

A doctor may break the confidentiality rule if he or she considers it to be in the person's best interests. As

Reflection Point 11

What would you do under these circumstances?

• A man rings to ask if his wife has attended clinic or surgery.

• A mother rings up to ask if her 14-year-old daughter is on the pill.

• A policeman asks if someone with particular injuries or identification marks attended accident and emergency or surgery.

a secretary you may be involved in these and similar actions; for example, in contacting the police or the Driver and Vehicle Licensing Authority (DVLA) so that your employer can give them information. As indicated in Chapter 3 it is the doctor's, not the secretary's, responsibility to divulge information. This might be in the person's best interests or in the interests of society as a whole. It may well be the doctor's decision to notify the DVLA when an epileptic continues to drive. If a serious crime has been committed then information may be given to protect society. A doctor should be obliged to notify cases of child abuse or neglect. In either case the doctor may have to justify his or her action in a civil court or in front of the GMC.

Examples of office procedures which might compromise confidentiality include:

• several people at the reception desk at the same time and able to hear each other's conversation
• the telephone within earshot of other people at the desk
• case notes, pathology, laboratory and X-ray results lying around in full view
• free access to the computer with patients' data (check that passwords are safeguarded and used correctly. See also Chapter 8 on using computers)
• fax machines placed in public areas (make sure that if you are sending confidential information by fax it will arrive at the right number and will only be read by the correct health care professional)
• calling across the waiting room (for example, it would not be appropriate to call out messages

about people's prescriptions, such as 'Your prescription for the pill is ready')
• putting confidential material in a waste bin; it should be shredded.

With the use of passwords and encryption of transmitted data, and protection from the Data Protection Act, it might be felt that everything possible has been done to protect confidential information within a computer system. The weak link in the chain is the human being. It is no use having sophisticated techniques if a secretary can be persuaded to hand over information by payment of a bribe or a promise of favours, even though this is illegal.

In some instances confidentiality is broken legally. There is compulsory registration of births, marriages and deaths. Wills become public knowledge. Income tax inspectors have access to information about our earnings. Doctors have to notify the authorities about certain infectious diseases.

For the benefit of their patients, doctors share information and pass it on to each other.

• When a person first registers with a GP, information is passed to the person doing the registration. This is passed to the PCT and details sent to the central register.
• Records are sent from the old GP to the PCT, then to the new PCT and finally on to the new GP and the secretarial staff. At all the different stages lay people are handling confidential information.
• When a person is referred to hospital, personal details are included with clinical information.
• In some instances, clinical information is open in a hospital referral form
• Secretaries concerned with costing and purchasing have access to clinical details.
• Results of tests and X-rays pass through non-medical hands.

Confidentiality and the Data Protection Acts

There is a great deal of information going around the NHS and other agencies, much of it within easy access of those who do not have the right to know. The Data Protection Acts are there to protect peoples' confidentiality, and they cover both computerised and paper records.

People have the right to see their own medical records. There is, however, an element of discretion; if the doctor considers a piece of information may harm the individual it may be withheld. Details of a third party would also be withheld.

Data is essential to plan and prepare developments. There has to be a balance between what is essential for an efficient health care system and preserving personal confidentiality. To reconcile these differences the Caldicott Committee was set up. The Committee established a series of rules for the release of information, including:

- formal justification of purpose for disclosure
- information transferred only when absolutely necessary
- only the necessary information used
- 'need to know' access controls
- all users to understand their responsibilities, comply with and understand the law.

A senior person, preferably a health professional, should be nominated in each health organisation to act as guardian responsible for safeguarding the confidentiality of patient information. This person is the Caldicott Guardian.

As a medical secretary, you are the guardian of a great deal of information. Do not be tempted to look up details about your family, friends or acquaintances out of mere curiosity. In some organisations this would be an act warranting instant dismissal. All health care information should only be seen by those who 'need to know'.

Always be vigilant about confidentiality. If you see places where there may be breaches, discuss the matter with your manager or employer. Always be on your guard. If in doubt, seek guidance. If you are aware that confidentiality might be threatened, check what the health professional intends. Confidentiality is referred to in the AMSPAR Code of Conduct, this emphasises just what a crucial aspect of your practice it should be.

It must be remembered that confidentiality continues after the death of a patient. Details may not be released, even after death, apart from the legal requirements of death certification. A doctor will discuss with close relatives the circumstances of a death. However, the doctor must be very careful not to reveal facts that the ex-patient would have not wished to be disclosed. For example, information about sexual indiscretions or drug use might be withheld.

Discrimination

In Chapter 3, we discussed some of the legislation that aims to prevent discrimination, but discrimination is also an ethical issue. When we were discussing justice and fairness earlier in this chapter, it was emphasised that everyone has equal rights to medical treatment, regardless of their race, gender or religious beliefs. Equally, these differences should be recognised and respected. As a medical secretary it is essential that you do not discriminate against anyone. Discrimination is illegal and unethical, and is in breach of professional conduct.

Discrimination can be overt; for example, a receptionist could refuse someone access to the doctor because she didn't like the way he looked or behaved. However, most discrimination is covert and sometimes people are unaware, at a conscious level, that their behaviour or actions are unjust and unfair. For example, many practice leaflets and notices might only be available in English and therefore information is unlikely to be readily available to people whose first language is not English.

Most hospitals will have a written policy regarding discrimination and some Trusts may have Equal Opportunities personnel. Try to find out the policy in your work area and read any leaflets that are available. Always be vigilant about your own attitudes, and try and be aware of how discrimination arises, and can therefore be countered.

ETIQUETTE

There are books of etiquette showing how to address a bishop or a knight, and how to lay a dinner table. This section is more to do with how we treat each other and show each other respect, irrespective of race, creed or social standing.

Reflection Point 12

You may think that discrimination is only about race, but there are many ways in which people are discriminated against. Women, children, old people, people with mental illness, those who are HIV positive can all be victims of discrimination. Think of ways in which access to health care services might discriminate against different kinds of people.

Many contacts with the health services take place over the telephone or over a reception desk. The initial contact may be a person's first contact with the NHS, the hospital or the practice. The manner of this introduction may colour the rest of the consultation or affect the attitude of the person on admission. Telephone skills, and other techniques of handling people, will be covered in Chapter 5. However, it is worth repeating that you should always be polite, give your name and ask in what way you may help. Do not keep people waiting too long without acknowledging their presence and apologising for any delay; preferably give some explanation for the delay.

Titles may be important to some people. It is worthwhile finding out if a woman prefers to be referred to as Ms, Miss or Mrs. Some people prefer to be referred to by their first name, other people will find this too familiar and be offended. Some people will prefer an even more formal approach and wish to be called Sir or Madam. You will only learn the correct approach by experience, so you should be prepared to alter your approach if it seems to be causing offence. It is best to use a more formal approach first, changing to a more informal approach when the barriers have been broken down. Among colleagues, the same techniques apply. An office manager may prefer to be called by his or her first name. Some doctors and employers may prefer the intimacy of first names.

There is often confusion, especially in hospitals, as to the correct title for a member of the medical staff. The rule is that surgeons are called Mister and the rest are called doctor. Most medical practitioners have separate degrees in surgery and medicine. Some countries, such as the USA, have a combined degree of MD and all medics are referred to as Doctor. Therefore, if you are in contact with an American surgeon, he or she will be referred to as Doctor.

MANNERS AND ATTITUDES

The use of the correct title is relatively unimportant. Manners and attitudes *are* important. In the section on autonomy we discussed how all people are entitled to respect, purely as human beings, irrespective of age, sex, colour, ethnic or religious group or social or economic class. It is one of the fundamental principles of the NHS that all should be treated equally according to need.

The scruffy unkempt man in front of you may be a

Reflection Point 13

Next time you ring up an organisation, listen to the telephone technique. Are you treated as a person? Is the approach brusque or condescending? How long are you kept waiting? Did you get irritated and frustrated?

Reflection Point 14

Next time you go into a bank, building society, travel agent or other business, observe techniques. How are customers treated? Are different customers treated with different levels of respect and etiquette?

Reflection Point 15

Refer again to the AMSPAR Ethics Code. Which parts of the code are specific to medical etiquette? Why is it necessary for AMSPAR to make this statement? Consider these statements when reading this section.

wealthy farmer, not a tramp. Even if he is a tramp, his medical needs could be very great and should be considered impartially. Appearances may be very deceptive. Attitudes may also be deceptive. The most aggressive person may be the most frightened person. The aggressive person under the influence of drugs or alcohol may well be pacified by a calm approach, by proper etiquette, and by not responding with aggression.

Tact and diplomacy are required in handling all people, but especially those who are acutely or even terminally ill. Tact is required in handling those who are concerned about their loved ones or have been bereaved. Treat everybody in the way you would prefer to be treated under those circumstances. Try to put yourself in their position. Above all, the AMSPAR Code states that you must 'at all times behave in a manner calculated to maintain respect and confidence of patients'.

MEDICAL ETIQUETTE

There are also issues of medical etiquette which are very relevant to your role as a medical secretary. Medical etiquette is primarily concerned with how health care professionals treat each other. As a secretary, you will be involved in these matters.

In general, except in an emergency, it is not ethical for a doctor to see another doctor's patient without the consent of the doctor. This is the basis of the referral system within the NHS and in private practice. One doctor must not charge a fee or obtain a fee from another doctor for a referral.

The GP is the holder of the total patient record and responsible for continuity of care. This is of great value within the NHS and does not apply in many other health care systems around the world. If a doctor has seen a patient of another doctor then he or she should inform the patient's doctor about the diagnosis and action taken. If one doctor refers to another, all relevant information must be made available. It may be a secretary's task to collect and send this information. A secretary could be of great help in checking that the necessary notifications and letters have been sent.

PROFESSIONAL CRITICISM

It is not ethical for one doctor to criticise the actions of another. If there is a risk of professional misconduct or negligence, contacting the appropriate governing body would be justified. Therefore, it would not be ethical for a member of his or her staff to criticise another doctor.

Criticism is sometimes indirect. A hospital doctor may say to a relative, 'We could have done more if the patient had been referred earlier'. There may be an implied criticism of the GP whose management of the case may have been quite correct. Even if this was in fact the case, it is not for another doctor to criticise. By extension, it is not correct for a member of staff to criticise another professional. This is not objecting to 'whistleblowing' or advocating a professional closed shop. In your role, you must beware of repeating comments you may have heard outside the practice, or of becoming involved in discussions with anyone about the practice of the people who work there.

ADVERTISING

Doctors do not advertise in the commercial sense. It is

Reflection Point 16

- You work for a private doctor and someone wishes to see your employer without a reference from another doctor. What should you do?

- A person starts to criticise a doctor who is not your employer. You know some of the criticisms may have some justification. Discuss how you would handle such a situation with your colleagues.

acceptable for doctors to give information in a practice leaflet or to notify colleagues that they are available for consultations. To suggest or even imply an excellence or superiority over colleagues is not acceptable. This principle extends to your role as a medical secretary and it is not acceptable for you to recommend any doctor or health professional to anyone in a way that might compromise other professionals.

PERSONAL PREJUDICES

Doctors must not let their own beliefs or views on a patient's lifestyle, culture or beliefs affect their judgment or any treatment given or arranged. If there is conflict because of personal beliefs between a patient and the doctor then the doctor should inform the patient of his or her right to see another doctor. This might apply when there is a request for contraception or termination of pregnancy, contrary to the doctor's own personal values. In these and similar cases the patient should be referred to another doctor. It is essential that the beliefs and opinions of any members of staff are not permitted to interfere with everyone receiving the appropriate medical care to which they are entitled.

The doctor–patient relationship is built on trust. Comments and actions by other members of the health care team can damage or even destroy that trust and do irreparable harm to the patient.

CONTINUITY OF CARE

Doctors are responsible for making sure there is continuity of care for their patient. In hospital this may mean a junior is responsible for the day-to-day management of a case, but the ultimate responsibility rests with the specialist. This is especially relevant to your role as a medical secretary, as you may have to be aware of who is on call for emergency admissions and who is deputising for the doctor concerned. In general practice, a partner or deputising service might be on call. You may have to find a locum for your employer. It is essential that you are aware of the deputising arrangements within a practice, whether a general practice or within a suite of specialists. The medical secretary's role is to ensure that relevant information is relayed to guarantee continuity of care.

CONCLUSION

To be an effective member of a health care team it is essential to know something of the ethical framework within which health care professionals have to work. Increasing demands, new techniques and resource limitation are altering the framework almost daily. Be prepared for new ideas and attitudes, but remember that the basic principles that we have discussed in this chapter should always inform the way you think and act in your role as a medical secretary.

Exercises

- Try and discuss some of the issues and reflection points raised in this chapter with colleagues and friends. Look out for cases that are reported in the media and discuss them too. Try and get as many facts as possible and try, as far as possible, to remove bias and prejudices when thinking or discussing the problems.

- Make a list of all the ways in which confidentiality can be breached. Think about the physical layout of work areas. Think about access.

- Think about the different forms of patient notes and information there may be – how do we safeguard them?

- Is there a practice/department policy laid down for these areas of work, such as confidentiality or discrimination? Where do you find it?

Further reading

Beauchamp TL and Childress JF 1989 Principles of biomedical ethics. OUP, Oxford
  This is perhaps the best textbook for anyone wishing to study medical ethics in more detail, but it is not light reading. It is the ethicist's 'bible'.
BMA 2004 Medical ethics today. BMJ Publishing, London
  This gives the BMA opinion on most subjects and is very useful for reference.
Caldicott report: www.doh.gov.uk/confidence/crep
Cohen SL 1993 Whose life is it anyhow? Robson Books, London
  This is a very readable account of some of the problems encountered in intensive care units.
Declaration of Geneva: www.wmw.net
Gillon R 1986 Philosophical medical ethics. John Wiley, Chichester
GMC 2001 Good medical practice. GMC, London
McDowell J, Stewart D 1988 Concise guide to today's religions. Scripture Press, England
Orme-Smith, Spicer J 2001 Ethics in general practice. Radcliffe Medical Press, Abingdon
Phillips, Dawson 1985 Doctor's dilemmas. Harvester Wheatsheaf, London.
  This is probably the most readable book on medical ethics.
Singleton J, McLaren S. 1995 Ethical foundations of health care. Mosby, Edinburgh
Tavistock Principles: http://bmj.com/talks/tavistock/
This site is presented as a slide show, and is a good entry point for finding many other related websites.

SECTION 2

Fundamentals of medical secretarial practice

Chapter 5

The qualities of the medical secretary

Tracy A Grafton

CHAPTER CONTENTS

OBJECTIVES

- To provide a broad overview of the role and qualities of the medical secretary
- To assist the reader to evaluate personal strengths and weaknesses
- To outline appropriate coping strategies
- To stimulate debate and discussion
- To promote professional behaviour and supply a code of conduct
- To encourage self-development.

INTRODUCTION

What do we mean by 'qualities'? The dictionary defines a quality as 'a characteristic, something that is special in a person or thing'. This chapter will examine a range of key characteristics of direct relevance to the work of a medical secretary. We present a combination of personal qualities and professional skills, all of which are desirable in a medical secretary. The chapter does not aim to provide an exhaustive list but rather a summary. From the premise that we all have highly individual characteristics, we will aim to highlight those of most value to the medical secretary in the workplace. Whilst reading, use the reflection points and scenarios to evaluate your own qualities. Identify any areas of weakness and list your strong points.

Working as a medical secretary can be a most rewarding and challenging experience, and improving your performance and capabilities will help you to become a valued member of the health care team. It is essential for all medical secretaries to become aware of their potential in order to contribute effectively to the care of patients and to achieve job satisfaction. A medical secretary is expected to perform a wide range of tasks competently and efficiently, and an office which runs smoothly will be a huge benefit to the organisation.

The majority of the qualities outlined in this chapter can be brought together under four general titles: confidentiality, cooperation, commitment and courtesy – the 4Cs.

CONFIDENTIALITY

The relationship between patient and doctor is based on a foundation of confidentiality and trust. Medical ethics and etiquette are fully discussed in Chapter 4, which demonstrates that the provision of health care is underpinned by a code of ethics. The medical secretary must uphold this code and maintaining confidentiality is an essential requirement. The Association of Medical Secretaries, Practice Managers, Administrators and Receptionists (AMSPAR) publish an Ethics Code which all members must observe. The first point of this code states that any information learned from a patient, the patient's record, a medical practitioner or correspondence must never be disclosed to any unauthorised person.

The medical secretary should never initiate unauthorised release of information and must remember that the prime objective is to provide a confidential service to each individual patient. This may create difficulties when dealing with a patient's relatives, who may be distressed, anxious and in need of information. As a medical secretary, you will frequently be the first point of contact for many of these callers and you will need skills to cope effectively.

This type of conversation will be a common occurrence in any health care environment. Your initial reaction should include attentive listening, noting the salient points of the conversation and empathising with the caller. What it should not include is any indication of the patient's condition or other personal information. This caller is looking for information which you cannot supply. The conversation should

Scenario 1

You receive a telephone call from the wife of a patient whose family are well known to you. You also know that the husband has elected not to reveal the extent of his illness to his family at present. The family have observed his decline and are very distressed to not have any definite information. His wife asks about her husband's illness. She asks you directly to reveal his diagnosis and becomes angry at the lack of information the family have had so far. She explains her worry and is obviously in a very emotional state.

What is your initial reaction to this caller? How will you answer her question? What type of assistance might you be able to provide?

be relayed to the medical practitioner who will decide what further action is required. Most of all, this caller needs to be listened to in a kind and respectful manner, but the patient's right to privacy must be maintained.

You may be working in an area where a member of staff (perhaps from your team) is under the care of one of the doctors you work for. Colleagues will be naturally curious about their diagnosis, care and treatment and it must be remembered that they are entitled to the same high level of confidentiality as any other patient. The same applies for a doctor who is off sick; the reason why is not necessarily for public knowledge.

Reflection Point 1

Identify two more examples of situations where you will be required to maintain confidentiality whilst dealing with enquiries from relatives. What external factors may compromise confidentiality in the workplace?

You have a duty to protect any patient-related information in your care. You should become aware of the external factors which may compromise confidentiality.

COMPUTERS

Most hospitals and practices will use computers to store patient information, and the subject of information technology is covered in Chapter 8. You will probably use a word processor to produce clinic letters, summaries and reports. During the course of your work, you may be called away from your computer at short notice to deal with other enquiries and events. When presented with interruptions you should, if possible, save the unfinished document and file it before leaving your office. Alternatively, the information can be protected by turning off the screen so that visitors to the office will not be able to see it.

Screensavers are a common feature with computer packages and whilst these offer privacy for whatever is on the screen, the use of 'unprofessional' looking screensavers reflects badly on both you and the organisation. It is important, therefore, that you think carefully before you customise your computer screensaver to show the latest Hollywood heart-throb!

Many hospitals and GP practices are now using email as a form of communication for sending in patient referrals and other patient-related correspondence. If this is the case in your particular work area, be extra vigilant about the email address you are sending letters to and, if in doubt, check with the receiver that this is an acceptable means of communicating patient information.

WRITTEN INFORMATION

Despite the introduction of computers, most patient information is still received and stored on paper. These documents are confidential and should always be treated with care. Incoming correspondence should be placed inside a file or folder before being distributed to the medical staff or other team members. If you are called away whilst using patient records, you should cover letters or close the medical notes before leaving them unattended. Staff medical records should never be left on an unattended desk and are normally filed in a separate area with restricted access (normally the Medical Records Manager in a hospital and the Practice Manager in a surgery will have access).

A 'clear desk' policy at night should be encouraged and used wherever possible to ensure that confidential papers and other items such as patient correspondence are locked away out of sight overnight.

TELEPHONE

The telephone is widely used in all health care environments. If conversations conducted via the telephone may be overheard by others, you need to be aware of a possible breach of confidentiality. When speaking to patients, ensure that your responses are appropriate if you are not alone. This is particularly relevant if you are working in a reception area as members of the general public may be queuing at reception to make appointments, collect prescriptions or ask for information. If you find yourself in this position, you should avoid using the patient's full name, address or telephone number as these may provide bystanders with enough clues to identify the person. If the call is a routine enquiry, this should not present you with too many difficulties. However, if the call requires more in-depth discussion, it would be preferable to transfer it to another telephone or to telephone the caller back to ensure a reasonable degree of privacy.

You must also be cautious when telephoning a patient as they may be at work or have visitors and may feel unable to speak to you openly. Under these circumstances an individual may appear uninterested, uncommunicative or obstructive. If contacting a patient on a mobile phone, again, it may be difficult for them to speak, either due to the environment they are in at that particular moment or because signal reception is poor. It should become part of your routine to check that the patient feels able to have the conversation before you continue.

MESSAGES

Leaving a message presents a further risk to confidentiality and should be avoided if at all possible. However, if you are contacting someone as a matter of urgency, restrict your message to your name, organisation or the name of the doctor you work for and telephone number and ask that the person contacts you. It may be beneficial to state up until what time you can be contacted. Also be aware that whoever is taking the message may ask you what your call is about and prompt you for further information, which you should never give. Answerphones are now common both in the workplace and in many homes so be aware that you can never be sure that only the patient will hear the message.

FACSIMILE MACHINES

As with answerphones, the fax has become a common method of communication and many practices and hospitals now use this as a routine method of communicating referral letters (particularly urgent ones), results and urgent clinic/discharge letters. It is important to check whether the recipient's fax is a safe haven (i.e. placed in a secure area). If not, ask that the recipient of the fax stands by the machine while you fax the correspondence through. Check the fax number and ask the recipient to ring you to confirm that they have received the fax safely.

CARELESS TALK

General discussions with work colleagues about patients should be avoided. Discussing patients with anyone outside the workplace is unacceptable under any circumstances. However, discussing individual patients' needs with colleagues is frequently necessary but should be undertaken at appropriate times in appropriate surroundings using appropriate language in a professional manner. You should ensure that the conversation cannot be overheard by anyone other than the members of the team who are involved in that person's care. If circumstances arise where you need to exchange information in front of others, do not identify the patient by name. It may be possible to use other general identifiers, such as 'The lady you saw first thing this morning telephoned to say...' or 'Your patient with the tumour from yesterday wants to talk to you again'. Each situation should be judged individually and if there is any doubt, wait for a more suitable opportunity.

COOPERATION

The following phrase is frequently used in job advertisements: 'must be willing to work as part of the team'. What exactly does this mean? An effective team is created when attention is paid to the attitudes, skills and qualities of the team members and the concept of an effective team is based on cooperation and communication. A team cannot be effective if its members do not cooperate to achieve their objectives and if communication is poor. The criteria for being a good team member are not easily measured but certain key characteristics can be found in all efficient teams.

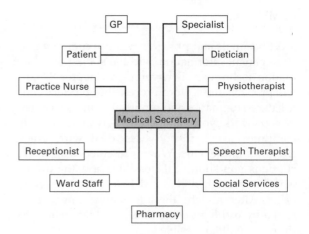

Figure 5.1 The medical secretary and the health care team

COMMUNICATION

The sharing of knowledge and information with other team members is a prime factor in effective teamwork. The medical secretary will often find herself at the centre of a health care team with responsibility for ensuring clear, accurate and appropriate communication of information (Figure 5.1).

The constituent members of a team will be determined by the individual patient's needs and will therefore by definition, be multi-disciplinary. Throughout the period of care, information will be exchanged between members of the team and this will often be facilitated by the medical secretary.

Scenario 2

One of the medical staff has requested that you arrange a team meeting to review the case of Mrs Sanders. This will be the second team meeting relating to Mrs Sanders. Consider what you need to do. Devise an action plan to follow. What information needs to be communicated? How will you achieve this?

Team meetings of this nature are common in both general practice and hospital departments. You should firstly have considered the date, time and

Scenario 3

At the case meeting, you were requested to take notes. A list of action points were identified for immediate attention. The physiotherapist had been unable to attend. The team leader is going away for two weeks and asks you to ensure the necessary follow-up action is initiated and to prepare a brief report to be available on his/her return.

What will be your first priority following the meeting? Identify all the tasks to be completed and devise an action plan to follow, giving yourself a timescale.

Box 5.1 Example of an action plan

ACTION REQUIRED	DEADLINE (Date)
Read notes and pass on relevant action points to physiotherapist	Within 1 day
Prepare minutes	Within 3 days
Circulate minutes	Within 5 days
Request feedback on action taken by team members	Within 10 days
Prepare brief report for team leader	Within 14 days

---

venue. Once these details have been finalised, information regarding the meeting needs to be conveyed to each team member, either in writing or by speaking to those involved. The information needed by the team at this stage can be referred to as the what, why, where and when. What is the meeting for? Why is it being held? Where and when will it take place? Notes taken at the first team meeting should have been circulated to team members before the second meeting, although it is advisable to have spare copies available at the second meeting along with the patient's medical records, including any relevant X-rays and investigation results. You should ask the person convening the meeting whether any further action is required in advance. Refreshments may be required, particularly if the meeting is to be held at lunchtime or early evening. Keep a record if any team

member is unable to attend. Check who will be available to take notes at the meeting or whether you will be required to attend.

You can see that you will be the key organiser of this meeting and that good communication practice is vital in this situation.

TRUST

All members of the team must feel able to trust their colleagues to carry out their duties and responsibilities in a competent manner. Teamwork breaks down when trust is absent from the relationships. Trust will be earned by demonstrating your reliability and organisation skills. In the case of Mrs Sanders' case meeting, the medical secretary was responsible for organising the meeting and for ensuring that all the appropriate personnel were informed. The team leader trusted that this task would be completed effectively.

The first priority following the meeting will be to prepare minutes/notes for circulation. In this case you should have considered the possibility that one of the action points identified at the meeting involves the physiotherapist. It would then be appropriate for you to contact the physiotherapist as a priority. An action plan can be written in a number of formats but a simple outline is provided in Box 5.1.

Action plans provide you with an easy reference guide for any task you are responsible for. You can check your progress without having to read through all the documentation and they will enable you to communicate the requirements to other team members more effectively. By following your action plan you will be able to provide the team leader with an informative report on the day he/she returns from leave. Your trustworthiness will have been effectively demonstrated. Being an active team member will enhance your feelings of job satisfaction as you will know that your contribution is valued and beneficial to patient care and support. Being a willing and able member of the team will identify you as a valuable asset to the organisation.

COMMITMENT

Anyone who contributes to patient care and support should invest a level of commitment and quality in the role they perform within the organisation; in other words, giving priority to the needs and wants of the organisation. The following character-istics are desirable in all medical secretaries and demonstrate commitment.

RELIABILITY

As previously discussed, the medical secretary will often work at the centre of patient care. As a result, colleagues, patients and external agencies will rely upon you to carry out your duties both competently and promptly. Being reliable means always taking appropriate action when asked, completing work within accepted and agreed deadlines and responding to enquiries as soon as possible. People who are invariably late, who do not meet deadlines, who do not respond to requests within acceptable timescales and who do not complete a task without being reminded are generally viewed as unreliable.

ACCURACY

As a medical secretary, one of the most valuable attributes you can possess is that of accuracy and this ability should be applied to every aspect of your work. One area of obvious relevance is the production of typed documents where accuracy will lessen the amount of time spent on corrections. Even the most accurate touch-typist can make errors. Proof-reading of all documents is therefore essential. Do not rely solely on the spell-check facility on your word processor as this will not identify words which have been correctly spelt but used out of context and many medical spell checkers do not offer a fully comprehensive stock of words. Use medical and English dictionaries, check the British National Formulary (BNF) for drug spellings and if you are unsure of the spelling of a person's name, check with their secretary/office. An effective, but time-consuming, proof-reading technique is that of reading the text out loud. Errors or omissions become more obvious when heard. Another useful tool is to read each sentence backwards, as this concentrates your attention on each word rather than on the overall meaning of the text.

Your work will require you to keep a variety of records, both manual and computerised. It is essential that you enter information accurately and check the details before closing a file or record. In a hospital, patients are allocated a hospital number at the point of registration. When accessing a system to find a patient record number, you will rely on the patient's surname, first name and date of birth. If the patient's surname is spelt incorrectly, the system will not be able to find the file. Apart from being time-consuming, this can result in the patient being registered twice and being allocated a second hospital number. If this error is not spotted at an early stage, it is possible for a patient to have two separate sets of medical records in circulation at the same time.

Another aspect to remember is that the information held on the hospital Patient Administration System (PAS) will be used nationally to look at spread, treatment and outcome of certain illnesses (e.g. cancer) and locally to plan and commission health care services between the Primary Care Trust (PCT) and the hospital, so the importance of accuracy cannot be over-emphasised.

As previously discussed, you will be using the telephone during your work. Most telephone conversations will require you to take notes/messages for future reference. Your method of recording this information must be reliable and accurate, as you may be receiving urgent investigation results, prescribing or medication information, or other clinical details. You will also receive cancellation of appointments and changes of address and contact numbers.

Scenario 4

Mrs Jenson telephones you to give her new address and telephone number. She has already moved but forgot to notify you in advance.

Other than the new address and telephone number, what other details should you request from the caller? Which records will need to be updated?

The most essential information you need is the caller's full name and correct spelling. On the telephone, what sounds like Jenson could in reality be Genson, Jensen or Jemson. If you omit to take the caller's first name, you could find yourself faced with an extensive list of Jensons to search through. It would also be a useful precaution to check the caller's date of birth to be sure of accurate identification. When you have taken the new address and telephone number, read the information back to the caller to check it is correct. A change of address needs to be entered on the computerised patient record, the medical notes and on any other medical records which are kept within your organisation. If the caller is notifying you of a forthcoming change of address, check the date that this becomes effective. Are they changing their GP as well? If so, ask them to contact you when they have registered with a new practice.

EFFECTIVE USE OF TIME AND PRIORITISATION OF WORKLOAD

As a medical secretary you will experience fluctuating workloads and you will be required to adopt appropriate time-management techniques to cope. Learning to use your time effectively and identify problem areas will help you to achieve more in the time available. Time is your most precious resource and you must learn to use it well. There will be occasions when you are required to work to a specific deadline and you should learn to plan and prioritise your workload accordingly.

SETTING PRIORITIES

An ability to organise your daily workload will assist you in meeting deadlines and, hopefully, keeping on top of your workload. You will be asked to complete a variety of tasks each day and it is important to realise that these will carry differing levels of urgency. If you work solely for one person, prioritising the tasks will prove relatively simple. However, most medical secretaries work for more than one person, all of whom will provide work requiring immediate or priority attention. Your dilemma will be what to address first. Priority setting is a skill we all use in our everyday lives and it is an organisational skill which can be developed.

You may have decided that finding the X-rays should be your first priority. You know the patient is due to go to theatre in the afternoon so you have a specific deadline. Alternatively, the urgent audio tape may have been your first priority, as you have no knowledge of the contents and the doctor concerned thought it important enough to be marked 'urgent'.

The incoming mail is clearly of secondary importance in this situation. This is a routine task and there is no set deadline. The list of messages will need to be examined and placed in order of priority, depending upon the content of each message. You might consider that the three patients have the most immediate need of your attention over your manager and the

Scenario 5

You work for two consultants, who share a team of junior staff. You have returned to work following three days' leave. Your in-tray contains the following:

- six messages: three from patients, one from your manager and two from drug company representatives

- an audio tape from one of your consultants, marked 'urgent'

- a file of incoming mail

- a note from your other consultant asking you to locate some X-rays for a patient scheduled for surgery that afternoon.

Consider this list. Decide the priority of each, giving an explanation for your decision.

When deciding the priority of a task, ask the following questions:

- What do I know?

- Is there an obvious deadline?

- Which has the most immediate need?

drug representatives. Alternatively, the message from your manager may need to take precedence.

If you organise your tasks in this manner you will ensure that you meet urgent needs and deadlines whilst making the best use of your time.

ACCEPTING RESPONSIBILITY

In your role, you may be presented with situations which require a greater degree of responsibility. These situations should be viewed as opportunities to develop new skills, to use your existing skills and to demonstrate your value to the practice or department. When busy, it is tempting to view additional responsibility with a negative attitude, considering only the impact this may have on your current workload.

An induction programme should be specific to the environment and the post of the new member of staff. Your list should have covered the following areas:

Scenario 6

A new clerical assistant has been appointed. Your manager asks you to plan an induction programme for this person.

Devise a list of topics around which an induction programme could be constructed. What personal skills will you use by accepting and completing this task?

- familiarisation with premises and facilities (e.g. toilets, kitchen, canteen, fire extinguishers)
- introduction to existing staff and description of roles
- supplying written protocols or procedures (e.g. fire drill, health and safety regulations, timetables)
- training on telephone, fax and photocopier
- introduction to filing systems
- provision of internal staff list and telephone directory
- training on computer systems.

To perform this task competently you will require effective written and verbal communication skills, time-management techniques, good judgment for priority setting and assessing the needs of the new member of staff, and the department.

It is appropriate at this point to warn you about the pitfalls of accepting too much responsibility. Always ensure that the allocated task falls within your area of skill and knowledge. Never be afraid of asking for further guidance or assistance from your manager, experienced colleagues or the medical team. Although you should be willing to become involved in new ventures, beware of allowing yourself to become overburdened with work.

QUALITY

Even in the provision of health care, quality standards are applied to ensure that the patient receives the best possible care and treatment. Along with clinical standards concerned with waiting and treatment times, many hospitals have also agreed standards with their medical secretaries that define acceptable response times to phone messages, clinic and discharge letters sent out within certain timescales, patient complaints to be acknowledged and responded to promptly and some even define the number of rings within which the telephone should be answered. It is the duty of the medical secretary to uphold these standards and to be aware that they are an important part of the patient's perception of the organisation as a whole.

Clinical audit has now become an integral part of clinical governance, the most widely accepted definition of which is 'a framework through which NHS organisations are accountable for continually improving the quality of their services and safeguarding high standards of care by creating an environment in which excellence in clinical care will flourish' (Scally & Donaldson 1998).

Exercises

Discuss these situations with your colleagues.

You notice that one of your medical secretarial colleagues has made a number of mistakes recently. One was concerned with entering incorrect patient details into a discharge summary and the other was wrongly informing a GP surgery that a patient had died.

- How would you deal with this situation?

- What may be the issues involved?

A number of patients have telephoned you and, in the general course of the call, it is evident that they are unhappy with the treatment received from one particular doctor on your team. Each patient is reluctant to put this in writing, saying that they 'do not want to cause a fuss' as the care they received from everyone else was 'first class'.

- What action (if any) would you take?

- At what stage would you raise it as a concern and to whom?

- What factors might influence the decision you take?

In the 1999 Health Act, the Government placed a statutory duty of quality on each health care organisation. Clinical governance is the way in which that duty of quality is turned into reality. It seeks to transform the culture, ways of working and systems of every health care organisation so that quality assurance, patient safety and quality improvement are an integral part of everyday work.

The medical secretary is often in a position to notice lapses in the quality of service provision and, where it becomes an area of concern, it is important that action is taken. Hospitals are now encouraging a more open, non-discriminatory reporting process for adverse incidents/events and unsatisfactory outcomes of care. Whistleblowing policies are in place in a number of health care organisations to enable staff to draw attention to these without fear of reprisals, and the NHS as a whole is working towards a blame-free reporting culture.

COURTESY

In this section we will consider those qualities which govern your relationships with people. Your interpersonal skills describe your reaction to and interaction with others. As a medical secretary you will be dealing with people from all sections of the community. Your colleagues and clients will demonstrate a variety of differing cultural attitudes and beliefs, come from varied social and economic groups, may suffer difficult domestic backgrounds and circumstances. The cornerstone of good interpersonal skills is to afford all people equal respect, care and consideration.

YOUR COLLEAGUES

As previously discussed, the medical secretary will often work at the centre of a multidisciplinary team of health care staff. You will have contact with many types of personality: some pleasant and helpful, others brusque or obstructive. You should demonstrate a professional attitude to all colleagues regardless of their position or status within the organisation. Acknowledge that each person has a contribution to make. Do not judge your colleagues by your own morals or beliefs. You should show tolerance and professionalism in the face of adversity. You should never allow personal feelings to influence your professional relationships.

YOUR CLIENTS

Your clients will include patients, relatives, external agencies and other health care workers. Always remember that you are representing your employer when dealing with clients. The service you provide will influence the client's opinion not only of you, but of the medical team and the whole organisation as well. You should display a helpful and pleasant disposition at all times. You must be non-judgmental, non-discriminatory and approachable. In medicine it is common to hear the term 'patient advocate'. A simple definition of this phrase is that an individual will act as a supporter or ally of the patient. The medical secretary will act as a patient advocate in many situations, particularly when a patient is trying to communicate information or requests to members of the medical team. You will be relaying information on behalf of the patient.

Reflection Point 2

Think of an acquaintance you do not particularly like. Try to analyse why this person provokes this reaction in you. Then think of someone you do like and identify why you like this person. How does your behaviour differ when dealing with each of these people?

In the main, your reaction to a person is based on your own standards of attitude and behaviour. There will be specific qualities that you admire and habits that you find irritating. In your personal life you can choose the people you spend time with. In your professional life, this choice is not always available to you. You will be required to work and have contact with people you do not like or admire. However, these personal feelings must be put to one side in order that you can perform your role effectively.

ASSERTIVENESS

Assertion can be described as the process of standing up for your own rights whilst respecting the rights of others by expressing yourself in direct, honest and appropriate ways. The aim of assertiveness is to satisfy the needs of both parties in any given situation. Assertiveness will assist you in coping with difficult situations at work such as:

- feeling anger or frustration
- disagreeing with seniors
- dealing with irate patients
- responding to unreasonable requests.

Your ability to be assertive should not be confused with being aggressive. Nor is it the opposite of being polite. Assertive behaviour is a skill which can be learned and improved. Being assertive will result in your becoming more effective in your job and will also improve your self-confidence. You will be taking responsibility for your behaviour, which will in turn allow you to become proactive rather than reactive.

Scenario 7

Your manager telephones you to say that a colleague has been sent home ill and asks that you cover the reception desk for the afternoon session. You are working on a lengthy report for one of the medical team to take to an important meeting this evening.

What is your response to your manager?

An assertive response would be, 'I appreciate the problem but at present I am typing a report which is required for the meeting this evening and I will not be able to help until it is finished'. A non-assertive response would be, 'Well, I am in the middle of this report but I suppose I could work on it over lunch instead'. An aggressive response would be, 'You must be joking, I've got this report to do and I can't possibly spare any time for you'.

The non-assertive response will leave you with difficult deadlines to meet, a feeling of frustration that you have been 'put upon', and anger with yourself for not fully explaining your own situation. The aggressive response will earn you a reputation of being unhelpful and obstructive and will leave you feeling very defensive.

To be assertive you must believe the following statements:

- I am in control of my behaviour
- I can change my behaviour
- I am responsible for what happens to me
- I can learn from any situation
- I can take the initiative to reach objectives.

We have examined the role of assertion in refusing requests, but assertiveness will be equally helpful to you when making requests.

When you wish to make a request, be straightforward. Do not apologise for making the request. Be direct, precise and provide a reason for the request. You must learn not to take a refusal personally by accepting the other person's right to say no.

HANDLING AGGRESSION

Dealing with aggressive or abusive people can be emotionally unsettling and lead to an undesirable confrontational exchange. When faced with an aggressive patient it will help you to remain assertive by remembering the following:

- their behaviour may be affected by pain or discomfort
- their behaviour may be the result of frustration
- their behaviour may be the result of severe anxiety
- their behaviour may be due to a recognised neurological or psychiatric disorder.

Scenario 8

You are manning the reception during a clinic. Owing to a shortage of medical staff the clinic is running behind schedule and several patients have been waiting for more than an hour. A patient approaches the desk wanting to know why he is being kept waiting so long. His voice is raised and he appears very tense. He unjustly accuses you of allowing other patients to go ahead in the queue and calls you inefficient.

What is your initial reaction? What is your response to the question?

In most cases, the individual will not be attacking you on a personal level, but you are supplying an easy target. They may have been building up their anger over a period of time and you are simply the face/voice of the organisation.

It is particularly difficult to deal with an aggressive patient in front of other people in an unusually stressful time. In a situation such as this, it is wise to take a pause before offering your response. Use an assertive tone of voice but do not retaliate or show anger. Do remember to put the patient's needs first. Be calm, concerned, confident and professional when you respond. If you are unable to provide the patient with an adequate explanation, seek further information or advice from someone more senior. Put yourself in his shoes and imagine how you would feel under similar circumstances. Add to this the possibility that he is ill or in pain and you can see why he is demonstrating aggression towards you, as the person representing the organisation.

HANDLING STRESS

It needs to be acknowledged that stress is ever present in our lives and is inevitable during times of increased pressure in the workplace. Stress is a normal human reaction to difficult situations and is sometimes described as the 'fight or flight' response. A small amount is beneficial, but too much stress can be detrimental to your health, state of mind and performance.

There are a variety of causes of stress in the workplace, some of which are listed below:

- long hours without proper breaks
- complex or time-consuming tasks
- rapid changes within the organisation or management structure
- unrealistic deadlines
- inadequate resources
- lack of communication
- fear about job security
- fear of being perceived as unable to cope
- developing new skills
- continuous interruptions.

You must become familiar with your own stress threshold and learn to recognise signs and symptoms which may be related to stress. Some of these are listed below:

- anxiety
- pounding heart
- inability to relax
- sweating

- indigestion
- depression
- weariness
- restlessness
- insomnia
- despondency
- moodiness
- moaning
- short temper.

In addition to the physical signs, you should be aware that your work performance could also be affected in the following ways:

- indecision
- poor time management
- absenteeism
- lack of humour
- low productivity
- increased frequency of errors
- apathy/disinterest
- poor presentation of written work.

There are a number of steps we can all take to combat the effects of stress. One of the most important is improving your physical health and lifestyle. You should be aware of the dangers of smoking, drinking alcohol, lack of sleep and poor diet. Pay attention to your diet and ensure you are providing sufficient amounts of appropriate fuel for your body. Taking regular exercise and being aware of your level of fitness will also help you to fight stress.

Relaxation techniques can be learned and employed as part of your normal lifestyle. Regular exercise is an excellent way to relax and promote well-being. Other physical activities may prove more rewarding to you as an individual, such as dancing, gardening or DIY. It is your responsibility to ensure that you always maintain an acceptable balance between work activities and leisure time. If your workload is consistently too large, admit that you are only human and seek further advice or help.

Learning to recognise excessive stress can be turned to your advantage. Examine the situation and identify the main source of stress, and then tackle the situation directly. Your assertiveness skills will help you in this task.

You might find the checklist in Box 5.2 useful: Adopt CARL as your coping strategy, or develop your own personal code, and take it with you into all working environments.

Exercises

You are an experienced medical secretary who has been employed in the same area/department for many years. The good news has just been announced that funds have been approved to increase the levels of staffing. The existing staff have long worked under difficult conditions with heavy workloads and your manager has invited you to contribute your views at a team meeting to discuss what the staffing priorities should be. Your workload is too large for one person and there are several areas of responsibility you would like to take on, but simply have not had enough time to do so in the past.

• How will you approach this situation? What kind of information and evidence will you present in order to influence the decision-makers to include additional secretarial assistance in the recruitment programme?

• How will you present this information? Plan your reasoning and ensure that you reflect the needs of the patients in your notes.

As a result of the announcement of an imminent local rationalisation of services, there is much speculation about the future of your hospital. Staff morale has fallen to a low ebb. Your manager comes to you to ask for your assistance in helping to allay staff fears about their future and ensure the team continues to function effectively.

• How will you react to this request? What information will you ask for?

• What suggestions would you make to your manager with regard to improving staff morale?

• How will you respond to colleagues who voice their fears to you directly? Examine the issues surrounding this situation.

CONCLUSION

This chapter has illustrated many of the personal skills and qualities that are desirable in an effective medical secretary. The scenarios and reflection points serve as exercises for you to highlight your own strengths and weaknesses and will provide you with ideas for future self-development. We have illustrated ways in which the role of a medical secretary can be extended with time and experience, allowing opportunities for complete involvement as a member of the team. The patient is at the centre of everything you do as a medical secretary and this should remain your main priority at all times.

The skills you bring to your work will enhance the

Box 5.2 CARL

• Communicate – recognise your limitations and ask when you need help
• Assert yourself – avoid conflicts and frustration
• Recognise stress – identify and tackle sources at an early stage
• Lifestyle – take responsibility for your health and protect your leisure time

service provided to each and every patient, provide your medical team with professional, efficient and reliable administrative support and supply you with a great sense of job satisfaction and achievement.

Further reading

Black K, Black K 1995 Assertiveness at work. McGraw-Hill, Maidenhead

Brem C 1995 Are we on the same team here? Allen & Unwin, Sydney

Fontana D 1989 Managing stress. British Psychological Society in association with Routledge Ltd, London

Haynes ME 1992 Make every minute count. Kogan Page, London

Peel M 1990 Improving your communication skills. Kogan Page, London

Pringle M (ed) 1993 Change and teamwork in primary care. BMJ Publishing, London

Sommerville A 1993 Medical ethics today: its practice and philosophy. BMJ Publishing, London

Time management, Stress, Hints on handling communications with difficult customers are all AMSPAR Guidelines

Wilkinson G 1993 Understanding stress. Family Doctor Publications Ltd in association with the British Medical Association

References

Scally G, Donaldson LJ. Clinical governance and the drive for quality improvement in the new NHS in England. BMJ 1998; 317:61-65

Communication

Sara Ladyman

OBJECTIVES

- To consider communication issues, such as confidentiality, affecting the medical secretary

- To focus on verbal communication: active listening, availability and appropriate level of information, checking skills, recording and relaying messages, suggestions for and emphasis on good telephone technique, including useful proformas and reflection points

- To focus on visual communication: dress code, body language and the working environment

- To focus on written communication: using the medical record, filing systems and best practice for preparing correspondence, examples of labels, proforma letters, managing and prioritising work

- To conclude with an examination of internal and external systems which can facilitate good communication, for example tracking systems, a short bibliography of useful books, departmental information dissemination, the internal mail systems, using fax and e-mail.

INTRODUCTION

The secretary's role is to relieve the medical team of the administrative workload of the department. A wide range of communication skills are essential to enable the medical secretary to be an effective member of the team providing patient care. Competence is necessary for verbal, visual and written communications. We will be addressing each of these areas and it would be helpful to refer to the Patient's Charter.

GENERAL

To communicate effectively with patients and members of staff you will need to systematically assess their needs and plan the response that best meets the individual's specific need.

All patients and staff with whom you come into contact should be treated politely, respectfully and in a helpful manner, regardless of their social standing, nationality, appearance or age. Familiarise yourself with the national and local Patient Charters and the rights of patients. Patients have a right to see or speak to their doctor and the effectiveness of this communication is influenced by the secretary's active management of the doctor's time. The secretary has to assess and prioritise queries and decide which can be resolved satisfactorily without a doctor's input and come within a secretary's responsibilities, and which messages must be passed on to a doctor ensuring all relevant information is available, such as the patient record, for the doctor to make an informed decision. Chapter 4 on ethics and etiquette, explores this in greater depth.

CONFIDENTIALITY

Patients have a right to confidentiality and there are some general guidelines you must be aware of when working in a health care environment. An understanding of these will form part of a confidentiality clause in the contract of employment and staff should have appropriate guidance and training to address confidentiality issues that may arise in the workplace, some of which will be covered in this chapter. In particular, the secretary must be aware and apply the principles and recommendations of the Caldicott review to improve the way the NHS protects and uses patient information, and the standards within the 1998 Data Protection Act for obtaining, recording, holding, using and disposing of computer and manual records. There should be written policies and guidelines wherever you work which encompass these standards, and if in doubt on any aspect of con-

fidentiality it is essential to seek clarification before taking any action regarding a patient. Some of the practical applications of these recommendations and standards are covered in this chapter.

Information should only be shared with staff or agencies outside your work area if it is appropriate to do so. In particular, written consent from the patient is required before information can be released to the patient or their guardian, police, solicitor or insurance company even when acting on their behalf. Release of information, and decisions on what can and what cannot be released, must be sanctioned by the patient's doctor, or doctors if they are being seen in different departments. There will be clearly defined procedures laid down for disclosure of information to external bodies and these should be readily available for reference.

INFORMING PATIENTS OF TEST RESULTS

As a rule the secretary is not responsible for informing patients of test results, even at the patient's request, unless a doctor specifically asks them to release this information. If the doctor asks you to contact a patient by telephone and inform them of a result this information must only be given to the patient, or the parent of someone under 14 years of age, and no one else. If a relative or parent of some one *over* 14 years of age asks for results, or indeed wishes to discuss their relative's medical care, they must be informed politely that it is unusual to disclose information to anyone but the patient and the doctor will have to decide whether this is appropriate. Clinical staff may choose to give results over the telephone although an appointment is usually made for the patient to meet with the doctor to discuss results and to agree a course of action. As a general rule always ask a doctor before disclosing any medical information to a patient, relative or external agency and make yourself familiar with the organisation's policy and procedures regarding this.

For general enquiries for information about chemists, dental surgeons, opticians and other local practitioners the secretary must not make personal recommendations to one particular practitioner. There should be a list available so patients can make their own choice. The secretary should avoid making personal recommendations or remarks about the ability and personality of doctors and other staff in their department.

Should a problem arise which cannot be resolved satisfactorily the secretary must use common sense and follow departmental guidelines for resolving com-

Box 6.1 Confidentiality

DO:
- clarify who is requesting information and justify the purposes of disclosing confidential information
- only provide authorised and minimum information required, on a need-to-know basis, direct to a patient, guardian or other agency
- if in any doubt as to the legitimacy of a person making a request, take their details, check these out, and seek advice from medical or senior staff if unsure how to proceed
- observe medical etiquette and understand and comply with the law
- keep to the facts and avoid expressing personal comments and opinions.

DO NOT:
- share information outside the department or workplace unless it is appropriate and necessary to do so
- collect information unless it is appropriate and is to be used
- pass comment on the ability of doctors or make recommendations
- release information to any third party unless a written request and written consent from doctor and the patient has been received
- leave messages on answerphones unless you have permission to do so; it is preferable to leave minimum information, a name, telephone number and message to call back
- inform a patient of results or other medical information unless a doctor has given express and clear instructions to do so, and never leave this information on an answerphone
- discuss one patient with another.

Box 6.2 Medical etiquette

GPs	Address the GP as 'Doctor...' followed by his or her second name, e.g. 'Doctor Smith'.
Consultant physicians	Called 'Doctor' followed by their second name, e.g. 'Doctor Smith'.
Consultant surgeons	Referred to as Mister (male) followed by their second name, e.g. 'Mister Smith'.
Consultant surgeons	Miss, Ms or Mrs (female) followed by their second name, e.g. 'Miss Smith'.
Professors	Called Professor, e.g. 'Professor Smith'.

plaints to ensure the matter is brought to the attention of the patient's doctor or appropriate member of staff so that remedial action can be taken if necessary. Some dos and don'ts for confidentiality are listed in Box 6.1.

VERBAL COMMUNICATION

The secretary is responsible for receiving and relaying oral and written messages between members of the medical team and patients, doctors, and all departments, both internal and external. Remember that the tone and intonation of the voice can posi-

tively or negatively affect the person's perception of the department and the outcome of their communication in terms of patient care.

It is also important to observe medical etiquette when speaking with doctors and nurses. The guidelines given in Box 6.2 will assist you; if in doubt ask for guidance.

A consistent and precise approach to taking and relaying messages is essential for the accurate and prompt resolution of queries. It is important to remember that all health issues raise major concerns in a person's life and can result in a patient experiencing feelings of fear, confusion, anger, frustration and lack of empowerment. These can be reasons for an apparent lack of comprehension and understanding of the organisation's administrative systems and procedures, and a degree of understanding and empathy is required with people who find themselves in this situation. There is a range of skills and tools that can be used to facilitate good communication with particular reference to patients and some are outlined below.

Reflection Point 1

As a medical secretary, you are one of the 'windows' of the hospital and what you communicate and how you communicate will colour the view patients and other staff have of your department and hospital.

LISTENING SKILLS

Active listening requires you to:

- focus on what the patient is saying
- repeat back what has been said to ensure understanding, and moderate the voice to ensure privacy
- allow the patient to say everything they have to say and to describe their symptoms fully, their duration, spelling of medication and so on
- be open, honest and clear and provide a positive response with a choice rather than just a negative statement. If they are unhappy with your response suggest their concerns are brought to the attention of the doctor or nurse as applicable and an appropriate follow up to their concerns made
- ensure your environment is kept free of unnecessary interruptions and distractions.

In addition to the message you should always record the following information from the caller and be clear they understand why you need the information and who you are going to share it with:

- first and second names
- date of birth and / or hospital or other reference number
- contact telephone number, when they will be available to take the call, whether this is in the workplace or home and, where there is an answerphone, can a message be left and how much detail
- note the date and time of the call
- address may or may not be required but is useful to assist with verification of the caller and to make a brief check against current hospital record information.

Always check any details that are unclear, even if the person leaving the message expresses irritation. It is far better to check details at the time of the message rather than take down incomplete or incorrect details which then require further action.

Reflection Point 2

What are some of the distractions which can get in the way of active listening? How can you minimise these?

Box 6.3 The international alphabet

A	Alpha	N	November
B	Bravo	O	Oscar
C	Charlie	P	Papa
D	Delta	Q	Quebec
E	Echo	R	Romeo
F	Fox-trot	S	Sierra
G	Golf	T	Tango
H	Holland	U	Uniform
I	India	V	Victor
J	Juliet	W	Whisky
K	Kilo	X	X-ray
L	Lima	Y	Yankee
M	Mike	Z	Zulu

AVAILABILITY OF INFORMATION

As well as receiving a full message it is important that the doctor has as much relevant information to hand as possible in order to decide on any action to be taken and to update the patient's written or computerised records. If there is a delay in obtaining written case notes a copy of the most recent correspondence may be helpful in the interim to avoid a delay in the doctor prioritising or acting upon the message.

CHECKING SKILLS

We have mentioned the need to check correct understanding when message taking. A useful tool to check spelling is to use the international alphabet (Box 6.3).

Read the message back to the caller to make sure you have the correct information, even if you feel confident that you have all the facts, and be clear on what follow-up action you will be taking.

RECORDING AND RELAYING MESSAGES

A spiral bound notebook is an essential tool for effective message management. Messages taken on scrap paper can easily be mislaid; a notebook provides a safer, lasting record for future reference if necessary, and messages taken in chronological order can be more easily prioritised for action. However, it must be remembered that notebooks

---

MESSAGE

DATE

TIME

TO

FROM

SURGERY / HOSPITAL

TELEPHONE NUMBER / BLEEP

PATIENT NAME

HOSPITAL / REF NUMBER

DATE OF BIRTH

ADDRESS *as required*

TELEPHONE NUMBER

MESSAGE

RE:

OUTCOME / INSTRUCTIONS *(as appropriate)*

Figure 6.1 Examples of message proformas which can be adapted for hospital or general practice use. They ensure a consistent approach is taken and information can be elicited clearly and concisely from the caller.

REQUEST FOR A WARD VISIT

DATE/TIME REQUEST

TO

NAME

POSITION

TEL NO/

BLEEP NO

PATIENT NAME

HOSPITAL/REF NO

CONSULTANT PATIENT UNDER

PATIENT ON WARD

DATE OF BIRTH

ADDRESS *(if applicable)*

ADMISSION DATE

PATIENT ADMITTED FOR

EXPECTED LENGTH OF STAY/DISCHARGE DATE *(if known)*

ABILITY TO ATTEND AN OUT PATIENT CLINIC VIA WHEELCHAIR YES/NO

HISTORY/CURRENT PROBLEM *(including MRSA status)*

Figure 6.1 Continued

are a potential source of confidential information and they should be kept in the confines of the office environment, and eventually destroyed.

Messages can be relayed either verbally or in writing, depending on their nature and urgency, and you will need to familiarise yourself with the times to expect doctors' visits during the week. This may depend on where the office is situated, and on the doctor's work commitments and preferences.

The majority of doctors carry hand-held bleeps or radiopages which can be accessed using the telephone system or the switchboard. Be familiar with doctors' preferences and availability for being contacted; for example, it would usually be inappropriate to page a doctor who is with a patient.

The following tools can ensure messages are received even when the secretary is out of the office or on the telephone.

All messages should be clearly and legibly copied into an A4 message book or diary. Alternatively, a white board or pinboard may be utilised for messages, though no patient-identifying details must be visible and the board should be in an area not accessible to patients. A typed or hand written message, with accompanying patient records as required, can be left in a doctor's pigeonhole or tray labelled for a doctor's attention. The message may be in the format of a proforma to assist message taking and two examples can be found in Figure 6.1.

Message proformas ensure that a consistent approach is taken to information gathering. Different proformas can be utilised for different types of call. For example:

- urgent appointment requests, which require as much information as possible for the doctor prior to receipt of the referral letter
- domiciliary or home visit requests
- Ward visit requests.

THE TELEPHONE

It is important to remember that, when you use a telephone, the person to whom you are speaking can only relate to your voice. They will be unable to observe body or facial expressions and the voice must clearly state the message. The language should be simple, clear and avoid the use of jargon and abbreviations. To avoid distortion, speak into the mouthpiece and not across it. Speak more slowly than in face-to-face communication, and pitch the

Box 6.4 Telephone services	
Call forward	To forward calls to another extension in your absence
Follow me	If you are in another office and wish to have all calls diverted to this extension
Ring back	To ring back from a number which is currently busy
Save	To save an external number you have just dialled
Conference facility	To add one or more parties to your two-way call
Pick up group	Ability to take calls at your phone from other telephones within your vicinity and hearing range
Page/Bleep	There will be a sequence of numbers you will need to ring to page a doctor, or you may have to go through a switchboard.

voice slightly lower. A smile on the face lifts the voice and sounds more agreeable. Remember that both parties in a telephone conversation will be unaware of the other person's surroundings and distractions. The caller is able to minimise these, but if there is difficulty in communicating because of background noise it may be better to bring the conversation to a close and arrange a more convenient time to speak.

Familiarity with the organisation's telephone system is essential, as these are usually programmed to provide some or all of the services shown in Box 6.4. It is essential to use the secrecy button when discussing a patient whilst that patient is holding on the telephone, returning to the caller frequently to let them know their query is still being processed and offering to take their telephone number and return their call if the wait for a response may be prolonged.

Check whether your telephone has the facility to make and receive external calls. When outgoing calls are made without switchboard intervention a number is used to access an external line, although this facility may be inaccessible before 9.00 a.m. and after 5.00 p.m. Alternatively, external telephone calls may be made via a switchboard.

Always respond to incoming calls promptly, even when busy with other duties. To avoid sounding abrupt on the telephone, or when feeling harassed, before lifting the handset, pause, take a deep breath and put a smile in your voice. Box 6.5 lists some guidelines for good telephone practice.

Whether the caller has come through to the department directly, or has been diverted via a switchboard, it is the secretary's responsibility to ensure the caller knows to whom they are speaking and that they have the correct destination, with an offer to transfer the caller when this is not the case.

It is courteous when transferring calls to speak briefly to the person who picks up the call, providing the caller's name and the reason for transferring them before replacing the handset. If there is no answer or an answerphone is switched on, the caller should not be diverted and the secretary should return to them and provide the caller with a choice of either leaving a message, ringing the department directly themselves, or transferring them to the answerphone to leave a message if they so wish.

Familiarity with the preferred terminology and house style for receiving incoming calls is important. In a hospital, this may involve giving the name of the department followed by your name, for example 'Dermatology Department, June Jones speaking, how can I help you?' or 'Mr Smith's secretary, how can I help you?' Similarly in a general practice, 'Southwest Health Centre, Dr Allen's secretary speaking, how can I help you?' or 'Southwest Health Centre, Barbara Evans speaking, how can I help you?' This should be a response to both internal and external telephone calls, as internal telephones can be linked to organisations outside your hospital. An informal 'hello' is unacceptable and does not promote a positive corporate image. An offer of help is a positive way to start communications.

Maintaining confidentiality is essential when using the telephone and it is important to remember this when the telephone is used so frequently in the workplace. If in doubt as to the credibility of the caller, take as many details as you can to corroborate their request and inform them that their call will be returned, enabling a check to be made and permission sought to release information as necessary.

ANSWERPHONES

A message should only be left on a patient's answerphone when permission has been given by the patient. If there is no alternative to leaving a message it is important to be aware that patient

---

Box 6.5 Tips and hints for good telephone practice

Receiving calls
- answer calls promptly.
- avoid keeping callers waiting – give callers the choice of being rung back if their query requires a search for information or consultation with other staff
- take the caller's name and telephone number in case they are cut off, and ring back directly if this occurs
- keep coming back to a caller who is on hold
- have a general knowledge or access to a list of staff, departments and their extension numbers
- when re-routing calls, ensure the called extension wishes to accept the call. If the call cannot be put through or there is no reply, give the caller a choice of ringing back, together with a telephone number, or ask if they wish to leave a message and pass this on
- do not be over familiar and avoid personal comments
- if a caller is cut off, ring them back immediately
- be aware of policy for dealing with abusive or unusual telephone calls
- end the call politely.

Making calls
- make a clear introduction and ensure it is convenient to speak
- plan what you are going to say and have all the information to hand with a list of points to raise
- dial the number carefully. If the wrong number is dialed, offer an apology
- give the name of the person you wish to speak to, or state the purpose of your call so you can be put through to appropriate person
- aways update and return calls, even to say the query has yet to be resolved
- be aware of costs – the use of mobile telephones, distance and length of call.

---

confidentiality could be breached because the message is accessible to others. It is inadvisable to leave messages on workplace answerphones. The message should clearly address the recipient, leaving a contact name and telephone number and a request to return the call at the earliest opportunity. Even when permission to leave a message has been granted by a patient, keep the message brief and keep details to a minimum.

In the office, an answerphone should only be used selectively as a tool to aid communication in the department. It is important that the doctor, via their secretary, is easily accessible to anyone who needs to get a message to the doctor member of the medical team. The constant use of answerphones can be frustrating for callers, especially if the message on the answerphone is out of date or inappropriate. It is advantageous to provide a number for callers who wish to seek advice rather than leave a message.

The following guidelines may be helpful when deciding how you are going to utilise an answerphone most effectively.

- Aim to use only when out of the office
- Avoid using when in the office except in exceptional circumstances, for example, during meetings or in exceptional circumstances when work priorities demand
- Provide timely response to messages by retrieving them at regular intervals through the day
- Ring caller(s) back as soon as possible to confirm receipt of the message and take more details as required
- Update the outgoing recorded message regularly, keeping it brief, indicating when someone will next be available and ensure the switchboard staff are aware of the arrangement
- Incorporate the organisation protocol for answerphone use.

VISUAL COMMUNICATION

This includes how staff present themselves personally within the working environment. It is important for all staff to observe a dress code. Some organisations provide their medical secretaries with a uniform or suggest a colour. If no such guidelines exist consider the impression given as a representative of the practice or hospital.

An identity badge must be worn at all times in the workplace as this is a patient charter standard. It usually forms part of an organisation's security strategy and is considered a disciplinary offence if not worn.

Non-verbal signals are as important as what we are saying and how we say it. Here are some areas where you should consider whether the non-verbal signals you are giving can be interpreted positively or negatively by the other person:

Reflection Point 3

A well-groomed and smart appearance can affect the patients perspective on the care they are to receive. Consider how you would expect a member of staff to be dressed should you have to attend for a doctor's appointment. Also, be aware of the practical considerations of dress. A medical secretary may need to travel some distance on foot on a daily basis as well as lifting, bending and stretching when looking for and moving case notes in the office.

- posture, positioning and proximity to the patient
- gestures, including body and head movements
- facial expressions
- eye contact
- mirroring the other person's body language
- taking account of environmental barriers such as reflective screens, sunlight, lack of privacy.

Reflection Point 4

Think about the positive and negative ways non-verbal signals can be interpreted by the receiver for each of the above.

WRITTEN COMMUNICATION

PATIENT CASE NOTES

In addition to the computerised Patient Administrative System (PAS) and systems found in General Practice, explained fully in Chapter 8 on information technology, the main source of information regarding a patient's care will be found in the patient's medical record or case notes. The primary medical record file should contain the information listed below, and reference will be made to the most recent clinic notation and test results as well as the patient's personal and demographic data, particularly when copy or audio typewriting correspondence.

A medical record usually includes:

- current identification sheet
- internal and external correspondence
- copies of discharge summaries following inpatient stays as appropriate
- history sheets/clinical notation for each visit
- operation and anaesthetic records (hospital records primarily)
- diagnostic test results, e.g. chemical pathology, haematology, ECG records
- X-ray results
- pathology results
- drug prescription chart
- labels with patient data.

It is important that every effort is made to ensure that correspondence and results are filed in the case notes promptly. Make reference to Chapters 12 and 16 for further details of patient case notes and their organisation.

When patients attend regularly, their case notes may increase in size and it may be necessary to have a secondary file containing non-current information to reduce the bulk of paperwork to be handled.

It is easy to become complacent and forget that an office contains many confidential documents. Generally, patients and relatives are discouraged from entering offices. It is considered more appropriate, for example, for the patient to meet the secretary in the reception or clinic area.

The office should be kept tidy, for reasons of health and safety and efficiency. Shelves, cupboards and filing cabinets must be appropriately and clearly labelled so that whilst patient records are secure in the office they can also be accessed if required for an emergency and are available routinely for staff. However, temporary and contract staff may have access to the office and it is important that confidential documents are locked away and a clear desk policy is in operation so that whenever possible patient information is not left on display on desk tops and is kept out of sight outside working hours. The secretary will also be aware of protocols concerning access to computers, including passwords and logging off when absent from the office to prevent unauthorised access. This is covered elsewhere in the chapter.

WRITTEN CORRESPONDENCE

Typewritten correspondence still forms the primary link between general practice and hospitals. The initial referral letter from the GP requests the hospital specialist's opinion and treatment plan. Once the hospital specialist has accepted the shared care of the patient, a letter follows each hospital outpatient visit to ensure the GP has current and accurate information available on a patient's episode of care. This information will include details of medication, test results and so on until the patient is discharged by the specialist to the GP's exclusive care. See Chapters 13 and 14.

It is therefore essential that any correspondence produced from audio, hand-written or shorthand dictation is accurate, complete, easily identifiable and filed in chronological order. Care should be taken inputting information to ensure accuracy and that patient details are up to date.

Whilst there may be a standard organisation format for letters, the secretary will have to become familiar with the format and house style of letters in the department. This may include the use of proformas and case note copies being colour coded to highlight them in the case notes. For example, with a diabetes clinic, copies of correspondence might be printed on green.

The patient's details form the heading of the letter; these must be prominently displayed so that the doctor can easily identify the patient. In addition, the following should be included:

- NHS registration number
- a reference comprising doctor's initials/your initials/record or case note number including site indicator if suitable e.g. 'SM/sac/MK 12 34 26'
- clinic date patient attended
- date dictated (if not the same as clinic date, optional)
- date letter typed
- addressee details
- signatory.

The letter is usually addressed to the doctor. If it is to a GP the letter can be addressed as follows:

Dr D Benson
Watling Road Practice
Watling Road West
Milton Keynes
MK12 5MM

If the letter is to a consultant physician the letter can be addressed as follows:

Dr D Watson (doctor's qualifications if used)
Consultant Gastroenterologist

Milton Hospital
Milton Road
Milton Keynes
MK12 5MM

If it is to a consultant surgeon the letter can be addressed as follows:

Mr D Watson (or Mrs/Ms/Miss Watson) (doctor's qualifications if used)
Consultant Gynaecologist
Milton Hospital
Milton Road
Milton Keynes
MK12 5MM

For the signatory's name, it is essential to check organisational preferences; for example, doctors may prefer to have their qualifications listed after their name (e.g. FRCS or MRCP).

It is usual for GPs to put their name only, for example:

Dr D Benson

For a consultant it may be acceptable as follows:

Mr D Watson
Consultant Gastroenterologist

See Figures 6.2 and 6.3 for examples of the layout for an outpatient clinic letter.

A copy of the letter should be filed in the appropriate section of the case notes; the most recent letter is usually filed on top of all previous correspondence.

As they form part of the patient's medical case notes, and so that they can be easily referred to, it is important that copies are correct and legible. They should usually be in no smaller than 11 point type to enable legible microfiche copies to be made in the future. The spell-check facility on the PC and proof-reading correspondence before it is presented for signature minimises the effort, frustration and inevitable delay when letters have to be corrected, reprinted and re-presented for signature. In addition, it is helpful to keep a personalised dictionary, entering unfamiliar spellings for future reference and to assist locum secretaries.

MANAGING THE INCOMING TYPING WORKLOAD

The following systems can assist in managing your typing workload effectively.

Doctors should be encouraged to speak clearly and slowly whilst dictating. This will result in fewer queries and inaccuracies in correspondence which will need correction and re-presentation for signature.

When the GP or hospital doctor dictates correspondence on patients attending the clinics they should be asked to:

- dictate their name and the clinic date at the start of the audio cassette
- keep case notes in an orderly pile, preferably in the order dictated
- dictate clearly and precisely.

Any problems must be brought to their attention as a great deal of time can be taken in trying to decipher unclear or indistinct dictation. Remember that the ease of transcription depends partly on the quality of recorded text. If there are problems these should be discussed sensitively with the individual concerned. A mutually beneficial method of working is important if the workload is going to be completed speedily and accurately.

You can assist by taking responsibility for the following points:

- Ask doctors to dictate urgent letters if possible on a separate audio cassette, perhaps using a dedicated handset, for transcription after clinic to save time locating one letter somewhere on the cassette to be typed urgently.
- Ensure that a supply of batteries and quality audio cassettes are available for the doctors, as old batteries and cassettes can cause distortion of dictation.
- Once an audio cassette has been used it should be sealed in an envelope and the doctor's name/initials and clinic date written on the envelope to minimise the risk of dictation being wiped, dictated over or lost.
- Case notes should be secured with a rubber band and attached to the clinic cassette envelope to reduce the risk of notes and cassette becoming separated.
- Place cassettes in chronological order of clinic dates for typing.

When correspondence is printed for signature it is essential that two copies are made and that one copy is filed in the case notes at the earliest opportunity, ensuring the notes are complete and current before leaving the office.

HOSPITAL HEADING

Ref: DW/sac/proform/44 44 21

Date: 10 12 --

Dr D Benson
Watling Road Practice
Watling Road West
Milton Keynes
MK12 5MM

Dear Dr Benson

AL GUPTA dob 21.07.--

9 SEED STREET, CLOVER GATE, MILTON KEYNES MK2 3DT

I regret to inform you that the above patient has failed to attend their outpatient clinic appointment on one, two, three occasions. (delete as appropriate)

A further appointment has been sent to the patient.

No further appointment has been sent to the patient and they have been discharged back to your care. (delete as appropriate)

Yours sincerely

Mr D Watson
Consultant Gastroenterologist

Figure 6.2 Example of a Did Not Attend outpatient clinic letter

HOSPITAL HEADING

Ref: DW/sac/proform/44 44 21

Date: 10 12 --

> Dr D Benson
> Watling Road Practice
> Watling Road West
> Milton Keynes
> MK12 5MM

Dear Dr Benson

AL GUPTA dob 21.07.--

9 SEED STREET, CLOVER GATE, MILTON KEYNES MK2 3DT

Your patient attended for .... surgery on 9th December ....

A review appointment has been arranged for ....

> Yours sincerely

> Mr D Watson
> Consultant Gastroenterologist

Figure 6.3 Example of a letter to confirm that surgery has been carried out

PLEASE RETURN THESE CASE NOTES AS SOON AS POSSIBLE TO:

THE DERMATOLOGY SECRETARY

LEVEL 1, OUTPATIENT BUILDING

EXTENSION 3658

CASE NOTE TRACKING CODE: SECDERM

Reason: Clinic dictation 4.4.--

THANK YOU

Figure 6.4 Example of a return label for case notes taken for another clinic or doctor's attention

Letters for signature can be kept in pristine condition by keeping them in folders labelled appropriately and placed in the doctor's tray or pigeonhole. Check departmental procedure as some doctors like to be paged or bleeped when their letters are ready for signature; others may expect you to make them available at the beginning or end of outpatient clinic sessions.

If there are indistinct words or passages on the cassette which you are unable to decipher you should keep the cassette with the case note(s) and clearly mark where the gaps are for the doctor to complete at the earliest opportunity.

Wipe audio cassettes clean when you are satisfied that the dictation has been transcribed, and that the audio cassette will not need to be referred to again, and rewind to the start of side one to avoid confusion with cassettes which are waiting to be typed. See Chapter 13 for additional information about audio dictation.

Occasionally, case notes have to be taken for other clinics before there is an opportunity to type the letters. Set up a system whereby whoever removes the case notes leaves a patient and GP label from the notes, or a note. These are left with the other notes and cassette waiting to be typed. In addition a label can be attached to the front of the case notes asking for them to be returned so that the copy of the letter yet to be typed can be filed inside. See Figure 6.4 for an example of a return label which can be attached to the front of case notes. Departments are generally familiar with this system and should use internal systems to return the case notes to you and not return to the main records store.

It may be possible within your department to use a number of proforma letters on your personal computer for some groups of patients.

For example, when patients fail to attend their hospital appointments it is possible to have a standard letter format (see Figure 6.2) to be sent to the patient's doctor and the patient. Another example (see Figure 6.3), might be a letter to confirm that a patient has attended for a surgical procedure in an outpatient clinic and no further details, unless there were complications, need to be mentioned.

PRIORITISING TYPING WORKLOAD

The working week will be determined by the doctor's/consultant's clinic timetable or GP's surgery sessions. A clinic timetable is therefore a useful piece of information to have displayed on the noticeboard; see Figure 6.5 for an example of a hospital department timetable.

In this example an influx of clinic work for typewriting can be expected on the Tuesday afternoon, Wednesday afternoon, Thursday morning, Friday afternoon and late Friday or the following Monday morning. The number of patients attending each clinic is in direct relation to the number of letters dictated, though sometimes more than one letter is required for patients being referred elsewhere.

The ratio of new to old patients is also important. New patient letters are generally longer than those for follow-up patients because they contain reference

DAY	MORNING	AFTERNOON
Monday	-	-
Tuesday	OUTPATIENT CLINIC Dr Peach, Consultant Physician Dr George, Registrar	-
Wednesday	OUTPATIENT CLINIC Dr Fisher, Senior Registrar	OUTPATIENT CLINIC Professor Robert Johns Dr George, Registrar
Thursday	-	-
Friday	OUTPATIENT CLINIC Professor Robert Johns Dr Fisher, Senior Registrar	OUTPATIENT CLINIC Dr George, Registrar

Figure 6.5 Example of general medical outpatient clinic timetable

Reflection Point 5

Using the information given in Figure 6.5, when would you expect to receive your incoming typing workload?

Reflection Point 6

What other factors influence the period of time that elapses before correspondence is sent, and which of these should you be familiar with?

to the patients' relevant past medical and social history as well as clinical findings.

It is therefore important that the secretary considers the clinic workload as a continuous cycle of transcription, presentation for signature and dispatch. It is unusual for medical secretaries to clear the transcription every day; typing should be prioritised daily and issues addressed, within secretarial control, which might affect the turnaround of work. Clarify when doctors visit your department for signing letters, whether they need to be reminded and inform new medical staff joining your department of systems already established.

Hospitals

What are the implications if a member of your medical team delays dictating clinic letters for patients who have attended an outpatient clinic?

- Case notes awaiting dictation are static in the department, taking up valuable space and time when searching through for case notes.
- Case notes may be taken away for other clinics and if the case notes are not returned promptly, or are sent back to the medical records department in error, a letter may be delayed or missed. This may result in your department or the contracts department being contacted by a GP surgery requesting confirmation of clinic attendance and treatment received, and financial penalties may be incurred.

General practice

If there are delays in letters being dispatched by general practice then this will result in:

- Delays for patients entering the referral system at the hospital, including the dispatch of an outpatient appointment. This may result in telephone calls and queries from patients enquiring about their forthcoming appointment.

HOSPITAL LOGO

NOTIFICATION OF CANCELLATION AND REDUCTION OF CLINIC

Clinics will only be cancelled/amended when authorisation has been given by the Consultant in whose name the Clinic is held. A minimum of six weeks' notice should be given:

CLINIC LIST IN THE NAME OF: _____

IF JUNIOR DOCTOR, STATE WHICH
CONSULTANT YOU WORK FOR: _____

DATE	PAS CODE	CANCEL NEW PTS/ F/UP PTS	REDUCE BY	SPECIAL COMMENTS OR REQUESTS e.g. 4 doctors rather than usual 5

DATE:

CONSULTANT NAME (CAPITALS):

SIGNATURE:

FOR APPOINTMENTS USE ONLY

CLINIC AMENDMENT/CANCELLATION

DATE RECEIVED

ACKNOWLEDGEMENT SENT

CHANGE COMPLETED

Figure 6.6 Notification of cancellation and reduction of clinics proforma

INTERNAL/EXTERNAL SYSTEMS TO FACILITATE GOOD COMMUNICATION

It is essential that the staff you work with are also able to find their way around your office, so it is important to label trays and pigeonholes clearly and to ensure that files and records are easily accessible.

In addition, it is important to keep up-to-date information available on the different procedures you use, as you will be absent at different times throughout the year. This will help minimise the disruption to the daily routine whilst you are away and there will be fewer queries on your return.

TRACKING SYSTEM FOR MEDICAL CASE NOTES AND X-RAYS

It is essential that a tracking system is used for patient case notes entering and leaving the department. Increasingly, departments are utilising the computerised Patient Administration System (PAS) and bar coding case notes for accurate identification and tracking. The most important information recorded is the destination of case notes and the date they leave the office. The majority of case notes are returned to the medical records department for general filing.

There will, however, be requests for notes to be taken to other departments or outpatient clinics and, if the tracking system is not updated the case notes will still be tracked to the department and considered the secretary's responsibility.

In addition, the comments section in tracking systems can be used to track notes to various locations in the department and assist in saving time when locating them. A system is only as good as its users, so it is important that medical staff and other staff using the office are made aware of the tracking system, have access to it and update it.

DIARY

The secretary will usually hold the doctor's diary, whether computerised or manual, and may be required to provide the doctor with a supplementary list of appointments contained in the diary on a daily basis. Whichever system is used, it is important that entries are updated, accurate and accessible and that, if the secretary keeps records, a check is made that they match. The secretary will need to clarify times the doctor sees medical representatives as they may have a regular slot in the diary. Similarly, details of regular meetings can be transposed into the diary.

Notification of cancellation/reduction of clinics

The secretary is usually the first to know when a doctor is going to take annual or study leave. It is advisable to ask the doctors from time to time what their leave arrangements are to be, perhaps leaving a message to do so in the bring forward file. In hospitals it may also be helpful to liaise with the medical staffing department, usually based within the personnel or human resources department framework, who manage a doctor's leave records.

It is essential that information about doctors' leave is passed on as soon as possible, usually in writing, to the appropriate staff, particularly those in charge of clinics so the necessary reductions or cancellations can be made to the clinic. This may necessitate rescheduling of patients already booked into appointments to other clinic dates.

When notification has not been received, or there has been insufficient time to contact patients, even by telephone or telemessage, this can have serious consequences and result in clinics over running, doctors attending the clinic experiencing a higher than normal workload, patients having to wait unacceptable periods to be seen or being turned away. This situation should be avoided at all costs.

Figure 6.6 shows a proforma which might be utilised instead of a memorandum and illustrates some of the information required by the appointments staff.

BRING FORWARD SYSTEM

You may utilise both computerised and manual systems to highlight work requiring immediate attention. A simple example would be to use a concertina wallet divided into the twelve months of the year. Correspondence, queries and items to be actioned at a later date can then be placed in the appropriate slot. This can be used in conjunction with a concertina folder divided into days of the month (1 to 31), transferring papers and reminders from one to the other at the beginning of each month.

Any bring forward system must be checked daily and relevant correspondence or messages retrieved and actioned accordingly.

HOSPITAL HEADING

Direct Line:

Fax No:

Ref: DW / sac /

Clinic: (enter date and then copy)

Typed: (enter date and then copy)

Dear

                                                                Yours sincerely

                                                                Mr D Watson
                                                                Consultant Gastroenterologist

---

Figure 6.7 Outline of a letter which can be set up on computer as a macro or glossary

COMPUTER SYSTEM

It is imperative to keep back-up disks of work held on computer and endeavour to carry out regular housekeeping, at least once a month, to erase any files that are no longer required.

Building up a glossary facility with doctors' names and addresses for quick and easy insertion into correspondence, and setting up macro outlines or autotext entries to format correspondence for each member of the medical team saves time and keeps keying to a minimum. Figure 6.7 shows an outline of a letter. Similarly, you can add medical terms to autotext and spell-check to make them as comprehensive as possible.

Chapter 8, on information technology, looks at computer systems in more detail.

REFERENCE BOOKS

Ensure you have ready access to reference books such as:

- medical dictionary
- general dictionary
- Monthly Index of Medical Specialties (MIMS) and/or British National Formulary (BNF) for checking the spelling of drugs (sometimes obtainable from the pharmacy, or your doctors can provide you with a recent copy)
- internal and external telephone directories
- medical directories
- folder of departmental and hospital procedures and protocols
- general secretarial information pertaining to the department.

HOSPITAL LOGO

Date:

To: _____

____   For your information/circulation

____   Please take appropriate action

____   As requested

____   I should be grateful for your comments

____   Please answer this for me

____   Please read and return

____   For your files

Dr S. Patel

WITH COMPLIMENTS

Figure 6.8 Example of compliment slip style action proforma

NOTICE BOARDS

Your notice board is a useful tool for quick and easy reference for yourself and colleagues. For a notice board to be an effective aid, all information displayed must be current and updated at regular intervals. It is helpful to display:

- useful telephone numbers and doctors' page/bleep numbers
- diagrammatic clinic timetable
- diagrammatic doctors' timetables
- lists of macros and glossary short forms available on your PC
- holiday timetables
- calendar.

It must be remembered that no patient-identifying details must be displayed on notice boards, for example operating or clinic lists of patients

CIRCULATION OF INFORMATION TO MEMBERS OF THE TEAM

When information has to be circulated, a proforma can easily be attached to a document with the appropriate action indicated for the receiver; see Figure 6.8. Similarly, proformas can be used to simplify requests and avoid confusion, for example a photocopying requisition form when this is carried out by another department; see Figure 6.9.

MAIL

All correspondence, including patient case notes, must be transported securely in sealed envelopes or bags. There may be a dedicated transport service for patient case notes in addition to the internal mail service for general post. The secretary will need to clarify whether mail is delivered to the department or has to be collected from a central point.

PHOTOCOPYING REQUISITION

Date requested

Department

No. of originals

No. of copies

Print 2 sides

Collated YES/NO

Other requirements

Figure 6.9 Photocopying requisition form which can be adapted accordingly to instruct staff on facilities available to them

Hospital patient case notes must never leave the Trust from which they originate, except in extraordinary circumstances. Once a written request for information and the patient's written consent have been received, the doctor will indicate whether all or certain sections of the case notes can be copied and despatched. The same applies in general practice, unless the case notes have been recalled, for example, for auditing or for dispatch to a patient's new GP.

Incoming mail

Mail should be opened regularly and sorted into items for action by the secretary and items for the doctors. Some doctors prefer to open, sort and prioritise their own mail. All mail should be date stamped once it is opened, as this commences an audit trail. All case notes should ideally be tracked into the department when they are received.

As with some messages, it is important to provide the doctor with as much information as possible to accompany a letter or test result, and this will usually necessitate locating relevant case notes for the patient indicated. If, however, case notes are unobtainable in the first instance, this should not delay bringing the letter to the doctor's attention.

Incoming mail for general practice usually includes:

- letters from hospital for patients who have attended outpatient clinic visits
- discharge summaries for patients who have been discharged from an inpatient stay in hospital
- test results.

Incoming mail for a consultant and his team usually includes:

- referral letters from general practitioners requesting a specialist opinion
- test results from the various laboratories.

Both may receive:

- requests for information from solicitors, insurance companies, other hospitals
- agenda/minutes of meetings
- pharmaceutical literature
- medical journals
- general correspondence.

Outgoing mail

Mail must be clearly and fully labelled with its destination. It can be helpful to print labels, and a facility on PAS can produce freetext labels for frequently used destinations.

Mail will usually have to be sorted into 'internal' mail, which is going to departments or internal organisations, and 'external' mail, which is collected by the Post Office for delivery. Patient case notes must be tracked to their destinations on PAS.

Mail is usually sent out second class unless first class is indicated on the envelope. It will be necessary to clarify how, when and where mail is collected and this will need to be from a secure place. Outgoing mail should be left ready for collection and despatched at the earliest opportunity.

There may be an internal transport link system between neighbouring hospitals and general practices where post bypasses the Post Office, thus saving postage costs and distribution time and preserving confidentiality.

DEPARTMENT LOGO

ADDRESS

TELEPHONE NUMBER

(Headed Paper)
FACSIMILE NUMBER

FAX

INFORMATION STRICTLY CONFIDENTIAL

TO   _____

FROM   _____

DATE   _____

NUMBER OF PAGES, INCLUDING FRONT SHEET _____

IF THERE ARE ANY DIFFICULTIES WITH RECEIVING THIS FAX PLEASE CONTACT

_____

(optional) Please fax the attached sheet to us as soon as possible to confirm receipt.

YOUR MESSAGE

(This fax is strictly confidential and for the attention of the indicated recipient only and must not be disclosed to any other party than the recipient indicated above. If received in error please contact the sender immediately, or telephone this number: .... Thank you.)

Figure 6.10 Example of a fax covering sheet

FACSIMILE COPIES

The fax machine is a relatively cheap way to send information and is very useful when information has to be relayed quickly. It is essential that care is taken in dialing numbers (confidentiality could easily be breached if patient information were transmitted to the wrong destination).

Some safeguards include:

- checking with the recipient of the fax to find out where it will be received, and deleting patient identifying details if appropriate or if in doubt that the receiving area is secure

Exercises

Discuss how you would deal with the following situations.

- An elderly patient's daughter telephones you to ask why her mother is attending the clinic as she is very worried about her.

- A patient telephones you and asks you to tell him the result of his blood test. He says he was told to ring you for this information.

- You receive a call from a friend of a patient who wants to enquire whether the patient is still an inpatient in the hospital.

- A solicitor's clerk telephones and gives details of a particular patient whom he says has given permission for her records to be released to him. He asks you to send the case notes to him urgently, as the patient's court appearance is imminent, and to clarify some specific appointment dates on the telephone.

- contacting the recipient just before you send the fax
- asking the receiver of the fax to contact you as soon as it is received, either by telephone or with an acknowledgement fax

A top sheet should always accompany the faxed sheets and Figure 6.10 provides an example.

E-MAIL

The use of computer networking to facilitate communication between hospitals and general practice is gradually increasing as more sophisticated hardware and software is introduced into the health care sector. However, the accessibility of information means secure systems have to be in place to protect patient confidentiality. Secretaries should familiarise themselves with local protocols and whether patient-identifying details such as name, date of birth and address can be sent on internal e-mail, or whether, for example, only case note reference numbers can be used to identify the patient. (See Chapter 8, on information technology.) As a rule, the Internet should never be used to transmit details of patients outside the organisation.

CONCLUSION

The role of the medical secretary is to process a constant and wide variety of incoming verbal and written data. The dissemination of this information may in turn be verbal or written. Accuracy, timeliness and appropriate disclosure of information is central to the smooth running of the department. The secretary provides an important communication link between the professionals sharing the 'hands on' care of patients, and may often be the first representative of the organisation with whom a patient will come into contact. How the secretary relates to patients and staff is of great importance if patients are to have confidence, from the outset, in the care they are to receive.

Chapter 7

Finance

Stephanie J Green

OBJECTIVE

- To enable the reader to appreciate the importance of finance in general practice and the role of specific administrative staff to monitor and manage it
- To assist the reader in understanding the sources of finance in general practice
- To explain the different demands which private practice will make of the medical secretary
- To provide a source of reference material including official publications and journals.

INTRODUCTION

This chapter is designed to introduce basic financial procedures and to discuss the measures by which income and expenditure are managed in general practice and in private practice. It should be obvious that the finances of a hospital will not be part of a secretary's normal role. However, if this is an area of work which fascinates, there is nothing to stop the secretary undertaking further training to extend experience and ability, in order to fulfil a different role or to find promotion in a different area of administration.

Financial management in medicine has become more complicated over the past few years and the changes in structure generally have made the employment of other professional people a necessity. This does not mean that the medical secretary will have nothing to do with financial affairs; whatever the involvement with income and expenditure, it is always important to understand the responsibilities attached to this area of work and the good practice which should be observed at all levels. It is true to say that medical secretaries who work in private practice will probably have more to do with the financial side of their work than a secretary working within the National Health Service.

GENERAL PRACTICE

In general practice, the financial control of the practice will lie with the practice manager, with the help of an accountant at times, depending on the needs of the practice. Financial work will include:

- regular checks on NHS claims for work – complete, correct and submitted on time
- control of petty cash
- administration of invoices and receipts
- salaries
- insurance
- PAYE for staff
- maintenance of cheque books and accounts. It is likely that in the future all accounts will be computerised – many are already.

The medical secretary may be involved with some or none of this work, depending upon the nature of the practice. However, there are financial tasks which may well be the medical secretary's responsibility. These are:

- Receipt of invoices or payments in the mail – these will need to be recorded in the relevant book and redirected to the practice manager.
- Invoicing accurately for work completed, in accordance with the standard fees list, e.g. requests for medico-legal reports. These are usually the responsibility of the medical secretary because of the use of specialist language within the report. A diary system will also be needed to ensure that payment has been received, especially as these reports may be part of lengthy legal debate and payment may therefore be long term.
- Invoicing for photocopying of notes requested by solicitors, once patient consent/authority has been given for the use of confidential material. Again, a proper record of this kind of work should be kept and a note of payments made.

Although we have mentioned areas of financial concern specific to the medical secretary, there are some general points that all staff working in general practice will need to remember in order to maintain an efficient system. Today, general practice has to be run like any other business, balancing income against all the usual outgoings and expenditure.

Reflection Point 1

Make a list of all the expenses involved with business premises you can think of. Then think of your own general practice or one where you have had work experience and add all the more particularly medical items.

THE NEW CONTRACT

The title used for the system of funding at the moment for most practices is General Medical Services (GMS).

This contract is expected to apply to all countries in the UK and will be negotiated nationally, but the contract will be with each practice, not with individuals. The intention is to reward practices that offer quality services to their patients. The more NHS work that is carried out by a practice, the higher their reward. This is a positive incentive for GPs to treat patients in the community for such items as minor surgery and to carry out diagnostic tests rather than send them to hospital, which is the principle of the primary care-led NHS. The hope is that there will be a focus on quality and a vision of a modernised service where personal care matters and patients will see the benefits of a wider range of services. The following points are at the heart of the new contract:

- It will allow doctors to control their workload by allowing choice in the level of service they will provide.
- Each practice will be given a 'global' sum from which they must manage their budget to provide essential and additional services.
- The Red Book of fees and allowances will disappear and will be replaced by the Blue Book.
- New work will be matched by new money.

Other health care professionals may be employed to provide services identified by the practice where appropriate. This will allow them to facilitate an improvement in the quality of service to patients while also allowing them to choose a level of service which could ease their workload pressures.

- They can opt out of 'out of hours services'.
- It provides for salaried GPs with flexible contractual arrangements. It also recognises the need for a career structure for GPs.

The service will be grouped into the following categories:

- essential services
- additional services
- enhanced services.

Practice budgets will vary depending upon a number of factors such as the number of patients on the doctors' lists, and whether it is a rural practice or an inner city practice for which special payments may be made. The common activities known as 'essential services' are included in the budget. Some examples of essential services are shown in Box 7.1.

Another source of income is from 'additional services'. These are items of care which have a special percentage target to be achieved by the practitioners if they are to gain the maximum payment for their work. At the moment claims under this scheme are for organised care of illnessess shown in Box 7.2.

Enhanced services are services to patients which especially allow practices to increase their budget. These items are shown in Box 7.3.

Other sources of income for general practice are:

- trainee practitioner scheme
- postgraduate education allowance
- education of medical students
- private patients
- insurance medicals
- cremation forms
- special driving licences and passport forms.

Some GPs take other appointments such as medical responsibility for a local company or for the police as police surgeon.

It is hoped that the new contract will allow GPs to benefit from greater and fairer rewards with improvements to their working lives. This is needed to revitalise and encourage GPs. At the moment there is a perception that the workload is unsustainable and therefore unattractive. By creating a new contract the Government hopes to solve this problem and introduce extra resources in exchange for reform.

Box 7.1 Some essential services

- Patient registration
- Child surveillance
- Contraceptive services
- Antenatal care

Box 7.2 Some additional services

Care of:
- Asthma
- Cancer
- Diabetes
- Chronic Obstructive Pulmonary Disease
- Epilepsy
- Coronary Heart Disease

Box 7.3 Some enhanced services

- Childhood immunisations
- INR testing
- IUD fitting
- Minor surgery
- Advanced patient access
- Phlebotomy
- Influenza and Pneumococcal vaccination
- Shared care with other professionals e.g. for the care of drug misuse

---

PERSONAL MEDICAL SERVICES

Since the NHS Act 1997 the government has piloted a different contractual arrangement for the delivery of general medical services by general practitioners, known as Personal Medical Services (PMS). GP practices may decide to adopt this new scheme and will hold its new contract with its PCT. PMS allows a certain flexibility to deliver identified care by the necessary health professionals within the general practice. On the basis of identified local need the practice can negotiate a contract with their PCT to address these needs and can work to cover previous inadequacies or inappropriate provision. Under the Act there is a right to return to GMS following an agreed notice period. The initial funding will be based on the funding the practice would have received under GMS in the previous year.

> ## Box 7.4 General and personal medical services
>
> ### General Medical Services (GMS)
>
> Care is delivered through a nationally determined contract
>
> Payment is as a global sum known as Minimum Practice Income Guarantee (MPIG) with three levels of service
>
> Income can vary
>
> ### Personal Medical Services (PMS)
>
> A range of services is specified with individual practices in locally agreed contracts
>
> The Commissioner (PCT) and Providers (GPs and Nurses) agree a total annual price as their budget. This may be paid monthly and increases financial stability
>
> Income is agreed in advance

PMS practices can bid for GMS enhanced services to increase their budgets. The main differences are displayed in Box 7.4.

PMS practices may develop their provision with PMS Plus to reflect the specific needs of their practice population and offer an enhanced range of services. PMS allows the whole health team to provide for the specific health needs of their patient population. It emphasises the need for quality of provision.

It is hoped that this flexibility at a local level will encourage GPs, as there is more flexibility and stability in their employment. Remember that there is a national shortage of GPs and the government hopes that this will help to alleviate this problem and enhance the working practice of doctors. Students should try to keep up to date with developments by listening to the news, reading reliable newspapers and reading medical journals whenever possible.

Reflection Point 2

Remember to ask about funding when you are in a general practice work placement. Whose responsibility is it? Which method of funding is being used by your practice? If it is a new contract ask about the changes that have happened and how decisions are made.

PRIVATE PRACTICE

In private practice there is more responsibility demanded of the medical secretary for the maintenance of accurate accounts. This will largely fall into three areas:

- The maintenance of patient accounts
- The maintenance of practice accounts
- Banking.

PATIENT ACCOUNTS

Each practice will have a list of set charges appropriate to the work of the practice. This will include the items shown in Box 7.5.

Patient accounts may be kept on a card index or more commonly now, may be computerised. The record for each patient will record:

- the date of the bill sent for each visit
- the date the bill was paid
- the date of any reminders sent.

When a patient pays his/her account, a note should be made of the method of settlement, i.e. whether through his/her own account, by cheque, or by an insurance company in that patient's name – this is often the case where patients are subscribers to a private health care plan or are covered in this way through their work.

PRACTICE ACCOUNTS

A well-kept accounts book will:

- assist an accountant in preparing accounts
- provide much of the financial information for annual audit
- provide necessary information for tax self-assessment.

The accounts book will have separate pages for expenditure and income. It is also useful to keep a separate book for recording cheques written on the account, with all the details noted. Remember that only the cheque number will appear on the regular

- New patients – this is a charge for a first appointment or for a re-referral. As 'history taking' will be involved, these appointments take longer than a normal appointment.
- Follow-up visit
- Special treatments
- Injections
- X-ray
- Charge for inpatient care, should the patient be admitted to hospital. In this circumstance, the medical secretary must always be ready to take note of the following:
  - the number of days in hospital
  - any treatment carried out
  - any inpatient visits carried out.

These items will be picked up and charged for when the discharge report has been made.

bank statement. It is easier to identify cheque details and to trace payments if you have made another more detailed record. All bills and receipts should also be kept as a back-up record.

Each transaction entered into an accounts book should be dated and entered into the relevant column. If the payment has been made by cheque, the cheque number should be entered into that column as well.

Some transactions are made automatically by the bank. These may be identified by particular initials such as:

- DD – direct debit
- SO – standing order
- TR – transfer.

With DD and SO, sums of money are taken out of the account on a predetermined date each month. This is always an arrangement which is made in advance with the full authorisation of the account holder.

TR applies to another arrangement made with the bank and authorised by the account holder. This is not strictly a payment, but a setting aside of money from a current account to a holding account in order to allow for certain bills to be paid on demand on regular occasions. This may be for payments such as income tax. When this demand comes from the Inland Revenue, the secretary must contact the bank

and arrange for the correct amount of money to be transferred back to the practice account in order to make sure that there are sufficient funds available to meet the cheque.

Reflection Point 3

How long will it take for the bank to complete this transaction? If you do not know – find out!

Figure 7.1 provides an example of a payments page from an accounts book.

BANKING

A special bank account will be held by the practice and with it an accounts book, as a record of all financial transactions undertaken.

As cheques arrive:

- record details on the patient's record
- enter into the paying-in book
- record in cheque record book
- bank cheques weekly.

As bills arrive:

- present the bill and 'made out' cheque to the person authorised to make the payment, ready for signing and dispatch before the over-due date arrives. (You may find that some practices require two signatories.)
- do not present all the bills at once – plan the payment over a sensible amount of time.

Remember that cheques written as payment from the practice must also be recorded with all details of the payee, the date and the cheque number.

Reflection Point 4

When a bank statement arrives it will only show you a cheque number. How will you trace your payments? What other record should you keep of your payments so that your accounts can be properly checked?

PAYMENTS ANALYSIS									SUNDRIES
RENT RATES AND INSURANCE	REPAIRS RENEWALS AND MAINTENANCE	SALARIES AND WAGES	PETTY CASH	BANK LEGAL AND ACCOUNTANTS CHARGES	DRESSINGS DRUGS AND INSTRUMENTS	TRANSPORT EXPENSES			

Figure 7.1 A payments page.

IMPREST £	DATE	DETAILS	VOUCHER NO.	TOTAL £	POSTAGE	STATIONERY	OFFICE . EXP	OTHER EXP.
5.80	1	Balance B/F						
44.20	1	Cash Forward						
	3	Stamps	123	15.00	15.00			
	4	Tea/Coffee	124	7.34			7.34	
	8	Taxi	125	6.30				6.30
	10	Magazines	126	4.30			4.30	
	15	Flowers	127	5.60				5.60
	18	2 Electric plugs	128	2.00			2.00	
	21	Rec' Delivery	129	0.55	0.55			
	28	Notebooks	130	1.00		1.00		
	30	Luggage Labels	131	1.50				1.50
		Total Spent		43.59	15.55	1.00	13.64	13.40
		Balance in hand		6.41				
50.00				50.00				
6.41		Balance B/F						
43.59		Cash						

Figure 7.2 A petty cash book page totalled and 'restored'

PETTY CASH

Petty cash usually refers to transactions which are made by cash payment. This is a system used to account for everyday small payments in most businesses, and staff in general practice and in many other areas of medical administration need to know how this works. If payment is made to the practice for a fee for a service provided, this is a different matter altogether and this should be kept quite separate from the day-to-day petty cash, and should be accounted for properly, with a description in the accounts book and full payment made into the practice account. However, in order to deal with everyday petty cash, a float of money of an agreed amount may be kept to enable small payments to be made for items such as postage stamps. This sum of money is often referred to as 'imprest'. It will often be kept in a petty cash tin with petty cash vouchers and a petty cash book in which to enter the transactions for each month. A petty cash voucher must be issued as an authority to make a purchase, and will be signed by a senior member of staff.

A petty cash book will be divided into columns to describe the expenditure. These headings will vary depending on the character of the practice, but may use such headings as 'post, stationery, office and sundries'. Once the imprest has been decided upon, expenditure will be totalled up regularly on an agreed date (probably monthly) and the sum needed to restore the imprest to its agreed starting amount will be withdrawn from the general account (Figure 7.2).

CONCLUSION

From this chapter, the medical secretary should be able to understand some of the complexities of financial management in general practice and appreciate the differences which may be found in private practice.

Exercises

- Find out how to write out a cheque accurately.

- What is an invoice?

- How can you use a credit note?

- When you are on work placement, make sure you find out how your practice deals with petty cash.

- Does the practice have a reference source for new staff? Is there one member of staff who is particularly responsible for finance? Is this a good or a bad idea?

Further reading

Harrison J 1996 Secretarial duties, 10th edn. Longman, Harlow
This book covers the general financial aspects of secretarial duties.
Lilley R 2003 The new GP contract: How to make the most of it. Radcliffe Medical Press, Abingdon

Journals and Periodicals:
Medeconomics (published by Haymarket Medical)
www.bma.org.uk/ap.nsf/Content
www.doh.gov.uk/pricare/pca.htm

Chapter **8**

Information technology

Barbara Sen

CHAPTER CONTENTS

OBJECTIVES

- To demonstrate the importance of information and information technology in today's NHS

- To describe the different kinds of information that you may be involved in creating or working with as a medical secretary

- To show how you contribute towards information gathering and management

- To highlight the importance of confidentiality and accuracy on your part in using information technology, including the provisions of the Data Protection Act

- To explain the type of procedures you will have to observe regarding accuracy and security of patient data and the computing equipment itself

- To describe developments in information technology in the NHS that you may become involved with in the future, especially communications.

Before you start reading this chapter, find a bank (or building society current account) statement or a telephone bill (one that has the calls itemised).

INTRODUCTION

We deal first of all with the role of information in

today's NHS and what plans the NHS Information Authority has for information technology (IT) and information. One key White Paper outlining the government's strategy for information in the NHS is *Information for Health* (Department of Health, 1998) which has implications for the day-to-day use of IT for everyone in the NHS.

Then we discuss how you may be affected by IT, first in a hospital setting, then in general practice.

Next we point out the major aspects of confidentiality and security of data wherever you are working.

In the longer term, IT brings the prospect of NHS-wide data communications and we deal with this towards the end of the chapter.

Because each institution has different procedures and because there is such diversity of computer equipment we have dealt with topics in a general way, trying to focus on basic principles rather than specific types of computer. We do, however, use some examples taken from actual practice to illustrate the possibilities of IT.

Reflection Point 1

This activity will help you appreciate how information appears in different forms. Take a look at either the bank statement or the telephone bill that we asked you to find earlier on.

If you have a bank statement, note how each individual transaction is recorded and all the transactions are added up so the final result is a *summary* figure telling you how much money remains in your account. The individual transactions are simply bits of *data* but the summary is *information*. Additionally, the information is sorted into columns of deposits and withdrawals.

If you have an itemised telephone bill you can see how the telephone calls are individually listed but also grouped into local and national calls as well as providing a total amount to pay. Again, the computer has collected all the information relating to calls at different times and to different destinations from your telephone and brought them together to make up your telephone bill.

In these examples a constant factor such as your telephone number or bank account number brings all these different individual bits of data together. In the same way these 'constants' or 'unique' numbers (such as the NHS number, which we discuss later on) are an important requirement for NHS information systems.

In addition, there is a short glossary of computer terms at the end of the chapter.

Reflection Point 2

Earlier on we looked at the example of a bank statement and how it provides information for the bank customer. But the tens of thousands of individual transactions for thousands of customers form the basis for a summary for use for managerial purposes. The bank manager is responsible for thousands of customers' accounts and wants to know who has overdrawn and so that he/she can order action. But the manager doesn't need to see every account or every transaction, just exceptions and a summary, all of which can be created by a computer.

At Headquarters level the management want to know how branches are performing in comparison with national averages and which are performing poorly and might need closing. They don't need to know about individual transactions but they need to summarise information created from those transactions.

This shows that at different levels of the bank's management different people need different things from the same information. In the same way different 'layers' of the NHS need different types of information.

THE ROLE OF INFORMATION IN THE NHS

Before you read further you may like to consult Figure 8.1.

To run today's NHS a vast amount of information is needed at different levels and for different purposes. The information has to be timely, accurate and relevant to each level of the organisation. This means

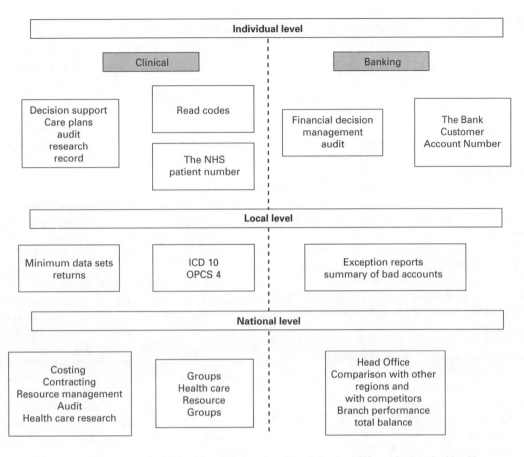

Figure 8.1 Information requirements at individual, local and national levels in the NHS and in a typical banking organisation

that the basic information about tens of hundreds of thousands of individual patient encounters with the NHS has to be summarised and codified so that different layers of information can be created for the different levels of authority in the NHS. As the level goes 'up' so the need for individual data diminishes and the need arises to summarise and group the information.

We will describe this, going from individual to national level.

INDIVIDUAL LEVEL

At the individual (and most important) level, clinical staff who treat the patient need to have access to individual patient information, to add to that information, and to share that information with other authorised professionals.

At this individual patient level there is a certain min-

imum amount of information such as name, age, sex, address and occupation (often called 'demographic' information). In addition, a record is kept of clinical activity associated with that patient. The problem for clinicians is to describe their activity in standardised terms that can be used by computers. In general practice special codes called 'Read' codes are used and are often entered directly into the computer by the doctors.

The Read codes are an agreed dictionary of medical terms that form a kind of 'language of health'. The terms are arranged in a hierarchy so that the

Box 8.1 Read codes	
H	Respiratory system diseases
H2	Pneumonia and influenza
H20	Viral pneumonia
H202	Pneumonia – parainfluenza virus

appropriate amount of detail can be chosen by the clinician. The example in Box 8.1 shows how it works.

The leftmost character defines the broad area, e.g. *Respiratory system diseases*. The more detailed descriptions are covered by characters further to the right. Because each character can be either a number 0-9, or an upper case letter, or a lower case letter, this gives each position 58 possibilities (the characters 'i' and 'o' are excluded). This means that there are over 650 million codes available to cover all sorts of terms.

The codes cover not only diseases and treatment but other aspects of care, such as the patient's occupation, what drugs were prescribed and preventative procedures.

Because different doctors use different clinical descriptions (e.g. a myocardial infarction may also be called a coronary thrombosis or heart attack) the Read codes have a vast number of synonyms so that whatever phrases are used, they all point to the same Read code.

The hierarchical structure of the codes allows for constant additions of new terms and synonyms as medical practice evolves.

In the hospital service ICD (International Classification of Diseases) terms are often used to categorise the diagnosis and OPCS (Office of Population Censuses and Surveys) codes are used to categorise the operations. The current versions are ICD 10 and OPCS 4.

ICD codes are used to describe diseases only. Typical examples of ICD codes are:

- Acute myocardial infarction   410
- Acute papillary muscle infarction   410.8

These codes are numeric only and they deal with levels of detail by using decimal points.

OPCS 4 codes describe treatments and operative procedures only. Example of such codes are:

- Ear operations   D01-28
- Drainage of middle ear   D15
- Radical mastoidectomy   D101
- Simple mastoidectomy   D104

These codes are often entered by specialised staff called 'coders' attached to clinical directorates and can be used to describe 'episodes of care', which are the basic units of hospital activity.

The computerisation of diagnoses and treatments facilitates medical audit: the practice of reviewing and comparing how patients with the same type of condition were treated and what the outcomes were. The latest version Read code (version 3) will be merged with SNOMED to form a preferred system of coding for the NHS. The SNOMED system of clinical terms is the preferred clinical terminology of the NHS. It stands for Systemised Nomenclature of Medicine and is a coding system allowing for the indexing of an entire medical record, and is the system chosen by the NHS for coding the electronic patient records.

LOCAL LEVEL

At local level, Primary Care Trusts and providers of secondary and tertiary care (mental health, acute and teaching hospital trusts within the NHS) need information to see how they are performing against set standards and to work out the cost of services as well as to give 'early warning' of unsatisfactory performance. Such standards include waiting list times for different treatments, cost per patient day and costs for different operations.

Computers can allow the terms entered at the individual level to be translated into the codes required for different purposes such as management information. At this level it is important to make this grouping for planning and costing but not necessary to have the detail that clinicians require for individual care.

Information technology allows the previously encoded information to be analysed quickly in many different ways and thus provides timely information – rather than requiring staff to fill in paper 'returns'. The codes such as ICD 10 for thousands of patients can in turn be translated into hundreds of groups of patients who require similar types of medical care. These groups are called Healthcare Resource Groups and, thus grouped, allow management to work out costings and compare performance.

Because there is so much information available about the patient and only a certain amount is actually needed for these purposes, health organisations use a 'minimum data set' containing only the basic demographic details necessary for their calculations. Amongst these health organisations, the newly formed Strategic Health Authorities (StHAs) take an overall perspective of the delivery of health care across a large population base or geographical boundary, e.g. Greater Manchester Strategic Health Authority.

NATIONAL LEVEL

The government has a statutory responsibility to make available information about overall numbers of patients treated nationwide and at what overall cost. This permits planning of new services, reviewing how existing services are going, and deciding what funds to allocate in the future. For example, average waiting times for treatments are an important measure of service level and have significant political implications.

At the same time, information at this level can be used to establish averages and standards, for example the cost per day of treating one patient.

This permits comparisons to be made between health service performance in different parts of the country and to highlight possible problem areas. It also allows international comparisons.

The role of information technology in all this is that it can greatly assist the communication of patient information, safeguard confidentiality and make the aggregation of individual patient records into useful statistical information much more quickly and accurately than before. It is, therefore, possible to take action to remedy unsatisfactory situations whilst the information is still current.

Because computers allow rapid sorting and transmission of information the possibility now exists for accurate information to be available to senior levels in the NHS without delay. The NHSnet is a secure wide area network (WAN) that has been developed exclusively for the NHS. It supports the sharing of information across health organisations. The NHSnet can be used for a range of information such as training and education, benchmarking services, ordering supplies and sending messages. Services available on the NHSnet are:

- Electronic mail (E-mail) – the ability to send messages and attached documents
- Electronic Data Exchange (EDI) – exchanging data between organisations e.g. pathology and radiology results
- Access to the NHSweb – an information resource exclusive to the NHS
- Remote support for clinical systems – system suppliers can give remote support
- Access to the Internet – access to the World Wide Web (WWW) through secure NHS gateways
- On-line patient bookings – booking patients in for treatment e.g. minor surgery.

THE NHS NUMBER

Now we will describe a particular initiative, which is crucial for the success of IT in the NHS, the NHS number.

The NHS number is a 10-digit number which replaces any previous numbers a patient may have had. In the past there were up to 20 separate types of number, none of which was suitable for computer use. The NHS number, which is now almost universally used by both hospitals and GPs, is more suitable for computer use. It allows seamless transfer of information between health care commissioners and providers for invoicing purposes because the number can be checked by the computer; for clinical staff new information such as test results will go directly to the right patient record. By 2005 all patients will have an electronic patient record (EPR) which will eventually replace paper records.

FOR HOSPITAL-BASED SECRETARIES

Most medical secretaries no longer use stand-alone computers. The majority of office computers are linked to the hospitals' computer network, making a vast range of computerised information services available to the user either over the hospital intranet (a network of computers within an organisation) or via the Internet. Most medical secretaries will find themselves using a Patient Administration System (PAS) containing the names, ages and addresses of all the patients plus episode history (gives demographic data), including those who are currently staying in the hospital.

The PAS is a very large and powerful database. A good example of a database is a telephone directory. Here, addresses and telephone numbers are stored in alphabetical order so that, if you know the name and initials, you can find the number.

A computerised database allows far more powerful arrangements of data so that when a logical question is presented to it, it can produce an appropriate output. So, for example, a *computerised* telephone directory would allow you to enter a telephone number and find out the name and address connected with that number.

In most hospitals the PAS is run by a powerful computer which is usually kept in a central secure location and which is connected by cables to a large number of computer terminals around the entire hospital site. This arrangement is called a 'network' and because it normally covers only one site it is typically called a local area network or LAN. The PAS usually covers all the inpatient work of a hospital as well as the outpatient department (see Chapter 13).

As a medical secretary you may have access to a computer terminal connected to the PAS. (You will require a password for this – we discuss this later on in this chapter.) You can extract information from the PAS such as:

1. Details about a patient's age and address, and some basic details about any episodes of care that patient may have had at the hospital, e.g. date and ward of admission; consultant in charge; diagnosis. Because this information relates to just one identified person we call it *individual* level.

2. The number of admissions in the past month for a particular consultant. Because this information is calculated from lots of *individual* records we call this *aggregate* information. Your work may involve you in extracting aggregate level information for your consultant or hospital management.

Scenario 1

At the Midshire Hospital Trust, consultant staff add patients to waiting lists whilst they are in the outpatient clinic by entering information directly into the PAS system. They can put a patient on particular waiting lists and designate them as 'urgent', 'routine', etc. The medical secretaries on the orthopaedic unit regularly print out the waiting lists by type of treatment or by surgeon. The list is divided into categories such as 'routine', 'urgent', 'soonest', etc. They can also print out the list by the patients' GP and PCT and which are Out of Area referrals.

You may also be required to enter information into the PAS such as admission dates and discharge summaries.

When you are entering information into a PAS you need to remember that the computer system remembers your identity and has an 'audit trail'; it

can trace which person entered, or viewed, a particular piece of information.

Most PAS systems allow different levels of access to different grades of staff. For example, non-clinical administrators may be locked out of information such as medical details and test results and you may find that you are not allowed to do certain things. For example, you may find that you are not allowed to modify a patient's NHS number or their diagnosis.

Because the PAS contains personal clinical information belonging to thousands of patients there are stringent security precautions.

You do not have to have access to the PAS to deal with information. For example, you may have access to a range of information sources and systems via the hospital network, for example word processing, spreadsheet and database programs.

Scenario 2

At the genitourinary clinic at St David's, a hospital in a large city, the secretaries keep a record of telephone enquiries on a computerised spreadsheet. The spreadsheet creates a graph which shows the range of problems dealt with by the unit (Fig. 8.2).

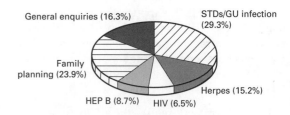

Figure 8.2 Telephone enquiries to the genitourinary clinic (week beginning 5 February)

GENERAL PRACTICE

Almost all primary care practices in the UK have some kind of computer system, so you are almost bound to find yourself using a computer in your practice. You will almost certainly find that the NHS number mentioned above has been implemented for all the patients.

Most consulting rooms and the reception desk usually use computers connected in a 'network'. These computers use programs specially designed for general practice and will handle:

- Basic or full patient records with name, age, sex and address.
- Records of drugs prescribed for patients. This is useful for printing out repeat prescriptions. Some programs can also warn of dangerous drug interactions.
- Recall systems for cervical cytology and children's immunisations. The computer automatically identifies certain patients by sex and age and prints out lists of patients who need certain treatments within a given time period. The computer may also print out standard letters inviting those patients to come for treatment.
- Tracking of additional and enhanced services under the new General Medical Services (GMS) contract from Primary Care Trusts. There is a move towards making some GPs employees of primary care trusts (salaried GPs) as opposed to independent contractors for the provision of medical services.
- Information for medical audit and research purposes. The GP can input special codes to record consultations and treatments for later analysis by the computer. By performing database queries it is possible to compare treatments and outcomes for patients with similar conditions.

 Scenario 3

In the Anytown practice, Dr Green uses her computer at every consultation. She enters the main aspects of the consultation (such as diagnosis, treatment given, drugs used) using special codes called Read codes.

Later on, she can perform a database query to search for patients with a condition or group of similar conditions.

For medical audit purposes, she can see the effect of certain drugs on patients with the same condition. Alternatively, if a warning has been issued by the Department of Health for a particular drug, Dr Green can get a list of all her patients given that drug.

The functions described above are often covered by an 'all-in-one package' from a specialist computer supplier.

Nearly all practices have a facility which combines computers and communications between GPs, Primary Care Trusts, and secondary/tertiary health care providers; the aim of this is to replace paper-based patient registration and transactions previously sent by post with an electronic system. Registrations and item of service details are entered by practice staff and gathered into a computer file for automatic transmission down the telephone line each evening to an electronic 'mailbox' run by a specialist computer company.

To send data down the telephone line a 'modem' is used. A modem takes the digital signal from a PC and modulates it into an analogue signal (sound). The receiving modem will then demodulate this sound signal back into a digital signal at the other end of the line.

The receiver computer dials in to the 'mailbox' and collects the claims. If the claims are accepted a message is sent back to the practice. Increasingly broadband connections are used to transmit information, which are faster and more efficient. Some broadband connections are by direct cable organisation to organisation.

If your practice has the communication systems described above then you may be involved in entering data. This requires you to observe a certain discipline when keying in information, e.g. not using abbreviations such as 'St' for Street. Data should be accurate, complete and consistent. You may have organisational conventions for data input that you have to follow. Being disciplined in data input enables you to retrieve the information more efficiently and effectively when it is needed.

Electronic communications are being developed nationwide with plans to add hospitals to the network of links and services such as on-line access to waiting lists. We cover this later in the chapter.

SAFEGUARDING THE PATIENT AND THE DATA

The latest NHS Executive's information strategy includes the statement that 'information must be confidential and secure, only available to those who need to know'. This section outlines basic security precautions which you will be required to follow, most of them required by the Data Protection Act 1998. The Data Protection Act 1998 replaces the 1984 Act. There are some key differences which include:

- Certain manual records (including all health records) are now covered, as well as electronic records.
- There is a wider definition of 'processing' which includes concepts of obtaining, storing and disclosing data.
- Access is permitted to all manual health records whenever made, subject to a few exemptions.
- Changes to the requirements of notification – now the Information Commissioner (previously the Data Protection Commissioner).

Box 8.2 Data Protection Act

The eight principles of the Data Protection Act 1998 (Schedule 1) say that data must be:
- fairly and lawfully processed
- processed for limited purposes
- adequate, relevant and not excessive
- accurate
- not kept any longer than necessary
- processed in accordance with the rights of the data subject
- secure
- not transferred to other countries without adequate protection.

The Data Protection Act covers the NHS. Box 8.2 lists the main provisions. (These have changed from the 1984 Act.)

Although senior management are responsible for registering your practice or organisation under the Act, everybody has responsibility for compliance with the conditions above.

Anyone processing personal data must comply with the eight enforceable principles of good practice. When you are responsible for handling personal data you will need to consider what information you handle and who you share it with. Following basic principles of good practice will help you to conform with the requirements of the Act. The main issues of concern are:

- Take security measures to prevent unauthorised or accidental access, alteration, disclosure or loss and destruction of information.
- Ensure the data is accurate and, where necessary, up to date.

We now discuss these points in more detail.

Restricting access to the computer system to authorised staff

This is normally achieved through the use of a password which you will have to enter before you can gain access ('log on') to programs containing confidential data such as a PAS. You need to observe the following precautions.

- Do not use your own name, middle name or nickname as your password. Some computers will reject a password consisting only of letters and may insist on you using more than four characters. Ideally you should use a mix of letters and numbers.
- Make sure that no one is looking over your shoulder when you are typing in your password. When you enter your password the computer screen will not display what you have typed but someone could memorise your keystrokes.
- Similarly, make sure that no unauthorised people can see the computer screen when you are viewing patient information.

When you have finished using the PAS you must 'log off' the program – each computer has different mechanisms for this. It is vitally important that you do this, even if you leave the room for just a few minutes, otherwise the computer thinks you are still there and will allow someone else to use it. Most computer systems automatically switch themselves off if they detect two or three minutes of inactivity, but you should not rely on this.

You need to remember that some computer screens go dark automatically to save electricity and to stop the screen from being damaged by 'burn in' – this is not the same as switching off or logging off.

Do not use someone else's password and do not let anyone know or use yours. When you first start work you will probably be issued with a temporary password which you will have to replace almost straight away with one that you think up. Finally, remember to change your password regularly!

ENSURING ACCURACY IS MAINTAINED

You need to be aware that it is much easier to confuse characters on screen and much harder to detect spelling mistakes. You need to be extremely careful when entering information into databases because the smallest mistake could mean that important test results and communications about a patient are misread or go astray.

Patients have the right to access electronic data held about them under the provisions of the Data Protection Act enacted in 1998 – so be careful what you put in, or are asked to put in – the patient may see it later. You should also be aware that patients are allowed to see their own paper-based record (see Chapter 12).

MAKING SURE THAT INFORMATION IS NOT CORRUPTED

Computer programs and the data they contain are at risk from corruption or damage from three sources.Be disciplined in checking, updating and renewing data.

Viruses

Whilst computers can be of great benefit, some destructive people make and distribute computer viruses which cause damage to computer systems.

A virus is a piece of computer code that can attach itself to a program and copy itself when the program is run. This enables the virus to be transmitted to other programs and also from one computer system to another. Viruses are often transmitted via e-mail or across the Internet.

The symptoms caused by a computer virus are: messages appear on the screen; data goes wrong; the computer takes longer to load and carry out commands. Viruses can seriously damage your data – which means that vitally important patient information and programs could be destroyed. Networks are particularly at risk because data is being passed rapidly around many computers.

The most common cause of transferring viruses is the use of floppy disks because they can easily be loaded into different computers. What this means for the medical secretary is that floppy disks containing 'shareware' programs or computer games should never be used on your work computer.

Your hospital or practice should have precautions in place against attack by viruses. Viruses can be detected by using a 'scanner' – a specialised piece of software. If you need to use a floppy disk at all, make sure that it is 'write protected' and that you test it with a 'scanner' program before copying data to your computer's hard disk or onto the network.

Viruses are strictly electronic in form and only affect computers but new viruses are being discovered at the rate of about 200 per month, so your 'scanner' software will need constant updating to stay effective.

Accidental damage

Although modern computers are very reliable they can be physically damaged like any other piece of machinery. So avoid moving the computer when it is in use, and make sure it is placed where no one can bump into it.

If information is stored on floppy disks, ensure they are stored safely in lockable, possibly fire proof disk boxes. Keep back up copies.

Computers and computer equipment, particularly keyboards, do not like having coffee spilt over them, so do not drink coffee at your desk!

Electricity supply faults

A lesser-known risk to computers is a sudden variation in the electricity supply. These are called 'spikes' or 'surges' and they can cause data to be corrupted. The electricity supply may even break down altogether. This makes it all the more important to follow the back-up procedures outlined below. If your computer is on a network there may be a special device for the central computer called an 'uninterruptible power supply' (UPS). The UPS is connected between the computer and the mains supply and acts as a kind of reservoir for electricity, keeping the supply at a constant level. The UPS also provides for a few minutes of battery power in the event of a total mains failure. Make sure your work is 'backed up' or saved frequently so the risk of data loss, damage or corruption is minimised.

PHYSICAL SECURITY

Computers and computer components are now a target for criminals. Often entire office blocks of computers are stripped of their valuable memory chips, or simply removed wholesale.

You will need to cooperate with procedures which may include bolting the computers to the desktop or actually locking them away in a secure room every evening, particularly lap-tops or note book computers.

MAKING BACK-UPS

Back-ups are copies of your data to devices that are separate from your computer. At the most simple level, for example, you can copy small amounts of data onto a floppy disk and store it in a drawer in your desk. The result is that if your computer has a virus attack, or is stolen, you can restore the data from the floppy disk.

In practice, back-ups are more complicated. Data is constantly changing every hour of every day, so most organisations will make a back-up every day or even every half day. This means that if disaster strikes only half a day's data is lost. Because there is so much data in hospitals and it takes so long to actually copy, special devices such as tapes or optical disks are used.

You may be asked to carry out back-ups and also to make sure that further copies of back-up tapes or disks are kept in a separate location – just in case the ultimate disaster happens and your building is damaged by fire.

None of these measures will work properly if you are working on a stand-alone computer and do not save your work frequently to disk. For advice on backing up your data consult with your local computer support services.

Reflection Point 3

You are a secretary in general practice. How would you normally tell everyone that Dr Green has had to take a day off today?

The all-important aspects of health and safety at work regarding seating and the VDU are dealt with in Chapters 3 and 17.

Sections of the Human Rights Act 1998 also impact on issues of privacy. The government also intends to introduce the Freedom of Information Act 2000, which will be fully implemented by 2005 and will allow for easier public access to information held by government departments.

OTHER DEVELOPMENTS IN IT

DEVELOPMENTS IN THE SHARING AND TRANSMISSION OF PATIENT INFORMATION

Mobile technology

Increasingly, mobile technology is being used to share and transmit health information. You may find that you are involved in its use. Examples of this could be the use of laptops to access a range of information sources needed to help patients, sending appointment reminders directly to patients' mobile phones, the use of Personal Digital Assistants (PDAs) which are small hand-held computers which enable the users to access information anywhere. If they are linked to a mobile phone then the functions are increased with the ability to access the Internet and email from anywhere. To get the maximum benefit from PDAs you can transfer data to other devices, other compatible PDAs or desktop computers. The use of mobile technology is subject to the same legal requirements with regard to data protection, so the same care must be taken particularly with patient information and details.

Linking primary and secondary care providers

The NHS number mentioned earlier is indispensable because it will ensure that information finds its way to the correct patient record. GPs will be able refer patients to hospitals electronically and even book outpatient appointments directly from their own surgeries. There are initiatives in the UK known as Referral Booking Management Systems (RBMS) and Tier 2 pilots that are looking at these developments. Remember, most GPs can already access pathology and radiology reports remotely from their secondary care providers.

The end result will be more efficient, accurate and rapid communications and a reduction in paperwork and time-consuming transcription of information.

Scenario 4

In the Whitely village practice the receptionist can use e-mail to pass messages to doctors seeing patients in the surgery without having to interrupt consultations. One of the doctors can send a message to everyone in the practice saying that one of the practice's patients has died.

National database of hospital places

This is in operation in some practices. It allows GPs to find out the range of treatments offered by hospitals around the country plus waiting times and costs. GPs access the database electronically. A similar postal system would involve postage and printing costs and would be quickly out of date. But because the electronic database is constantly updated, the information is always accurate.

The development of intranets and use of the Internet

The Internet gives access to a huge amount of health information which is used increasingly by patient and health professionals. Most health organisations have a health librarian or IT trainer who will be able to give advice on how to access this huge information source effectively. Even if you use the Internet regularly, information professionals have a great deal of professional tips that can safe you time and effort. Searching the Internet can be very time consuming. Anyone can publish anything on the Internet. Care must be taken to ensure the credibility of information accessed via the Internet especially when it is health related. To give the wrong information could be dangerous. Question what you are reading. We will look at effective use of the Internet in more detail in Chapter 9.

If you work in a hospital, you should be able to gain access to the Internet via your hospital Intranet. The intranet is a network of computers which is exclusive to an organisation. It can be used to give you access to a range of shared information sources such as the PAS system, email, hospital protocols, and newsletters. Sharing knowledge in this way can be termed as 'knowledge management'. Organisations use knowledge management as a tool to share all the valuable information that is held with the organisation which can be used to manage effectively.

SUMMARY OF KEY ISSUES

- Information technology now plays an extremely important part in today's NHS. This has only become possible in recent years with the increasing power and cheapness of computers and their ability to communicate rapidly via telephone lines or specialised cables.

- Developments in mobile technology are also increasing and provide health staff who need to work in different places with the ability to com-

municate easily and access a wide range of information from where ever they are.

- The strategy of the NHS Executive is to create a patient record that is accessible wherever a patient is treated. In addition, they want information in the NHS to be person based – so that information about health service performance is generated as a by-product of patient care rather than as an end in itself.

- However, all this needs accuracy, otherwise the data will be meaningless and may harm the patient. It also needs confidentiality and this is all the more important because so much medical information can be made available.

- It also means that data has to be compatible for it to be shared between computers. This highlights the need to speak the same language, hence the development of the NHS number and the investment by the NHS Read codes and Healthcare Resource Groups.

- What this means for you, the medical secretary, is that confidentiality and accuracy are vital when working with computers.

Exercises

- Find out if your hospital or practice has written guidance about data protection.

- Find out which clinical coding system your hospital or practice is using.

- Dr Brown tells you that he needs to look up a few patients' details but has forgotten his password. He asks you to 'log in' with your password and then allow him to use the computer. How would you respond to his request?

- One item of information on the minimum data set is the patient's postcode. What possibilities for medical research do you see for using the computer to sort information using the postcode?

- What possibilities can you see for management in using postcode information?

CONCLUSION

Information technology is one of the most powerful developments in today's NHS. However, powerful things can be destructive. For example, if patient information falls into the wrong hands or is lost then the damage can be catastrophic. Data has to be safeguarded against accidental loss or destruction by viruses and you need to be aware of, and cooperate with, the precautions taken by your hospital or practice. Above all you must guard against unauthorised access and use of patient information.

RESOURCES

For free leaflets and publications on NHS Information Management initiatives, including Read codes and the new NHS number, contact:

NHS Information Authority
Aqueous II
Aston Cross
Rocky Lane
Birmingham B6 5RQ
Tel: 0121 333 0333
Fax: 0121 333 0334
URL: http://www.nhsia.nhs.uk/

KEY TERMS

AGGREGATE LEVEL INFORMATION

This is statistical information that relates to groups rather than to individuals. For example, a list of wards with average lengths of stay would be aggregate level, because it is made up of a large number of individual recordings for each patient's length of stay. Another example would be numbers of emergency admissions to different hospitals.

AUDIT TRAIL

For computers, this is a way of tracing an exact history of when and by whom each new piece of information is entered into the computer system.

CODER

For management and clinical purposes, details of patients' diagnosis and treatment need to be entered onto a computer so that they can be analysed. Computers cannot handle medical terms because they can be ambiguous (for example MI could mean 'myocardial infarction' or 'mentally ill') or because there is no consistent terminology (for example, athlete's foot might be described by a doctor as 'tinea pedis'). So diagnoses have to be converted into unambiguous identifiers. Coders are members of health staff whose job is to enter the correct clinical codes (such as ICD, OPCS and Read codes) to cover each patient's encounter with the hospital or health unit.

DATA PROTECTION ACT

The purpose of this Act is to protect the rights of individuals about whom data is obtained, stored, processed or supplied. They may find out information about themselves, challenge it if appropriate and claim compensation in certain circumstances. Data users, such as Primary Care Trusts, must be open about their use of data and follow sound and proper practices.

DATABASE

An organised collection of information rather like a card index or telephone directory except that the computer's database is far more sophisticated and powerful.

DEMOGRAPHIC INFORMATION

This is information that refers to basic domestic details (e.g. name, sex, age, address, occupation) about a person rather than detailed clinical information.

EPISODE OF CARE

This is now the basic statistical unit of clinical care in hospitals and was one of the recommendations of the Kröner report on health service information.

The episode of care usually begins when a patient is transferred to the care of a new consultant. This allows statistics to be recorded in a uniform and accurate way.

GP LINKS

This is a system for allowing electronic transmission of information between general practices and NHS Support Services. This will speed up patient registration and de-registering procedures and claims for item of service payments, besides reducing clerical effort.

ICD (INTERNATIONAL CLASSIFICATION OF DISEASES)

These classifications (published by the World Health Organization) are used to code each patient's diagnosis, normally on discharge. Because they are standard throughout the world they can be used for comparisons of health problems between different countries. The current version is ICD 10.

INDIVIDUAL LEVEL INFORMATION

Information which can be related to individuals' individual entities. A good example of individual level information is a telephone directory because each record (i.e. a name, an address and a telephone number) is about an individual.

INTERNET

The Internet is a collection of separate networks worldwide connected together via a set of communication protocols. It was originally used for military and academic communications but is now a standard worldwide method of communicating. The Internet is not owned by any single organisation. World Wide Web sites are connected to the Internet. The NHS has its own websites. Some of these sites have limited access to those outside the NHS – this is to protect sensitive information.

INTRANET

An intranet is a communication system between computers, usually within an organisation. Information can be shared over an intranet.

Intranets are usually located on a local area network (LAN) and often have portals or gateways to other networks or the Internet.

KNOWLEDGE MANAGEMENT

There are many definitions of knowledge management. It is essentially a process through which organisations generate value from their knowledge assets. Such assets are shared throughout the organisation. Knowledge management (KM) is not just about IT, it is a wider concept and permeates the organisation's philosophy and structure. However, the visible face of KM is often delivered by Information Technology, perhaps via an organisation's intranet.

LAN (LOCAL AREA NETWORK)

A network is a number of computers connected together and sharing information. A local network means that all the computers are in the same building or on the same site. So, for example, a computer system on a large hospital site encompassing many buildings would be called a LAN.

LOG IN (ALSO SOMETIMES CALLED LOG ON)

The process whereby an individual keys in details about his/her identity into a computer system so that he/she can interact with that computer system. This process will often include entering a password known only to that individual.

LOG OFF (ALSO SOMETIMES CALLED LOG OUT)

The process whereby a user of a computer system tells the system that he/she is ceasing to use it. It is important to log off when leaving the computer, even for a few minutes.

MAILBOXES

A mailbox is a kind of electronic pigeonhole where people can send you electronic messages. Your mailbox must have an 'address' unique to you, such as your name or initials. Usually you will need to enter a password into the computer to read the messages in your mailbox.

MINIMUM DATA SET

This refers to the basic information about a patient that is necessary for contractual procedures in the NHS. It consists of a range of basic demographic information about the patient, details of the service provider, the consultant to whom the patient was referred, the referring clinician, the ward details, GP name, GP's correspondence address, GP's code. There are different minimum data sets for different encounters with the NHS, e.g. outpatient visits and emergency treatments.

NETWORK

A number of computers connected together (usually by special cable) and sharing information.

NHS NUMBER

A number which will uniquely identify each user of NHS services. This number will apply wherever the user is in the UK and whichever branch of the NHS they use. This will enable important clinical and demographic information to be available to authorised staff throughout the UK. Unlike previous numbering systems, which had 22 different formats, the NHS number will be designed for use with computers.

OUT OF AREA TREATMENTS (OATs)

These have replaced Extra Contractual Referrals (ECRs) and relate to one-off specialist episodes of care carried out under the NHS for a patient outside their home area and not covered by existing service agreements. It may also cover emergency treatment for holiday makers requiring emergency treatment.

Financial adjustments will be made with the health care provider and the service provider who carried out the treatment.

OPCS (OFFICE OF POPULATION CENSUSES AND SURVEYS)

This refers to classifications of surgical procedures (e.g. procedures that require the services of a surgeon and an anaesthetist) carried out on patients. The current version is OPCS 4.

PAS (PATIENT ADMINISTRATION SYSTEM)

These are networked computer systems that make patient information available to authorised staff at numerous terminals around a hospital. This speeds up the creation and interchange of clinical and statistical information.

READ CODES

A set of codes for accurately describing a wide range of clinically relevant information and used mostly in primary care. The codes were designed from the start to be used by computers and were created by a practising GP, Dr James Read. The latest version of the Read codes allows for sophisticated analysis by computers.

SCANNER

A device (similar in function to a modern photocopier) for converting the information in paper-based documents and images into digital form. They can then be stored, manipulated and transmitted by a computer.

SHAREWARE

Computer software that users can make use of for a trial period to see if they like it before electing to pay for a full licence to use the software. These programs may contain viruses and should not be used on NHS computers without the authority of senior staff.

SNOMED CLINICAL TERMS

SNOMED CT is the preferred clinical terminology for the NHS. SNOMED creates a single unified terminology to underpin the development of the Electronic Patient Record. It supports consistent, quality, structured data entry.

SPIKES

A sudden momentary increase or variation in the mains supply voltage which can occur from time to time without warning. The data in computers can be lost or corrupted by these sudden variations in the normal electricity supply voltage.

SURGES

Surges are similar to spikes (see above) but because they are of much longer duration and the energy concerned is greater, they are more liable to cause permanent damage to both the data and the computer and its associated equipment.

UNINTERRUPTIBLE POWER SUPPLY (UPS)

Computers rely on electrical power to process information. If the mains supply to a computer fails, or changes suddenly (see 'Surges' and 'Spikes' above), a computer will lose vital data in its electronic memory. The UPS is a device which ensures continuity of supply of power to the computer. Generally, it is the central computers or 'fileservers' in a health building that are connected to a UPS because they store vital data.

VIRUS

A virus is a self-replicating computer program that can cause loss of data and seriously harm computer systems. They are created by individuals with malicious intent and can be passed on by failure to use correct computer procedures. The most common cause of virus 'infection' is the use of floppy disks containing unauthorised software such as computer games on NHS computers.

WAN (WIDE AREA NETWORK)

These are networks that connect computers on more than one site and over a large area. For example, a network that connects several health centres and hospitals is a WAN.

WRITE PROTECTED

This refers to information in a computer file, drive, or floppy disk. It means that you cannot amend the information already existing by, for example, copying or saving new files. The protection can be achieved by physical means (such as sliding a small plastic catch on a floppy disk) or by software.

Further reading

Gilles A 2000 Information and IT for primary care: Everything you need to know but are afraid to ask. Radcliffe Medical Press, Oxford

Johns M 2002 Information management for health professionals. Delmar, USA

Tyrrell S 1999 Using the Internet in healthcare. Radcliffe Medical Press, Oxford

References

Data Protection Act 1998. Chapter 29. [online] http://www.hmso.gov.uk/acts/ acts1998/19980029.htm
Department of Health 1998 Information for Health. NHS Executive Leeds
Freedom of Information Act 2000. Chapter 36. [online]

http://www.hmso.gov.uk/acts/acts2000/20000036.htm
Human Rights Act 1998 Chapter 42. [online] Available. http://www.hmso.gov.uk/acts/acts1998/19980042.htm
Information Commissioner. [online] http://www.informationcommissioner.gov.uk

Chapter 9

Using your PC

Barbara Sen

OBJECTIVES

- To explain what you can achieve with your Personal Computer (PC) other than churning out plain correspondence by using enhanced word processing, spreadsheet packages, database software, presentation software or organisers

- To warn you about the pitfalls you may encounter when using your PC with office packages

- To explain some of the benefits of using the Internet to support your work

- To warn you of some of the pitfalls of using the Internet.

INTRODUCTION

We will be concentrating on what you can do with a conventional office package such as Microsoft Office, Microsoft Works or Microsoft Worksuite. Moreover we will be concentrating on things that you can achieve with a few hours of practice, assuming you already have some computer basics.

Firstly we will discuss briefly why there is a need to enhance your documents in today's NHS, with the aid of some examples which we will refer to throughout the chapter.

Then we go into detail of how to set about creating your own enhanced documents and introduce you to some simple steps that will help you achieve a good result.

We give some brief 'health warnings' about getting carried away with it all, and we outline some pitfalls to watch out for and give you some hints and thoughts about the cost and time implications involved. Finally, we look at the benefits and problems of using the Internet for your work.

Throughout the chapter there are examples which we ask you to examine closely.

WHY ENHANCE THE DOCUMENTS YOU PRODUCE?

COMPUTERS HAVE IMPROVED

In recent years, the cost of computers has dropped considerably, yet their speed and capacity has increased enormously. This means that modern computers are able to handle sophisticated graphical displays that help you organise your document's appearance on the screen. You are no longer limited to alphabetical characters but can include graphics and can see how your document will look on the printed page before you actually print it, enabling you to carry out work to a high professional standard.

PRINTERS HAVE ALSO IMPROVED

In the last few years, printers have come down in price. A decent laser or laser printer can now be purchased for around £350. Another sort of printer known as an 'inkjet' printer can be bought for about £200. This means that good quality text and graphics can be produced from your desktop computer. Combined printer/scanner/faxes can give you a great deal of flexibility in the way you manipulate your document and manage information. Photographs, diagrams and documents can be scanned and incorporated into your documents to add interest and give a polished result to the documentation you produce.

SOFTWARE IS EASIER TO USE

Software publishers now take a lot of trouble to ensure that their programs and their manuals are more 'user-friendly' than they used to be. This means that you don't need a degree in computer science to use their advanced features. If you need help, within the NHS there is a commitment to life-long learning and you should find a range of courses available from your IT trainer, library, education department or human resources department, which will enable you to build and develop your existing IT skills.

THERE IS MORE NEED TO COMMUNICATE

In today's NHS there are increasing demands for clear communication and transfer of information, both between the service and patients, and within the service itself. The NHS is expanding its active exploitation of knowledge management (see Chapter 8). There are, therefore, numerous possibilities in this area for using your computer, some of which are listed below.

For general practices to communicate with their patients:

- the practice leaflet
- the annual practice report
- patient group newsletters
- posters (Figure 9.1)
- websites

For hospitals to communicate with their patients:

- patient awareness of hospital services, particularly as new services are constantly being created or modified which are different from 'traditional' patterns of care, e.g. a 'drop in' psychology clinic
- patient information before admission for outpatient procedures such as day surgery or X-ray
- outpatient information, e.g. information about a genitourinary clinic (Figure 9.3)
- patient questionnaires (Figure 9.4)

For managerial purposes within the NHS:

- timetables, schedules and duty rosters (Figure 9.5)
- project planning
- form design
- management reports
- staff newsletters (Figure 9.6)
- temporary signposts and labels.

It is crucial that patients are given information that is relevant, up-to-date, correct, and meets the organisation's legal obligations. You should always liaise with your Patient Advice and Liaison Service or PALS. Your local PALS may be based within either your local hospital or your primary care

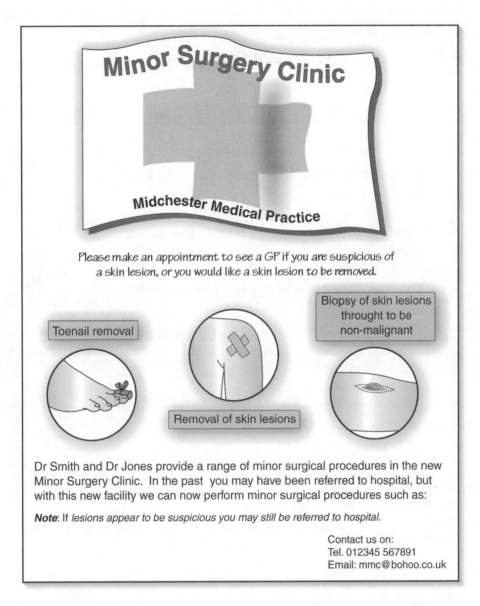

Figure 9.1 A general practice poster. This has been produced using Microsoft Word and clipart, different font, italics, text boxes, borders and shading techniques.

Reflection Point 1

Consider a situation where you could produce a creative document using your PC.

trust. The NHS also produces a patient information toolkit (Department of Health 2002) to guide you.

BENEFITS OF ENHANCING YOUR DOCUMENTS

1. *Interesting layouts.* You can make your documents more dynamic by including text in columns, importing graphs, tables etc., depending on the purpose of the document (Figure 9.6).

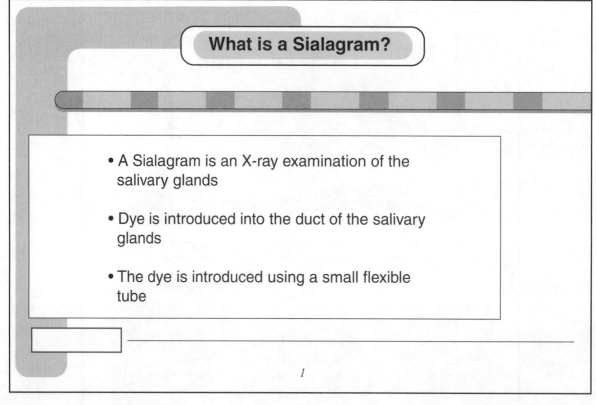

What is a Sialagram?

- A Sialagram is an X-ray examination of the salivary glands

- Dye is introduced into the duct of the salivary glands

- The dye is introduced using a small flexible tube

1

Figure 9.2 Powerpoint presentation

2. *Different type styles.* You have access to a range of interesting and stylish fonts which, if used well, can add interest and focus to your document.

3. *Savings in time and money.* On layout costs for simple documents, and for short runs of certain documents such as clinic timetables, or labels for temporary purposes.

4. *Greater control over the process.* Unlike sending rough drafts to a printer and getting back something that doesn't *quite* do what you wanted, you can experiment with different layouts and designs and go through several versions until you are satisfied with the outcome.

How it can affect the medical secretary

- It means that you can become more involved in the managerial and public relations side of your work and can broaden your computer skills.
- It also means having to allocate more of your time trying out the more advanced features of the computer programmes available to you.

HOW TO GET STARTED

A very important point for you to remember is the aspect of design. Before you rush into detailed work on a document, there are some aspects you need to consider.

CONSIDER YOUR AUDIENCE AND THE MESSAGE

- What is the document for?
- How is the reader going to use it?

For example, a work of fiction doesn't need an elaborate design because the reader becomes absorbed in the narrative. But sometimes when you are trying to convey a lot of factual information the reader may find it boring, even though it may be important that the reader understands and acts on this information; for example, the instructions in an admission letter will usually be very important, and so a layout that draws the reader's attention to the

The newly built Midtown clinic offers a range of services specifically to your sexual well-being. All these services are free and confidential.

The following services are provided:

- Information and advice or sexual health

- Screening for sexually transmitted diseases

- Counselling

- Psychological assessment and treatment

- Cervical smears

- Colposcopy

- HIV testing, counselling and care

- Hepatitis B testing

This service is an open access service. This means that you do not have to be referred by your GP.

We suggest that you make an appointment. You will usually take about 2 hours to complete your visit to the clinic.

No information will be released (not even to your GP) unless you give your consent.

How do I make an appointment?

You can make an appointment either in person or on the telephone at any time during clinic open hours.

Monday	9.00–5.30
Tuesday	9.00–5.30
Wednesday	2.30–7.30
Thursday	10.00–5.30
Friday	9.00–4.00

What will happen when I visit the clinic?

This will depend on why you have come to the clinic. However, you will always receive an initial examination by the doctor. If you need a test or treatment this will be arranged and may be carried out by nurses. Health advisors will be available to discuss ways of promoting good sexual health. Clinical psychologists are available if you need more specialised counselling.

How will my visit to the clinic be followed up?

You may have a problem that requires you to visit the clinic again. In some cases results of tests can be given to you by telephone.

Where is the clinic?

The clinic is in Broadway Road, just to the left of the main Midtown Hospital site.

How do I get to the clinic?

The clinic is easy to get to by public transport. Bus numbers 23, 11 and 49 all stop outside the hospital.

Please see the map overleaf.

Figure 9.3 A leaflet for a sexual health clinic

significant points is desirable.

Another example is where you provide information in a newsletter (Figure 9.6). Here the user can assimilate information in short bursts, so an 'active' layout is necessary.

Considering your audience will guide you in which layout to select.

CONSIDER THE LAYOUT

Your document doesn't *have* to be plain A4. You could fold it in two. Or you can fold it in three (a gatefold), but remember that the inside fold has to be a bit smaller (about 4mm) than the other two leaves. Of course, folding means a lot more work in finally producing the document.

Will your document be double sided? This may be so if you adopt the gatefold layout described above. Most printers have the option to print on both sides of a sheet of paper. If not, you can get around this if you have a photocopier that can do double-sided copying. You need to beware of text 'showing through' onto the other side, so the quality of paper used is important.

White space is important. It is not good enough to create a plain slab of text filling the whole page. White space is needed to define important text such as headings and to make the page more attractive to the eye.

If your text is in columns, you may need to decide about the lines between the columns. It is probably best to have lines between different articles and white space *within* an article (Figure 9.6).

PATIENT QUESTIONNAIRE – MIDTOWN SEXUAL HEALTH CLINIC

Please answer the following questions in the boxes provided:

1.   **Age** ☐

2.   **Gender**   Female ☐   Male ☐

3.   **Your postcode or the area where you live** ☐

4.   **Your occupation** ☐

5.   **How did you find out about the clinic?**   From:

Your GP ☐   *A friend* ☐   *Hospital* ☐

Partner ☐   *Magazine* ☐   *Leaflet* ☐

Telephone ☐   *Internet* ☐   *Other* ☐

Thank you for taking the time to complete this questionnaire.

Figure 9.4 A questionnaire. These are 'text boxes' with no content. These boxes can be copied and pasted from position to position. The font has been changed to proportional to give a more polished appearance.

Dr\Month:	Feb	March	April	May	June
Smith	Medical	Medical	Surgical	Surgical	Elective
Brown	Surgical	Surgical	Elective	Medical	Medical
Green	Ortho	Ortho	Medical	Elective	Surgical
Gray	a\leave	Medical	Ortho	Ortho	Elective
Note: Changeovers take place on the first Monday of the month.					

Figure 9.5 A duty roster: Junior House Officers' Rotation. Using tables function in Microsoft Word

Reflection Point 2

Look at the questionnaire in Figure 9.4. Note the use of 'text boxes' of different sizes. These can be copied and pasted from place to place. Can you think of other applications for this, e.g. creating forms?

Reflection Point 3

Figure 9.3 shows one side of a gatefold leaflet. This was produced using Microsoft Publisher with columns and text boxes. Can you think of some other applications for this kind of layout?

Reflection Point 4

Look at the poster (Figure 9.1) and consider how the generous use of white space emphasises the opening question and the subsequent short paragraphs.

Reflection Point 5

Look at Figure 9.5 and think of some other management purposes that the 'Table' feature could be used for, e.g. room allocations, clinic timetable blanks.

60-65 characters (approximately 10 words to the line) is uncomfortable to read. Moreover, the eye gets tired and it has further back to travel to the beginning of the next line, which it has to struggle to locate.

Avoid full justification. It may look fine on official correspondence but within the columns of a newsletter it can make 'rivers' of white and can look rather ponderous. Use left justified text but consider using your word processor's hyphenation facility so that words get split up. This fills up the line space more.

Don't make margins too narrow for your printer. Some printers, such as laser printers, have to have a 0.5 centimetre margin all around the page, and some printers need a 2.5 centimetre margin at the top. If the document is going to go into a plastic folder you need to allow extra margin space on the left for the binding. This space is often called the *gutter*.

Remember, for documents intended for patients, that your readers may have poor eyesight or may be colour blind. Don't expect patients to be able to read text in grey panels, for example.

CONSIDER HOW YOU WILL GROUP THE INFORMATION

Paragraphs organise information into groups and give the eye time to pause, besides providing a ref-

It doesn't have to be difficult working with columns. For example, the basic newsletter layouts in Figure 9.6 were created in a few minutes in 'Microsoft Office' using the 'wizard' facility. The wizard facilities give you a range of creative options which allow you to create complex documents quickly using the wizard templates.

Don't make the lines too long. The eye reads in *groups* of characters, so anything longer than about

Midshire Surgical Department

Surgical Unit Update

Volume 1, Issue 1   MARCH

Deadline for the April issue is 14th March. Contributions to Jane Smith, Editor Public Relations Dept. Trust HQ

Inside this issue:

WAITING TIMES DOWN

We've met our target!

We are pleased to announce that our waiting lists are below 12 months for all categories within our directorate. The graph opposite shows the progress that has been made in the last year.

"This shows that our improvement in services to the public is being maintained" said John Black, the Unit's Clinical Director, as he toured the wards congratulating the staff.

He continued, "We want to aim for a target of 6 months maximum over the next 2 years. This will be a priority for the management team to plan for."

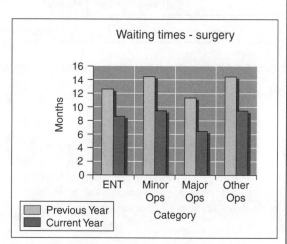

The reduction in waiting times was achieved by sweeping changes to the ways in which resources are used. The operating theatre maintenance sessions were moved to evenings and weekends to free up an additional 4 sessions. In addition a dedicated theatre was used for emergencies only.

Confidentiality

Last Thursday a page from a patient's medical record was found left inside the photocopier on level 4. This represents a serious breech of our basic responsibility towards our patients. We ask all staff to be on their guard against leaving confidential documents lying around where they can be seen by non-medical or non-hospital staff.

For guidance on our responsibility with regard to the Data Protection Act 1998 please refer to the hospital internet help page. The eight principles of the Act are clearly laid out. Further guidance can be obtained if needed from John Smith, Risk Manager, Planning and Development.

Figure 9.6 A page from a newsletter

erence point to return to. They also break up 'forbidding' slabs of text.

Different types of information can go in different parts of a document, as you can see in the example of the genitourinary clinic (Figure 9.3) where different boxes are used for this purpose.

Consider the use of the tables facility to do layouts. The example in Figure 9.5 was created using the Microsoft Word table feature. Similar results can be created using spreadsheet packages which can be used effectively to manage budgets and other data.

CONSIDER WHAT PAPER YOU WILL USE AND ANY FEATURES

Most laser paper is not very thick and may look flimsy for some types of document. However, thicker paper may not be accepted by your printer so it is best to check first before ordering expensive paper.

If you decide to use a paper colour other than white, try to choose a pastel colour – they are much easier to read from than a dark colour. If you are producing documents on acetates or overheads remember to check that the acetates are the right quality for the printer or photocopier or they may jam in the machine, melt in the photocopier, or the ink may not dry.

CHOOSE YOUR FONTS

With today's computer software you have a choice of interesting and creative fonts.

A font is a design for a set of characters. Box 9.1 shows a number of different fonts. Fonts can exist in different *point sizes*. Point size 12 is the standard for most correspondence So if you select a point size of 12, each character will take up about one sixth of an inch – we say *about* because in fact the point size is *not* based on the size of the character. Instead it is based on the block that the character would be mounted on if it were an actual printer's character. What this means is that different fonts in the same point size may take up different amounts of line.

The most usual point sizes you will work in will be 10 or 12, with 14, 18 or 24 being used for headings.

Beware of using too many fonts in the same document, even though you may have lots of fonts at your disposal. The result will look like a case of 'fontitis'! Instead, use a maximum of two or three fonts per document and use different point sizes for the more important paragraphs and headings, or vary the look by using **bold** or *italics* as in Figure

9.1. For example, a heading can be two point sizes bigger than the body of the text and the text for a quotation could be two point sizes smaller. Also, do not be tempted into using very small font sizes. This can lead to lines that are too long. When producing slides for presentations, use a large clear font. Small fonts will not be able to be seen from a distance (see Figure 9.2).

Fonts can be 'serif' and 'sans serif'. Serifed fonts have finishing strokes at the end and look more elegant. Research suggests that serifed fonts are easier to read because they give the eye more 'clues' about the characters. So use a 'serifed' font for the body of your text and reserve the sans serif fonts for titles, footnotes and introductory paragraphs.

When choosing fonts you have to consider if they will photocopy well – some fonts copy particularly badly when in italics.

Avoid using a lot of capital letters. They are fine for titles or headlines or OCCASIONAL emphasis but not for whole sentences or paragraphs.

Also, you should avoid long amounts of text in italics. Italics work best in *contrast* with plain text.

- Blobs can be tempting and useful for making a list of 'bulleted' points, but if you use them, make sure they are all the same size.

White on black text can be powerful for titles and short bursts of text but make sure your printer can support it. The next best thing is bold black on grey (Figure 9.5).

CONSIDER GRAPHICS

You don't need to go overboard on graphics. Just one or two icons or drawings can balance the text, emphasise points and invite the reader in (see Figure 9.1). You can use the clip art provided with the program, or maybe your hospital or practice has its logo available as a computer file. For example, if you work within the NHS then letters and other documents should incorporate a corporate logo in the header, and this can be printed from the computer rather than on pre-printed paper. The NHS corporate 'logo' is mandatory. Guidance on how to use the NHS logo is available in *The NHS Identity Guidelines* (Department of Health, 2002).

Although we have mentioned that you can make use of clip art libraries, you should not overdo the artwork so that it looks too fussy and overwhelms the text.

Box 9.1 Different fonts, all 12 point

Font type	Appearance
Arial	The Essential Medical Secretary
Baskerville Old Face	The Essential Medical Secretary
Comic Sans MS	The Essential Medical Secretary
Garamond	The Essential Medical Secretary
Marydale	The Essential Medical Secretary
Verdana	The Essential Medical Secretary

Using graphics can also brighten up a presentation and help hold the audience's attention. In such programmes as Microsoft Powerpoint you can also include animation in your work. Again, be careful not to overdo animation techniques as they can have the opposite effect and distract the viewer.

Figure 9.6 shows the use of a graph generated in another program and imported into the text.

If you want to include photographs, you can scan them into your document. If you do use a photo or an image don't forget to give it a caption – but don't tell the readers what is obvious from the picture; e.g. *not* 'Building work in progress on the West Wing' but 'West Wing – £4 million budget'.

Beware of breaching copyright with graphics. Most clip art is free if you are only producing a small quantity of the document and are not selling it. However, photographs and cartoons that you copy from books and magazines will require permission from the copyright holder. Be careful too with items taken from the Internet, some things are copyright free, but not everything, so do check before you use it. Being able to access information freely on the Internet does not mean it is not someone else's intellectual property. Beware, too, of location maps which may originate from Ordnance Survey, who are very strict about copyright.

CONSIDER YOUR WRITING STYLE

You need to modify your style according to your audience and the document.

Reflection Point 6

- If your laser printer can print 4 pages per minute, how long would it take to print 1,000 copies? And how many reloads of paper would you have to do if the paper tray only holds 50 sheets of paper?

- Consider also the cost of producing copies. For example, if the cost of a toner cartridge for a laser printer is £50 and it lasts for 2,500 copies what would be the cost (excluding paper) of laser printing 1,000 copies? How does that compare with photocopying costs (nominal cost of 3p per copy)?

- In newsletters you will find it difficult to write headlines – use of present tense seems strange but past tense is stranger!
- Remember that for patient information your writing needs to be clear and active and reassuring for the patient. See Figure 9.3, where the information the patient needs to know is clearly structured.
- 'Publishing' text calls for extra care and it will be worth checking your wording on a willing volunteer to check that the message has been understood. You also need to make sure that your text is correct clinically.

- When producing presentations, avoid being too 'wordy'. Use key phrases that the presenter can talk around.
- If producing web pages, pay attention to the headings you use and the layout of your information. How you word things affects how the search engines pick up on the information.

GET SOME FEEDBACK

Try a rough sketch layout first and if you are not sure about how different fonts and shaded panels appear, create a page with examples of different shade intensities and font and line sizes, and show it to your colleagues.

It is always a good idea to get feedback on your ideas and your work before printing or copying (Box 9.2). The first time you do print, print out in draft quality. You will find this selection in your printer options. It will save time in printing and ink. Ink cartridges are very expensive for good quality printers and cost between £22 – £80 depending on your printer. You will make the cartridges last longer by printing in best quality only for final documents.

Box 9.2 Getting feedback

- Try reading your text out loud. This is a good way of revealing 'nonsense writing', which can arise if you cut and paste text carelessly.
- Get reactions to your layout from colleagues.
- If the document is meant for the public, get advice from your PALS (Patient Advice Liaison Service) before publishing the document.

Box 9.3 Quality assurance is important

Misinformation can
- Mislead
- Undermine
- Be problematic
- Be dangerous

Quality information can
- Support
- Educate
- Improve
- Be beneficial

A WORD OF WARNING

Although software is a lot easier to use these days, you still need time and training to learn some of the advanced skills. Do not be tempted to imitate the layouts of daily newspapers or magazines – it takes highly skilled layout experts to create these. Instead try to detect what aspects of their designs seem to work and think about copying just one or two of them. It's easy to go 'over the top' and forget that the purpose of presentation is to enhance the content and not to distract from it.

If you want best quality layout and paper then you have to consider using a commercial printer. Here you can use your word processing skills to prepare rough layouts for discussion amongst your colleagues so that less time is spent by the printer in expensive layout work.

CONSIDER THE TIME COST OF PRODUCING MULTIPLE COPIES

Local photocopying costs can be reasonable for short runs but above a certain number it might be cheaper to use a commercial printer. Take the trouble to make back-ups at frequent intervals of documents you are working on. You may spend hours on layouts, only to lose them if your disk gets corrupted or someone accidentally overwrites the file. It's a good idea to save your work under different version numbers (e.g. 'newslet1.doc; newslet2.doc, etc.) so that you can always return to a previous version if you are not happy with your latest version.

Also, you should make the most of your work by saving settings, blank 'templates', etc., so that they can be reused later. (A good example is the gatefold leaflet in Figure 9.3.) Alternatively, you could use the 'styles' facility to store and reproduce your work.

WEB PUBLISHING

You may want or need to publish your work on an intranet or the Internet so that a wider group of people can have access to it. There are specialist software packages to help you do this called web publishing software such as Dreamweaver or Microsoft Frontpage. Electronic publishing uses a special computer language called HTML (Hyper Text Markup Language) which allows the document to be active via an intranet or the Internet. You will need permission to publish on your intranet or to publish on the Internet on behalf of your organisation. All NHS organisations have a 'webmaster', who has specific responsibility for developing, organising and publishing information on the organisation's intranet or website.

USING THE INTERNET TO HELP YOU IN YOUR WORK

The Internet is a worldwide communication tool that can be useful to you in the course of your work in a number of different ways:

- To obtain or publish educational material
- As a communication tool
- To access to information to support your work, your colleagues or your clients e.g. patients.

Even if you use the Internet regularly you may not know how to use it effectively. Library and information professionals have expert knowledge which they are generally very willing to share. It is worth checking with your local health library to see if they have a course to help you enhance your skills. Here are a few tips.

ACCESSING THE INTERNET

There are different tools to help you access the Internet: search engines, meta-search engines, directories, information portals or gateways.

Search engines

These are tools that help you search for information on the Internet. You will find that you get different results, or 'hits', when you use different search engines. This is because the search 'robots' work in different ways when they 'crawl' around the web. One of the most popular search engines is called Google (http://www.google.co.uk).

Technology changes so fast, you may find that loyalty to a single search engine is misplaced. There is a website (http://searchenginewatch.com) that reports on the reliablility and speed of search engines.

Meta–search engines

These are special search tools which employ a range of search engines to process your search for information. For example the meta-search engine

Dogpile (http:www.dogpile.com) searches a range of ordinary search engines simultaneously. It then presents the results from each search engine in a list. This is the 'meta-data', a collection of data.

Quite often the 'hits' are arranged in an order that the search engine calculates as being relevant to your enquiry. This order is called 'relevancy ranking'. Meta-search engines are good for retrieving large amounts of information quickly.

Directories

Although directories don't initially seem different to search engines, they work differently because humans index the web-sites rather than robots. This is better in some ways, but human indexing is a slower process so you might not get so many 'hits' or such recently indexed sites with a directory as with a standard search engine.

Portals or gateways

As the names suggest, these tools are gateways to information. They are often subject specific so you are not searching the whole of the web. One good example for health information is OMNI (www.omni.ac.uk). Quite often the information is validated before it is added, so that you can be assured of the quality of the information.

Because anyone can publish anything on the Internet, it is very important that you are careful about the information you access, especially when dealing with health information. The wrong information can be dangerous. Again, there are a number of tools available that can help you evaluate information on the Internet (e.g. Internet Detective http://sosig.ac.uk/desire/internet-detective.html, and Quick http://www.quick.org.uk). Until you get used to looking critically at the information you find then it is wise to use one of these tools. They will give you a range of questions to ask, to check if the information is accurate, current, authoritative, objective and covers the right material at the right level for the user. The Internet is prone to pranksters, jokers and Internet criminals: it is wise to be aware of this and to examine the information you retrieve carefully. *Incorrect information can have serious implications.*

SUMMARY

- The word processing package contains many features that allow you to enhance a document to increase its attractiveness to readers.
- You need to plan your approach to producing your document so that it suits its purpose and its audience.
- In particular, you need to consider layout, margins, fonts and the use of graphics. Look at other people's efforts and try to 'take the design apart' and then reproduce what appeals to you.
- Take time to develop your skills, taking advantage of training opportunities that may be available within your organisation.
- You may wish to publish your document electronically as well as in printed format. Your web master will help you with this.
- The Internet hosts a vast range of electronically published information which can help you with your work. However, much of the information will not be relevant to you. You need the skills to filter this information and to be able to evaluate its quality.

CONCLUSIONS

You have the tools to produce documents which can improve communications between health service workers and between hospital or practice and patients.

In particular, posters, reports and patient information can be generated on your computer instead of being sent to the printer. The result is that your hospital or practice retains more control over the layout

Exercises

Obtain a patient leaflet or patient guidance notes. Try asking a friend to read your leaflet and then ask them which points are clear and which are difficult to understand.

Try searching on the Internet for 'Patient Information Leaflets'. Use the search engine Google, the meta-search engine Dogpile and the information gateway OMNI. How many 'hits' do you get with each one? Look carefully at a selection of the resources you have found using each search tool. What can comments can you make about the scope and quality of the information you have found?

and content and can easily change it and save costs.

But you need to play it safe and avoid fancy layouts. Just use a few techniques at a time and you will gradually build up a range of new and useful skills. Exploiting opportunities on the Internet or via your organisation's intranet can help you in your work, increasing access to the documents you produce and enabling you to share knowledge and information.

FURTHER READING

In any high street book shop you will find a wide range of 'how to' books about using computer software. Choose books that you find easy to follow and are within your price range.

References

DoH 2002 Toolkit for producing patient information. Online. http://www.doh.gov.uk/nhsidentity/toolkit-patientinfo.pdf

DoH 2002 The NHS Identity Guidelines: The NHS logo. Online. http://www.doh.gov.uk/nhsidentity/logo.htm

Dogpile [online] http://www.dogpile.com

Google [online] http://www.google.co.uk

Internet Detective [online] http://www.sosiq.ac.uk/desire/internet-detective.html

OMNI [online] http://omni.ac.uk

Quick [online] http://quick.org.uk

Searchenginewatch [online] http://searchengine watch.com

Chapter 10

Clinical equipment

Stephanie J Green

OBJECTIVES

- To discuss some aspects of the general environment
- To describe the clinical environment, including the care and storage of equipment and instruments
- To explain the importance of sterilisation and the sterile field
- To provide an overview of commonly used instruments and emergency equipment.

INTRODUCTION

Most medical secretaries like to know and understand about particular areas of care so that they can work more effectively within the team. This will not necessarily stop at the administrative and secretarial side of work, but will naturally extend into other areas of professional care. Indeed, there may be times when to know what a particular instrument or pack looks like will be most useful should clinical staff be unavailable. However, the overall care of both the premises and equipment may well be a shared responsibility: this will vary from one workplace to another but it will certainly apply to private practice.

THE GENERAL ENVIRONMENT

Both hospitals and general practices employ domestic staff to cope with day-to-day cleaning, but it is important for staff to realise that dust may be contaminated by pathogenic organisms. This danger has been drawn to our attention both by professional staff and indeed by the Minister of Health who has introduced 'modern Matrons' to our hospitals to try to combat the spread of infection by introducing tighter controls on issues like cleaning. It is most important, therefore, that cleaning staff perform a thorough job and a work schedule may be devised in order to try to achieve a high standard of care. However, all members of the team need to be aware of these considerations and should ensure that the whole patient environment is clean and dry, thus inhibiting the multiplication of pathogenic organisms. Every area of the building, including the staff common room, needs to be kept as clean as possible. Particular care needs to be given to clinical areas. This is best carried out when patients are no longer present. Problems should always be reported and these may also draw attention to general maintenance which requires attention. Needless to say, attention will have been paid to the planning of all areas and surfaces, so floorings and coverings should all be hard wearing and easy to clean. In some instances, such as after a spillage, it may be necessary to be able to clean a surface with chemical cleaners. (See Chapter 17.)

The typical environment that patients will encounter, whether in hospital or general practice, should have a variety of different areas, including a welcoming and comfortable waiting area, an office which is well planned for its purpose and close to the reception area, and treatment and consulting rooms. Although all will have different characteristics, none should be intimidating to the patient and attention should be given to details such as blinds or screens to allow privacy, a mixture of lighting – bright and directable in clinical areas, softer and warmer in counselling or waiting areas, and toys for children, which should be washable and relatively quiet. Even the way in which furniture is arranged should be considered, with chairs placed to the side of a desk, rather than in front, as this is considered to be less confrontational and intimidating to patients. The safe exit of staff in cases of aggression also needs to be considered, so obstructions within clinical and reception areas should be avoided.

THE CLINICAL ENVIRONMENT

Although nurses will mainly be responsible for the work carried out in the treatment rooms, we all need some understanding of what is safe and acceptable in such important areas. These principles are relevant to both general practice and hospital work.

Ideally a treatment area should have:

- Enough space to allow treatment or minor surgery to take place
- Space for consultation and paperwork
- A preparation area
- Storage areas.

It is usual for a screened couch to be provided, along with the necessary linen, in any consulting area. Adequate lighting to enable examination to take place must also be easily available; this can be of the flexible variety and may be wall mounted or on a movable base. Some form of desk or writing surface must also be provided and, with it, storage facilities for a variety of forms and other paperwork and space for a computer system. Trolleys may also be used during clinical procedures, so adequate space needs to be allowed for them.

As far as preparation goes, this will depend upon the variety and extent of procedures that are to be carried out. However, it is considered best practice to separate used (and therefore dirty) instruments and equipment from clean areas or sterilised equipment. In the hospital context this can be readily achieved and increasingly in general practices this is the accepted mode of practice, especially where minor surgery is a regular occurrence or a developing feature. Where new premises are being built or adapted for primary health care the regulations governing the separation of clean and dirty areas will have to be observed.

Reflection Point 1

Think of two areas in a doctor's surgery you have visited, either as a patient or as part of your work experience. What impression did you take away with you and why? What might you like to change or improve and how would you try to achieve it?

Find out about the role of 'Modern Matrons'

STORAGE

We have mentioned the need for adequate storage in the treatment room. This will generally fall into three areas:

- Lotions
- Dry goods
- Vaccines.

Lotions

These should be stored separately from any other goods and adequate stock control should ensure that they are always within their shelf-life. Lotions may include saline or chlorhexadine sachets and distilled water. Surface cleaners may be used. This cupboard should be lockable.

Dry goods

These tend to fall into either clinical or non-clinical categories and so might usefully be kept in separate cupboards or storage areas. Some examples are given in Box 10.1.

Vaccines

A selection of vaccines used in treatment, which will require refrigeration. There should be a regulating gauge inside the refrigerator to enable correct storage to take place; this is especially important for vaccines. Expiry dates should be checked regularly and the refrigerator should be lockable. Other vaccines not requiring refrigeration should be stored separately in a lockable dry cupboard.

It goes without saying that any piece of equipment used in the treatment area must be cared for efficiently, whether it is a piece of electrical machinery such as an ECG machine, a specific surgical instrument, or a simple pupil torch. Many of these instruments and machines are extremely expensive and regular maintenance is of utmost importance, both to keep them in efficient working order and to prolong their working life wherever possible. Some machines require regular specialist maintenance, which should be booked in the diary in

---

Box 10.1 Dry goods

- Stationery
- Forms
- Paper couch roll
- Non-sterile gloves and household gloves
- Disposable protective aprons – plastic
- Sterile packs and dressings – these need to be kept in a dry area and a check kept on expiry dates
- Syringes and needles – a full supply of all sizes
- Specimen and blood bottles – a variety of different bottles will need to be stocked – these are often colour coded
- Suturing material – this will depend on the extent of work undertaken
- Examination equipment – this will obviously vary from hospital to general practice and specific items are listed later in this chapter
- Surgical instruments – checks should regularly be made on the state of repair and working order of instruments. Cleaning, preparation and sterilisation of these articles is usually a nursing task, but there may be occasions when other staff need to stand in when there is a crisis. In these cases, relevant health and safety recommendations must be adhered to and great care taken that the job is done thoroughly and efficiently

---

advance. Many will require special parts or spares, which should be kept in stock for use when necessary.

All pieces of equipment should be stored carefully; this includes the ordinary bulbs and batteries which are essential to so many pieces of equipment and so easily overlooked.

CLINICAL PROCEDURES

Although all clinical procedures will generally be carried out by professionally trained staff whether nursing or medical, it is useful for the medical secretary to understand the principles by which they work and the practicalities that are involved, including some of the pieces of equipment which are used. This section of the chapter will look at:

- The sterilisation of instruments and equipment by autoclave
- Maintenance of the sterile field and aseptic technique
- Commonly used clinical equipment.

Reflection Point 2

How might you ensure that equipment is properly looked after?

STERILISATION BY AUTOCLAVE

Autoclaves are special pieces of equipment in which instruments are sterilised. They will vary in size depending on where they are to be used. Hospitals have a whole department devoted to the safe care and sterilisation of surgical equipment, called the CSSD (Central Sterile Supply Department); they use several very large autoclaves. Doctors and dentists may use smaller 'table-top' versions, but all must meet British Standard specifications. However large or small they are, they all work on the same principle of steam under pressure. Items can be sterilised by such a process providing the correct temperature is maintained for the correct length of time, and this equation will vary from one machine to another. Machines using high temperatures will require shorter periods of time to be effective than machines operating at lower temperatures. Sterilisation by autoclave is considered to be the most efficient and the safest method in use.

Autoclaves need to be packed properly to be effective, and must not be over-packed since the steam must be able to meet all surfaces. They should also be put through a regular check run to ensure proper function. They should be serviced regularly, according to the manufacturer's recommendations, probably two or three times a year. Each time the machine is serviced it should be recorded. Obviously, any medical secretary who finds that it is necessary to use such a piece of equipment should make a point of becoming familiar with the particular machine before attempting to use it. There is further reference to the use of clinical sterilisation and infection control in Chapter 17.

THE STERILE FIELD

Any instrument or dressing that is to be used in any form of clinical procedure, be it surgery or a surgical dressing, must be sterile. In order to maintain this situation it is necessary to use what is known as aseptic technique. The word 'asepsis' means 'without microorganisms', and in using this technique, the risk of contamination by harmful microorganisms is avoided.

After any item has been sterilised ready for use in any procedure, it can then only be handled by someone who is wearing sterile gloves or using sterile forceps if aseptic conditions are to be maintained. It is also important that surfaces on which sterile packs are to be laid are also properly prepared, free from general dust and dirt, and uncontaminated by other people or articles close by. Of course, in most cases, the nursing staff will take charge in all of these areas, but it is valuable to have a proper understanding of all the implications involved in these procedures, should help be required or where there is an expectation for the medical secretary to be involved. If these principles are understood and adhered to, secretarial staff can be a help rather than a hindrance.

CLINICAL EQUIPMENT

In this section we shall consider some of the more usual instruments and pieces of equipment medical secretaries may encounter in their work. Most medical secretaries would like to familiarise themselves with the names of equipment in use, in order to avoid confusion, waste of time and embarrassment in an emergency, and of course to enhance their own knowledge!

Reflection Point 3

Consider how you would plan this area of a health centre to include these areas of work, and what your priorities would be.

Diagnostic instruments

Box 10.2 lists the main diagnostic instruments; some may also appear in the list of equipment used for treatment.

Treatment instruments

Some of the instruments listed in Box 10.3 will be used daily; others will only be used for special procedures.

Reflection Point 4

Think about what might be needed in a doctor's bag.

Box 10.2 Diagnostic instruments

- Thermometer (Figure 10.1), digital ear thermometer
- Stethoscope (Figure 10.1)
- Sphygmomanometer – with both adult and paediatric sized cuffs (Figure 10.1). This may be electronic
- Tongue depressors – disposable
- Peak flow gauge
- Auroscope or otoscope – with a variety of sizes of ear pieces (Figure 10.1)
- Ophthalmoscope (Figure 10.1)
- Sight chart – Keeler
- Scales – both standard scales and those used for weighing infants
- Height measure – this is often attached permanently to a wall
- Specula
  - nasal
  - vaginal – these are usually Sims or Cusco and may be disposable
- Swabs
  - throat and ear
  - high vaginal
  - wound
- Cervical smear – cervix brush
- Cytobrushes – if previous specimen was found to be inadequate
- Ring pessaries
- Specimen containers – various
- Urine testing equipment
- Gloves – disposable and ready sterilised
- Lubricant
- Proctoscope

- ECG machine – these come in a variety of sizes and those used in general practice may be portable. They may also be computer compatible (Figure 10.2)
- Fetal stethoscope or sonic aid

- Patella hammer (Figure 10.1)
- Tuning fork
- Pupil torch
- Tape measure
- Cotton wool balls
- Sterile needles

} These pieces of equipment are used in neurological examination

- Syringes and needles
- Mirror

Box 10.3 Instruments used in treatment

- Aural syringe – this is electrically operated
- Scissors – a variety of size and type
- Diathermy/cautery

Instruments used for minor surgery or for suturing:
- Tooth dissecting forceps
- Spencer Wells forceps
- Disposable scalpels – with a variety of blade sizes
- Sponge holders

Instruments used in the insertion of IUDs:
- Uterine sound
- Volsellum forceps
- Cuscoe's speculum
- Scissors

- Curetting spoons
- Probes
- Clip removers and stitch cutters

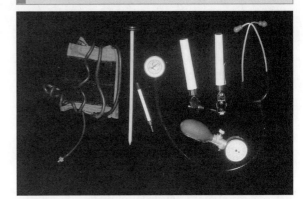

Figure 10.1 Diagnostic instruments. From the left: sphygmomanometer, patella hammer, thermometer, stethoscope, auroscope, ophthalmoscope

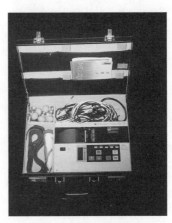

Figure 10.2 ECG machine

Box 10.4 Emergency equipment

• Airways – adult and paediatric – Brooks design
• Laryngoscope
• Endotracheal tubes
• IV giving sets
• Various drugs to be given by injection, such as hydrocortisone and adrenaline
• Syringes and needles
• Oxygen masks in a variety of sizes and an oxygen cylinder

Reflection Point 5

Do you know where the resuscitation equipment is kept in any of the places you have been to on work experience?

There is an increasing tendency to use 'single use' instruments in general practice and in some outpatient departments. These are usually made of plastic and should be disposed of after one use. Instruments which are likely to fall into this category include basic forceps.

A variety of pre-packed disposable sterile blades and sutures should also be available.

It may be considered necessary to keep a small supply of oxygen available in a cylinder and many general practices have a supply of nebulisers available for cases of severe asthma.

Conversion charts are also useful.

Emergency equipment

Emergency equipment is also necessary in order to resuscitate patients who have collapsed, perhaps due to anaphylaxis. The items listed in Box 10.4 should be readily available and preferably kept together ready for such an event.

In some general practices it is the policy for each member of staff to have responsibility for a particular consulting room. This will include overall monitoring of basic cleaning and the restocking of forms and equipment, and may include the clearing of used instruments at the end of a surgery. The treatment room will be the responsibility of the practice nurse. In the hospital environment this will also be undertaken by nursing and auxiliary staff.

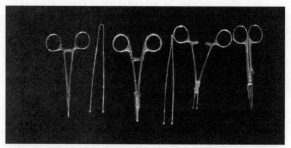

Figure 10.3 Instruments used for insertion and removal of sutures.

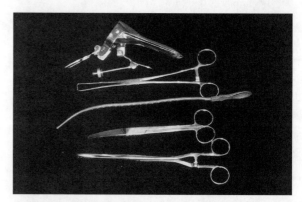

Figure 10.4 Instruments used for intrauterine contraceptive device (IUCD) insertion. From the top: Cusco's speculum, volsellum forceps, uterine sound, scissors, sponge holders.

CONCLUSION

When you have finished studying this chapter, you should have a better idea about the responsibilities held by other members of the team with regard to clinical activity. You should understand more about some of the procedures being carried out, and feel more prepared to be involved should the need arise.

Exercise

Try planning waiting, reception and office areas to allow patients and staff to benefit from a well thought through environment. Consider patient and staff needs. Consider how you would protect confidentiality.

Further reading

Medical secretaries and students who wish to further their understanding of the clinical environment in either hospital or general practice may like to take advantage of many books written for nursing education. You may find the following useful:

Clarke M 1991 Practical nursing, 14th edn. Baillière Tindall, London

Hampson GD 1994 Practice nurse handbook, 3rd edn. Blackwell Scientific Publications, Oxford

Jeffree P (ed) 1990 The practice nurse. Chapman and Hall, London

The reader should also remember that many professional magazines and journals will have relevant and interesting articles, which may be a useful source of information. These include:

Pulse

The AMSPAR Magazine.

SECTION 3

The secretary and hospital practice

Chapter 11

Personnel

Tracy A Grafton

CHAPTER CONTENTS

OBJECTIVES

- To identify principal health care staff groups and their roles
- To illustrate liaison between these groups and the medical secretary
- To highlight the importance of effective communication and teamwork.

INTRODUCTION

In any health service, whether public or private, community or hospital based, the care delivered will be reliant on many diverse teams of staff cooperating effectively to provide a high standard and efficient level of care. As a medical secretary, you will be an essential component of the delivery team. In a general practice environment you will be a member of the primary care team providing a key point of contact for the other team members (see Chapter 16 – The Working Practice). You will also be required to liaise with a wide range of external organisations and individuals. In the secondary care environment, a variety of teams will exist and will be called upon at different times to deliver a service to each individual patient. You will form part of the support structure which allows the medical and nursing care to be effectively delivered. You will also be a key liaison point for members of each patient's primary care team. Through this chapter we will aim to demonstrate the range of personnel who are involved in patient care and support, and the way in which primary and secondary care teams are linked to form an extended team to ensure the patient's needs are fully met. Members of the PCT are fully described in Chapter 16, so only brief reference will be made to individual functions in this chapter. It is worthwhile noting that the NHS spends more on staffing resources than on any other category of expenditure.

Reflection Point 1

Whilst reading this chapter, reflect upon the pivotal role played by the medical secretary in ensuring good communication is maintained between departments and health care personnel and note the recurring theme of effective teamwork throughout the text.

TRUST HOSPITALS

Trust hospitals are individual or groups of hospitals operating under their own management structure. Each Trust will manage its own finances, contracting, staffing and both day-to-day and strategic management issues. The Trust is controlled by the Board, which will include a chairperson, five executive directors and five non-executive directors. The five executive directors will all be full-time employees of the Trust and will by statute include the Chief Executive, Director of Finance, Director of Nursing, a Medical Director and one other, such as the Director of Corporate Affairs. The Board is accountable to the Secretary of State via one of the newly created Strategic Health Authorities (SHAs). The management structure of each Trust will vary depending on the size of the organisation and the range of services offered. Areas of responsibility will be divided into sections known as directorates which typically reflect specialties, for example, surgery, medicine, diagnostics and, depending upon the size of the organisation, the number of directorates within each hospital will vary. Each Directorate has its own business/general manager, senior nurse, budgets and support teams. Generally speaking, medical secretaries are now responsible to their individual business manager within their particular directorate. A full

description of the management structures of Trust hospitals appears in Chapter 2, The National Health Service today.

STAFF GROUPS

MEDICAL STAFF

This term is used to describe all doctors working within a health care organisation. Doctors, like many other professionals, must train and progress up the career ladder whilst working. 'Consultant' is the most senior title applied to medical staff in most hospitals, although the academic title of 'Professor' denotes particular seniority within a specialty in some university teaching hospitals. Each consultant will have a team of junior doctors working under his or her care, often referred to as a 'firm'. The consultant in charge of each firm is ultimately responsible for the performance and ability demonstrated by all members of the team. Teaching forms a large part of the remit of a consultant. Traditional titles of medical staff are listed in Box 11.1, in order of seniority.

Box 11.1 Medical staff

Consultant/Professor
Staff Grade/Hospital Grade
Specialist Registrar (SpR)
Senior House Officer (SHO)
Pre-Registration House Officer (PRHO)
Medical Student

Other university-employed medical staff will be known by other official titles such as Professor, Reader, Senior Lecturer and Lecturer.

Recent reforms have altered the traditional system by incorporating senior registrar and registrar grades into one 5-year specialist registrar (SpR) training programme, which, once completed, enables the SpR to apply for Consultant posts. Some hospitals may also employ general practitioners, who are given the title of clinical assistant, on a session-only basis. These doctors will be informally attached to one or more consultants to assist with specific outpatient clinics or diagnostic sessions, for example endoscopy. In addition, Staff Grades, who, for whatever reason have not attained the level of Consultant, hold a career grade post which is just short of Consultant status.

NURSING

Nurses form the single largest group of staff employed in any hospital. They are employed on a complex system of titles and grades and are shown, in descending order of seniority, in Box 11.2.

In addition to the 'hands on' practitioners listed in Box 11.3, most hospitals will employ a senior nurse in each Directorate to oversee the nursing services. They will also have a Director of Nursing or Chief Nurse, which is a board level appointment.

In most hospitals the work of the nursing staff will be supplemented by health care assistants or auxiliaries. These individuals are not specifically trained to undertake nursing skills but can perform a variety of supporting tasks in a clinical environment.

In every clinical area you will find a team of nurses: wards, intensive care units, outpatient clinics and theatres all require nursing staff with specialist skills. Since 1992, once nurses have successfully completed their basic training they are entitled to use the designation Registered Nurse (RN).

Those individuals who qualified prior to 1992 received the designation Registered General Nurse (RGN). These people may now choose to use the title Registered Nurse (RN) if they wish to do so. This has replaced the previous qualification system of SRN (State Registered Nurse) and SEN (State Enrolled Nurse).

In most hospitals, nurses' uniforms or belts will identify their grade or seniority. The use of elaborate hats is now less common but previously these were also an indication of a nurse's grade or status. In recent years the traditional view of the nurse as the 'doctor's handmaiden' has been dispelled and they are now appropriately viewed as professionals in their own right, bringing a range of specialist skills, nurse-led services and expertise to the care of a patient, which complement the skills of the medical staff, and other health care professionals.

RNs have the option to continue their studies to specialise in one particular field. Examples are the qualification of RSCN (Registered Sick Children's Nurse) or RMN (Registered Mental Nurse). Those employed in the operating theatres will be required to undergo a variety of additional study programmes

Box 11.2 Staff in order of seniority

Clinical Nurse Specialist
Senior Sister
Sister/Charge Nurse
Senior Staff Nurse
Staff Nurse
Enrolled Nurse
Health Care Assistant (HCA)
Student Nurse

such as anaesthetic training to become experts within that area of work. The Royal College of Nursing now offers advanced training for nurses to become Nurse Practitioners. These practitioners are empowered to provide diagnoses, prescribe suitable treatments and refer patients on for other services. At the time of writing, consultant nurses are currently being introduced into hospitals. These nurses are at the pinnacle of the nursing career structure: they have special academic and management expertise and will provide a professional leadership role to teams of one or more junior nurses across a range of specialties. Their role will also include carrying out minor operations and prescribing drugs and treatment. One of the complexities in the nursing profession is that there are so many titles and roles and, apart from those shown in Box 11.2, some hospitals will also have nursing lecturer practitioners, modern matrons, nurse managers and nurse researchers.

The nursing and medical staff work very closely to ensure patient care is of a high quality, both when given as an inpatient and on an outpatient basis. The nursing staff need to communicate with the medical team frequently and this will often be done through liaison directly with the consultant's medical secretary, particularly when the medical staff are unavailable or difficult to contact. The medical secretary needs to be able to converse effectively with all levels of staff, and attention to accurate recording of information and detail is essential. It is also important that the medical secretary is aware of the consultant's whereabouts at all times so that he or she can be found quickly in an emergency or urgent situation. The medical secretary must also learn how to judge when to 'find' the consultant, and when matters can wait until the consultant is freely available. If there is ever any doubt as to the urgency of a situation, the medical secretary should always demonstrate caution and contact the consultant immediately, unless prior experience dictates otherwise.

ADMINISTRATION AND CLERICAL STAFF

A very large group of staff come under the general heading of 'administration and clerical'. Medical secretaries are included within this group, along with medical receptionists, ward clerks and medical records clerks. Medical receptionists will be found working on the reception desk of an outpatient clinic and will be responsible for recording patients' arrival at the clinic and for making follow-up clinic or investigation appointments. They will also be involved in preparing medical records for clinic and ensuring that the medical records are sent through to the clinic area in a timely fashion. Ward clerks, sometimes referred to as ward coordinators or administrators, will be based within a ward working with the nursing staff to ensure patients' records, results and X-rays are available and in order. They will often be involved with making follow-up and discharge arrangements for the patients and for liaison with the admissions office on a daily basis. Medical record clerks or assistants are usually based within the central medical records library and will work as part of a team under the supervision of a medical records officer or manager. Their role varies from hospital to hospital, but generally, they ensure the correct storage, recording and filing of all patient-related documentation and respond to requests from hospital staff for medical records (including for research projects). They will prepare and check clinic lists and retrieve notes for clinics, search for and file results, arrange follow-up appointments and generally assist the medical records officer in the smooth running of the department. Much time is spent searching for and filing case notes, which are usually housed in huge filing areas operating a numerical system. Each patient is allocated an individual hospital number and set of notes at their first attendance at a hospital. These are then kept and used for every future visit or admission. The role of the medical records department is further explored in Chapters 5 and 12. Medical records clerks will also undertake general repair and maintenance of the records folders as they pass through the system. Clerks may also be required to staff the clinic reception desk as part of their normal job description.

Other medical administration staff will be found working in specialised areas such as the admissions office, supplies, patient services, transport office, radiology department, clinical coding and medical audit.

Whilst all require basic office skills, each will develop specialised knowledge and skills in their own particular area of responsibility and may have the opportunity to achieve formal qualifications such as the Clinical Coding Certificate offered by the Institute of Health Record Information and Management (IHRIM).

PROFESSIONS ALLIED TO MEDICINE

There are a large number of specialist staff who are referred to as PAMs (professions allied to medicine).

- Physiotherapists or physical therapists: assisting in rehabilitation and providing advice on appropriate exercise for those with orthopaedic conditions, general injuries, sports injuries, those recovering from surgical procedures or medical conditions, and the elderly.
- Occupational therapists: working with those who are permanently or temporarily mentally or physically disabled, to enable them to cope with everyday tasks and to learn new skills.
- Speech and language therapists: providing treatment for all types of speech and communication problems afflicting the hearing impaired, trauma patients, the disabled, children and

Reflection Point 2

The list below contains many different departments within a hospital. What members of staff would be in each?

- Speech and language
- Rehabilitation
- General outpatients
- Oral surgery and orthodontics
- Diagnostic imaging
- Audiology
- Blood tests and pathology samples
- Restaurant
- Chapel
- Boardroom
- Dietician
- Antenatal clinic
- Social services department

adults with speech impediments and those learning to speak following major surgery to the larynx or oesophagus, and those recovering from strokes or other medical conditions.

* Dieticians: providing individual dietary advice for patients suffering from specific food allergies, obesity, swallowing problems, malnutrition, kidney disease and other medical conditions. They also provide information on healthy eating, and safe alcohol consumption, in general.
* Chiropodists/Podiatrists: provide expert advice on the care of feet, which may be particularly important to diabetics, the elderly and those with circulatory problems. They also undertake gait assessments and other related tasks.
* Pharmacists: responsible for dispensing drugs via the pharmacy in all hospitals, for both outpatients and inpatients. They will also provide drug information. Each pharmacy will be managed by a senior pharmacist.
* Social workers: responsible for coordinating the needs of patients who are to be discharged, either to their own home or to another environment, such as a hospice.
* Radiographers: working with the team of radiologists providing a range of radiological investigations.

All PAMs undergo specific professional training and will gain recognised qualifications before being able to practise. Their professional status will be governed by their own professional body, e.g. the College of Speech and Language Therapists.

TECHNICIANS

This term covers a range of specialist staff, some of whom are described in Box 11.3.

MANAGEMENT

We have already outlined the Trust Board and senior executives but these individuals will be supported by a team of middle and first line managers, administrators and secretaries to ensure the management of the organisation as a whole is well maintained and cost-effective.

HUMAN RESOURCES

The personnel department is now commonly referred to as 'human resources'. It will normally be headed up by a director of human resources and will be supported by a team including a deputy, human resources advisors/managers, a secretary and clerical staff. In some hospitals, individual directorates will be assigned their own human resource advisor who will provide help and support on human resource issues. The work of the human resources department will include staff retention and recruitment, handling industrial relations issues (including disciplinary and grievance procedures), workforce planning and information, job evaluation, liaison with payroll, and the management of the appraisal process for all staff ensuring a link through personal development plans (PDPs) to the training and development strategy, the development of family friendly policies and procedures (for example, flexible working) and formulating local policies on pay and conditions of service. Within the HRD there is also a staff training and development department, supported by the introduction of the NHS University, which is to be established during 2003. The aim of the NHS University is that staff training and development will be flexible and accessible, ensuring transferable skills across the NHS. This is seen as a high priority and forms one of the key objectives of the *NHS Plan*, promoting high quality and lifelong learning through renewing and extending skills and knowledge. It is envisaged that through this structured programme of training and development, jobs traditionally hard to recruit to will become more attractive. Staff training and development also includes organisational development which is involved with the culture, values and philosophy of the organisation.

Also included in the function of human resources is medical staffing, which is led by a medical staffing officer. This department looks after the recruitment of medical staff (including locum doctors), monitors sickness and annual leave amongst the medical staff, the management of medical rotations and adherence to working time regulations for staff (*The New Deal for junior medical staff*).

FINANCE

Each NHS Trust has financial autonomy and employs a team of staff dedicated to its financial management. The finance department has to ensure that legal and statutory financial requirements are met, along with general accounting principles (GAP). A director of finance is responsible for this area of work, assisted by a team of accountants, account clerks and administrative staff. Generally, the finance function is divided into two:

1. Financial services: Deals with sending out and payment of invoices, the production of financial accounts, financial management of charitable funds, the hospital cashier (who looks after patient monies and travel re-imbursements) and financial control of any capital programmes.
2. Management Accounts: Deals with the production of budget statements for directorates/departments, budgets, long term financial planning, capital planning and financial advice to budget holders. A management accountant is usually assigned to each directorate.

The audit function in the past has been provided in house, but is now more usually outsourced through a consortium arrangement with other Trusts, Primary Care Trusts (PCTs) and/or Strategic Health Authorities (SHAs).

Some large Trusts also have a payroll function, but many now contract this out.

CONTRACTS

One of the key changes brought about by the intro-duction of Trusts and PCTs was the setting up of a system of funding health care, which is commonly referred to as the purchaser/provider split. A hospital can be both a provider of care and a purchaser. The hospital will provide care as requested by a PCT but may also need to purchase additional services from other hospitals, both NHS and independent. For example, one hospital may need to purchase the services of the radiology department of another hospital where a highly specialised investigation is required, such as a magnetic resonance imaging (MRI) scan.

Where providing services to patients is concerned, a service and financial framework (SAFF) is agreed between the purchaser (the PCT) and the provider (the NHS Trust) based on the level of patient activity which has been calculated to take place (using previous years' activity). The SAFF will also include adherence to nationally set targets for waiting times, clinic appointments etc. The provider is paid on a monthly basis and patient activity is monitored via the Trust's computerised Patient Administration System (PAS). However, many Trusts have found that they treat more patients than has been agreed in the SAFF with no extra funding to cover this, and have therefore subsequently been faced with rationalising treatment in other areas to ensure budgets are not overspent.

To try and streamline the old Extra Contractual Referral (ECR) system, and make it less bureaucratic and time consuming, Out of Area Treatments (OATS) now replace ECRs for those patients falling outside of a SAFF. The Trust's treatment of patients from outside their area is costed out and monies are top sliced off each individual purchaser and sent to the host purchaser. Unfortunately, this system works on a two year delay of payment and many Trusts still find the system laborious and time consuming.

Reflection Point 3

- Consider the issues which relate to the opinion that we have a 'postcode lottery' when it comes to NHS treatment. How do these compare with the original premise for the creation of a National Health Service in 1948?

- Consider the arguments in favour of a business approach to NHS funding.

HOTEL AND CATERING STAFF

This category of staff provides support services such as cleaning, linen and laundry, sewing and repairs. The catering staff (led by a catering manager) are employed to provide a wide range of food services for patients, staff and visitors and will normally work in shifts. There will usually be a hotel services manager employed to ensure these services are available and of a high standard whilst remaining within set budgets. Typically, this group of services is now contracted out to private companies.

PORTERS

Porters provide an essential link in the chain of service delivery. They will be managed by a head porter or portering manager and their duties are diverse. Apart from assisting with the movement of patients from department to department or from ward to theatre and the transport of specimens, equipment and gas supplies, they will often assist in providing a secure environment for the staff and visitors to the hospital. They may also be involved in receiving, sorting and delivering mail, and for ensuring all out-going mail is franked and despatched. Porters will normally be employed to work on a shift system, including nights, to ensure the service is available 24 hours a day, 7 days a week. They also assist in ward/departmental moves and the moving of heavy/large equipment (for example, beds).

MAINTENANCE STAFF

The hospital premises are usually maintained by a team of workers employed in the estates department. This team will comprise carpenters, painters, plumbers, electricians and general workers. As many hospitals in the UK are still housed in old premises, the work of the estates team is of vital importance in ensuring that the hospital remains a safe environment for patients and staff alike. They will undertake the majority of repairs and redecoration as and when required, although most major refurbishment projects are generally contracted to outside companies.

In many Trusts, the non-clinical services (for example, portering, estates, linen and laundry, hotel services) come under the umbrella of the 'facilities department', led by a facilities manager or director.

Scenario 1

Mrs Andrews, aged 79, has been an inpatient under the care of a consultant endocrinologist for a 48-hour period of observation and monitoring. She is diabetic, suffers from arthritis and is blind in one eye. The consultant requests a nutritional assessment, a mobility assessment and a full blood screen as part of her treatment.

Which members of the health care team, other than the doctors, will be involved in her treatment and assessment?

You should have listed at least some of the following personnel: dietician, catering staff, nursing staff, physiotherapist, phlebotomist and social worker. All of these people will contribute to the required treatment regimen.

Scenario 2

Following a satisfactory assessment period, Mrs Andrews is pronounced fit for discharge. Two hours before her transport is due to collect her to take her back home she trips over a loose floor tile in the bathroom and sustains a blow to the elbow.

What follow-up action will need to take place as a result of this accident?

Your thoughts should have included:

- consultant in charge to be informed
- physical examination by doctor
- possible X-ray of arm
- completion of an incident/accident report form
- enquiry into how accident happened
- report loose floor tile for immediate repair
- possible need to postpone discharge from ward
- contact next of kin to inform them of situation.

If Mrs Andrews' discharge from the ward is postponed, who needs to know?

Once you have deliberated this question, you

should see that there are many individuals who may need to be updated on the current situation. The patient's consultant or his/her medical secretary must be informed. The transport officer needs to be told so that if official transport has been arranged, this can be cancelled. The patient's relatives will need to be contacted as soon as possible. The admissions department will need to know that the bed is not being vacated as expected, as they may have to cancel the admission of another patient to prevent a wasted journey. The patient may also have an assigned social worker who will also need to be kept informed. It may also be necessary to advise the patient's GP by telephone that the patient is not being discharged home, particularly if a home visit has already been organised. It is possible that the medical secretary may be required to undertake some or all of these communications.

CONCLUSION

In this chapter we have examined a number of staffing groups to be found within a health care environment, outlining the who, where and why. It is important to note that staff from all these groups may be found working within both primary and secondary care. Each member of staff has an important function in the delivery of health care services, whether they are involved in direct patient care or in a supporting role. As recipients of health care, as we all will be at some point in our lives, we will rely on the efforts and expertise of an extensive network of professionals and support staff who will work together to ensure an acceptable level, and quality, of care.

Exercises

- Find out what other specialist nursing qualifications are available by further reading and contacting recognised nursing bodies and associations.

- Through further reading and group discussion, make a list of professional bodies responsible for the training and conduct of PAMs in the UK.

- On your work placement or at your place of employment, find out who is responsible for training and development within the organisation. What development opportunities do they offer which might be useful for medical secretaries? Do they actively promote the attainment of professional qualifications?

As a medical secretary you have a duty to familiarise yourself with the staff and services available within your place of work. Ensure that you obtain a copy of the in-house directory detailing the names, departments and contact telephone numbers for all staff. Nurture good working relationships with all other staff. You should also ensure that your colleagues are aware of who you are, how you can be contacted and what the full extent of your role is. Your aim should be always to make a worthwhile contribution to the service received by the patients. In this way you will help to create an environment conducive to effective communication and promote your own value as a member of the team.

Useful websites

www.nhsuniversity.nhs.uk

www.nhs.uk

Further reading

Irvine D, Irvine S 1996 The practice of quality. Radcliffe Medical Press, Oxford

Pringle M (ed) 1993 Change and teamwork in primary care. BMJ Publishing, London

Chapter 12

Medical records

Grizelda Moules

OBJECTIVES

- To examine some important aspects of patient notes including the ownership of hospital records, the length of time that they should be kept and means of accessing them
- To explain the different methods of compilation and storage of medical records in the hospital environment
- To highlight the importance of confidentiality and accuracy in all record-keeping activities
- To outline the most important forms used in hospital
- To describe the role of audit and the part you need to play to ensure accurate information is recorded, with particular reference to research purposes
- To show how you may need to oversee the needs of other secretarial staff or assistants.

INTRODUCTION

This chapter focuses primarily on medical records in the hospital environment, but also covers the important documentary links between hospitals and GPs. One of its key themes will be the importance of confidentiality and accuracy in all record-keeping activities.

PATIENTS' NOTES

The ICRS (Integrated Care Record Services) is aimed at collating all aspects of patient records together, and planning is underway to integrate all aspects of records of care, particularly those in electronic form, in the future. As this is quite difficult to implement, because there are a variety of different methods being used in primary care, it is probable that separate hospital medical records will continue for some time yet until a common system is implemented.

OWNERSHIP OF RECORDS

Any records that are in writing are made up of the following two elements:

- the physical paper on which the words are written; and
- the information contained in them.

Within the NHS, the records belong physically to the NHS Trust or hospital and ultimately to the Secretary of State.

The records of *private patients* belong to the health professional with whom they have a contract.

This ownership is unusual in law in that the 'owner' has a custodial responsibility, but is unable to sell or dispose of records. It is also an obligation that the 'owner' has to provide patients with access to them under the Access to Health Records Act 1990. All those who are aged 16 and over have the right to see any of their case notes which were created since November 1991. This is described later in this chapter.

There is a *duty of confidence* whereby the contents of records should not be disclosed to unauthorised parties. It is important that hospitals make arrangements to ensure that records are kept securely. There needs to be an overall policy on confidentiality and security.

CONFIDENTIALITY AND SECURITY OF RECORDS

The Caldicott Committee Report on the review of patient identifiable information was published in December 1997 and is concerned with protecting patient confidentiality and security. The report found that compliance across the NHS with the full range of confidentiality and security arrangements was inconsistent and that action needed to be taken to raise awareness.

The report identified 18 principles and suggested that it was essential for all organisations to evaluate their current performances across a wide range of confidentiality and security measures. This information should then be used to highlight areas where improvement is needed as well as providing a benchmark for evaluating progress over time. There should be appointed a network of Organisational Guardians to facilitate and to manage this work.

Subsequent audits of progress have often found that further education/training of staff in aspects of confidentiality and security is still needed. Policies such as the following can be considered.

- It should be ensured that all staff are made aware of the importance of high standards of confidentiality and security with regard to patient records. All staff members employed by the NHS need to sign a confidentiality statement. It is also important to consider the position of other people, such as volunteers or other workers not normally directly employed by the NHS, who may have access to data.

- It may be necessary to improve the physical security of records. In addition, with regard to computer-held records, it is important to ensure that unique passwords are used, and kept secret by their owner. Many other measures may need to be considered with regard to computer-held records and levels of access to them.

- Notes should not be taken out of the hospital.

- Computers should not be left unattended, particularly when logged on, as they are open to anyone else using them. Sometimes automatic log-off, which can cut in if a screen is left unattended, is not appropriate, as, for example a physician may have left the computer to examine a patient. If the automated log out occurs it can prevent subsequent access by other computer users.

- Measures such as ensuring that the medical records department is a 'closed library', i.e. only open to specific medical records personnel by means of an electronic entry code, are very successful. This prevents other staff trying to find records and taking them without leaving any record of where they can be found. Normally medical records staff will complete a 'tracer card' of a noticeable colour, which gives details of the date, patient name and number

Scenario 1

A hospital has chosen to retain the following categories of case notes for longer than usual. Would you recommend including the same categories or would it be appropriate to add or omit any in your own environment?

Categories of notes which should not be destroyed

- War pensions
- Brain tumours (severe head injury)
- Very severe accidents (road traffic accident, etc.)
- ANYTHING hereditary (e.g. congenital heart disease)
- Pathology
- L2 Leukaemia
- Haemophilia (hereditary) – also Christmas disease, von Willebrand's disease
- Radioactive iodine in thyroid cases
- Septal defects
- By-pass surgery
- Pacemaker (cardiology)
- Unusual cases or rare ones
- Jehovah's Witness (blood denial)
- Self discharge – mainly ward cases
- Overdose – can destroy if once only and if not followed up by psychiatric clinic – MORE than once – keep
- Cone biopsy – gynaecology – check carefully
- Colposcopy
- TOP (termination of pregnancy) – destroy (keep if more than one)
- Unusual blood group
- Sickle cell
- Basal cell carcinoma – use own discretion
- Asbestosis

Could possible reasons for keeping these records include teaching purposes, data for research, potential injury or insurance claims?

How should they ensure that these notes are not destroyed after the usual period? Why do you think they may need to retain them?

Reflection Point 1

Having seen the criteria for retaining records, what do you think a hospital might choose to include as other categories of case notes to be retained for longer periods? What reasons could there be for retaining these case notes?

and department to which the notes have been sent. Unauthorised staff are also prevented from mis-filing the returned records back to the wrong location. Closed libraries often result in far fewer records being difficult to locate.

RETENTION

The period of legal retention depends on the purposes for which the patient records are to be used. Currently, the Department of Health recommendations as on HC 1999 053 (www.hsc/1999/053) are that medical records should be retained for the following periods:

Primary documents. To be retained for a legal minimum period (case note folder, identification sheets, discharge letters/summaries, referral letters, history sheets, operation sheets, nursing records, anaesthetic sheet).

- Obstetric records: 25 years, or 10 years after the death of the child (but not the mother) if sooner.
- Children and young people: until the 25th birthday, or 26th if an entry was made when the patient was 17, or 10 years after a patient's death if sooner.
- Mental health records (Mental Health Act 1983): 20 years after no further treatment is considered necessary or 10 years after a patient's death if sooner.
- All other patient records: 10 years after the conclusion of treatment, patient's death or patient's permanent departure from the country.

Secondary documents. To be retained for locally agreed periods (mount sheet, pathology reports, X-ray reports, drug sheets).

Transitory documents. To be retained for locally agreed periods (temperature, pulse, respiration, blood pressure and fluid balance charts).

It is recommended that until further advice is received, computerised patient records are retained at the site and in the form in which they were originated for the period of time for which they were originally required in that form, e.g. during an inpatient stay.

It is important that hospitals should set out a clear policy for the retention and destruction of records. To do this, it is necessary to refer to the *Department of Health Circular* HC (1999) 053, issued in 1999, for guidance in determining their policy. It is essential that sufficient training is given so that staff are able to ensure it is fully implemented.

Additional categories which a hospital may choose to retain often cover the following categories:

- records of patients involved in a legal case
- records of patients involved in a drug trial
- records of patients who have had open heart surgery
- radiotherapy / cancer records.

All other records may be destroyed after the 8th year after the last date of the last episode of care, unless notes are marked 'DO NOT DESTROY'.

COMPILING NEW NOTES

Reflection Point 2

What steps can you think of taking to ensure that the correct patient's details are recorded prior to them attending their hospital consultation?

- Check all details from hospital referral forms or letters are entered correctly, or check details if the referral has been made by online booking.
- Send patients a form to complete and bring with them when they attend. Ensure that patients are informed of the reason why this data is needed.
- Go through details with patients when they attend for their appointment, having asked them to arrive a little early to allow time for this to take place.
- Ensure the patient has been asked to give their consent to having their records held electronically and that an alternative method of storage of records is available should they not wish

them to be stored in this form. This is a major policy decision, which you will need to check with the particular Trust by whom you are employed.

Ensure that this can take place as confidentially as possible. Ideally the patient should be able to give information out of the hearing of others attending a clinic.

Do not repeat information unnecessarily from telephone calls as this can easily be overheard by others and can be a direct breach of confidentiality.

Be aware of the possibility that patients may have difficulty with reading and writing. A possible way of them avoiding saying this directly can be that they have 'forgotten their glasses'. They may also have difficulty in hearing or in understanding English, so be sensitive to these needs. Many hospitals are able to provide interpreters or people who can assist with sign language when needed. The GP should alert the hospital if he or she knows of these needs, but is not always aware of them. It is worth noting that in the UK 8.7 million people are deaf or hard of hearing, 7.3 million people have literacy difficulties, 1.7 million people are visually impaired and 1 million people have learning difficulties.

Remember to update information. It is important to update any changes in patients' details. These may include changes of name, title, address, telephone number and GP and / or GP address. It is quite possible that just one detail may change at a time and this can mean that data is lost from the hospital record or that it is mis-filed or never reaches the correct GP. From the clinical side it is also important that medical staff are updated and informed of any changes in medication. Inaccuracies in medication are potentially very serious. When the patient has been seen at the hospital, a clinic letter will be sent to the GP. As the IHCR develops, the electronically held information about the patient should be transferred more easily so that the clinic letter, as well as discharge summaries, should be able to be incorporated directly into the GP held records. This should help eliminate errors in filing and assist rapid location of particular information.

PROTOCOL FOR REGISTRATION OF PATIENTS

A protocol needs to be agreed for patient registration, and several steps need to be followed. This is covered in Chapter 13 on the outpatient department. The referral may be made through the online booking system but otherwise all details should be supplied on the (Blue) GP referral form (HMR 3) or on a referral printout letter. Sometimes both types are sent and Trusts often generate an electronic form of the standard referral letter, which is often directorate specific. Some data may be able to be entered in automatically, but it is very important when working in general practice to ensure all details are given. If you are working in general practice, you can find a reference to a hospital number at the beginning of either a letter from a clinic or sometimes from a laboratory test result. Make sure these relate to the hospital to which the patient is being referred.

Babies now are given a unique NHS identifying number which they will carry throughout their life and which can be used in the form of a barcode.

In the medical records department, firstly the referral (if not online) needs to be approved. Providing that the patient has not previously been registered at the hospital, and does not have the new national identifying number, a pre-registration hospital number will be allocated and a hospital record file prepared. The allocation of a number is usually made on a computer and the method must ensure that the specific number is unique to that patient, so that even if several clerks access the computer simultaneously, the number allocation is controlled. Patients will be sent a questionnaire to complete and to bring with them when they attend for their first appointment.

The PAS computer database should be able to identify a set of hospital records from the details given. It is important to check that these relate to the right patient, particularly when several people may have the same name. In cases where details may have changed, such as GP and address, a note should be made and attached to the records or recorded on screen so that clinic reception staff can check that these are the right notes.

Normally patients will be allocated a hospital number on their first attendance at a hospital and this number may be specific to that hospital, or may be used within a specified group of hospitals. This is a particular case where GP staff can help tremendously. In whichever situation you are working you need to try and quote the current hospital number accurately and draw attention to any changes of name, address or GP. It is also worth identifying any different hospital numbers, which may have been used previously at the same hospital, so that all details on that patient can be amalgamated.

Reflection Point 3

How could you try to ensure all the data on a patient is kept up to date?

Possible ideas: Incorporation of reminder notices in the waiting room or at reception desk.

PROTOCOLS AND CHECKLISTS FOR RECEPTION/NURSING STAFF

It is advisable to compare previous letters from the GP to see if they include different addresses or other information. Such changes of data need to be checked with the patient to see what is accurate, e.g. they may have been staying at a temporary address.

The patient may be encouraged to bring a current repeat prescription card or even the bottles of medicine themselves for a first attendance or when changes in either dosage or medications are made. Notes of drug sensitivities or allergies should also be recorded.

POCKET GUIDE FOR JUNIOR DOCTORS

This idea may help to encourage junior medical staff to help to maintain a good quality of patient record. The Welsh Medical Records Forum has designed a pocket guide in the form of a card. The importance of the medical records is emphasised and the doctor's responsibility towards them is outlined. The advice includes the points listed in Box 12.1.

Reflection Point 4

- Do you think this guide is a good idea? Why/why not?

- What points would you suggest adding or changing to this list?

- Which other categories of staff do you think could benefit from such an aide-memoire?

Box 12.1 Patient record guidelines for junior B

- The case notes must not be removed from the hospital.
- The patient must be identified on all documents.
- All entries must be written legibly, in black ink, dated and signed.
- Electronic entries must be dates and attributable to their author.
- Consent forms must be completed and signed.
- Test results must be signed and dated when seen.
- Discharge letters must be timely, neat and accurate.
- Senior staff need to check coding of diagnosis and procedures.

COMPILER RECORDS

A record should be kept of who compiles this information. Data entered on computer during or after a hospital consultation *should be automatically attributable to the health professional who entered it*. This would normally be part of a computer audit trail and for this as well as other reasons, it is important that staff do not borrow or use other people's password identifiers.

In the case of manual records, initials may be used, but these should be readily decipherable and there should be a means of tracking them back to their originator.

ACCESS TO NOTES

PATIENT ACCESS TO THEIR MEDICAL RECORDS

The Access to Health Records Act 1990 allowed all people over the age of 16 to see their own case notes created since November 1991. This is unless a clinical case is made for access being denied. Access to any records created before that date is at the discretion of the physician involved.

Following the Data Protection Acts of 1984 and 1998, patients have a right of access to any information held about them on computer. Applications have to be made in writing to the holder of the record and the application must be processed within 21 days. Applications for access are usually dealt with by

medical records staff. Record holders who supply information are entitled to charge a fee and may also charge for copying and postage.

HOW IT WORKS IN PRACTICE

A patient who wishes to have access to his or her notes may be asked to complete a request form. This form will ask for the person's identification details and will require the person's signature. In the case of a person under 18 a responsible adult needs to certify that the child understands the nature of the application. The young person will need to sign an authorisation of release of any personal health records relating to him or her.

The application will then go to the consultant concerned and, if approved, the notes will be prepared.

Reasons why details may not have to be released include:

- if the information identifies a third party
- if legal issues are being considered by solicitors
- if the information is thought to be potentially mentally damaging
- if the information was recorded prior to the Data Protection Act of 1 November 1991.

Patients may also ask to see their records during a consultation. It is recommended that when a patient is accessing notes, someone who has the appropriate expertise and ability should be present to 'explain' where necessary.

This situation may change with patient-held smart cards or patient-held notes. Currently maternity patients often keep a set of obstetric notes with them, which are passed back to a health care professional a few weeks after the baby's birth. Similar records for child care may be held parentally to encourage partnership of care between parents and health care professionals. A booklet prepared by the Medical Protection Society *A simplified version of the 1998 Data Protection Act* for use by clinicians is available.

CLASSIFICATION FOR FILING

THE CONTENTS OF THE MEDICAL RECORD FILES

On the outer cover of the record, the name of the hospital is printed. In addition, the patient's name is written, usually with the surname first and the hospital number in a position so that it is prominent when filing. It is likely that there will be increasing use of bar-coding to identify patient records and new babies are now allocated bar-coded identification for their records. It is also helpful to put a patient identification sticker on the outside, so that should two patients with the same name be attending the same clinic, they can be readily differentiated, while aspects of confidentiality are also maintained.

Inside the medical record envelope there should be the following items.

Patient information sheet. This should include the patient minimum data set and additional information, which is also often kept on computer.

It should be possible to print this out and to attach it at the front of the records. It is a good idea for it to be glued inside the front cover so it is easily accessible to anyone reading the records and is a recognised place for data to be updated. There should be plenty of room for changes of detail, such as address or GP, particularly in areas of a fluctuating population. It is very important to keep the records up to date.

Other details that should be included here are:

- telephone number
- details of religion
- next of kin
- details of known allergies or hypersensitivities.

Reflection Point 5

What other details should or could be included here?

The patient questionnaire. This may have provided a source of useful information and could be included in the record and used to complete data held on the computer. Another questionnaire may be used to ask for details of medical history. If it covers general information, it may be included at the front, perhaps on a colour of paper that can be easily identified. Other questionnaires may be included in a departmental section (see 'Specialty coding', below).

Stickers. These should give basic patient details (name, address, GP, date of birth, etc.) and should be included in the notes. It may well be your job to ensure that they contain current information (and relate to the right patient). If they have run out or

need updating a note could be put on the front of the records before they are returned to the medical records department.

History sheets. These should be included here, if not already within the departmental sections (see 'Specialty coding', below). They should be headed with patient details or a **sticker**. The question as to how the history sheets are stored varies. In some cases these are chronological, from the top downwards (like a book), in others the most current (and most relevant notes) are kept at the top. The latter method is often used in general practice for history cards. The sheets may be held together with treasury tags or with a flexible plastic device, which clips into place and holds the notes tightly, but is sometimes difficult to open and close.

X-ray reports. These are often stored at the back of the notes on a set of single pages and are attached by a sticky strip. Some hospitals report that they stop sticking after a while and can fall off. Some recommend glue, others suggest staples.

Pathology laboratory results. These are stored in a similar way to X-ray results, but are particularly likely to accumulate with some patients. They may need to be 'culled' from time to time and an agreed protocol for this needs to be in place. It may be your job to alert the doctor to the situation that the notes are getting full or that information is at risk of being lost. It may be that a summary of results is required at some stage, and in some cases computer-held results can provide a summary printout easily. A graphical representation may also be provided to show a pattern over time, perhaps of levels of hormone in relation to the use of a particular drug. The order in which these sections are arranged can vary between hospitals.

Nursing records. While a patient is an inpatient, records will be kept of the nursing care and this is incorporated in the notes in a separate section.

Specialty coding

This can be a very effective way of distinguishing between the notes of different departments. Each department is assigned a different colour for a dividing folder, e.g. dermatology notes may be kept within a green folder and orthopaedics within a red one. The name of the department and consultant are then stamped on the front of this section and if a particular questionnaire relating to that treatment has been completed it can be included at the beginning of that section.

History sheets should also be stamped with the department and consultant's name, and headed with the patient's details (on label where possible). This can save time when the consultant or other doctors wish to see the patient's progress with a particular condition, without necessitating them reading through a perhaps considerable amount of notes relating to other complaints.

A possible drawback of dividing the case notes by department is that this method does not allow the notes to be totally chronological of all that relates to the patient in hospital, and consultations in other departments may shed light on what could be an interrelated condition. A particular effort may need to be made to look at other notes or to question the patient about other illnesses for which they are being seen. From a medical secretary's point of view, division of the notes does facilitate the location and maintenance of notes relating to a particular department within the patient's records.

Whatever the method used for filing within the record, it is important that this is consistent, so that everyone knows where to look for the information they need.

It may also be necessary for you to let the medical records department know if the notes have become badly torn or are just too big to be kept together effectively. In some cases notes need to consist of more than one volume. If it is not possible, for clinical or other reasons, to cull the notes further, they may be stored and clearly labelled as a series of volumes and stored in a special area for large notes.

FILING OF MEDICAL RECORDS

Within a medical records department records awaiting filing should be stored in the order in which they will be filed to enable rapid access should they be required. Records should not be kept in cupboards or on shelves where they would be difficult to locate when needed should an emergency situation arise. It is also important that this applies in your own office. Alternatively records in clinic bags may be kept in the order in which patients were seen at the clinic. Inclusion of a clinic list in each bag can be invaluable in the location of these files.

DOB index

A method of cross reference back to other details such as date of birth, name and address is essential to check that a hospital number has not previously been allocated, and to enable records to be located when the hospital number is not specified or not known. This used to be in the form of a series of cards filed in order of date of birth, then alphabetically by surname. This method is sometimes occasionally used in small hospitals, but generally, nowadays such data is normally accessible electronically either by entering in the name of the patient or via clinic dates.

Systems of filing

Medical records in general practice are usually filed alphabetically by the patient's surname, but in a hospital, where large numbers of records are held and there can be many patients with the same name, numerical filing systems are preferred.

Hospital numbers are allocated chronologically. The number is often of six figures. In some hospitals, usually smaller ones, straight numerical filing may be used. This has the advantage of being easy to understand, but may result in mis-filing through transposition of numbers; for example, a record with the number 324558 may be filed as 325458.

One of the main drawbacks of this method of filing is that the part of the filing area which has most activity and needs to be available to the most staff at once is that of the newest records, which in this case would have the highest numbers and would be filed next to each other.

To prevent such bottlenecks of use occurring, other filing methods have been introduced.

Terminal digit filing system. The terminal digit system is a popular method of filing health records in hospitals. It relies on locating records by use of the patient's hospital number. A record number of various lengths can be used but often six-figure numbers are used. A six-figure number can be divided into three pairs of two numbers, which may be written with a space between each pair.

The terminal digit filing system is easy to operate and efficient in the use of space in the records department, but does require some training. The last two digits of the record number are termed the 'primary digits', the middle two are the 'secondary digits' and the first two (on the left of the number) are the 'tertiary digits'. For example, with the number *67 80 54*, *67* are *tertiary* digits, *80* are *secondary* digits and *54* are primary digits.

Box 12.2 Number arranged by terminal digit	
56 87 90	98 99 41
57 87 90	99 99 41
58 87 90	00 00 42
59 87 90	01 00 42
60 87 90	02 00 42

Box 12.3 Terminal digit filing using a nine–digit number

For the number 571-02-64-39, the group could be divided as follows:

57102	64	39
Tertiary digits	Secondary digits	Primary digits

The tertiary digits would then be filed sequentially. So the next ones would be:
57103 64 39, 57104 64 39, etc

In the terminal digit file there are 100 primary sections from 00 to 99. Each individual record is filed in straight numerical order according to its *tertiary digits*.

When filing a record, you would look at the primary digits first (remembering that these are the last two, on the right of the number). On finding the section for those primary digits, you need to look at the secondary digits next. On finding that part, the record should be filed in straight numerical order according to the terminal digits, i.e. the first two numbers.

Examples of file numbers arranged this way are given in Box 12.2.

Should an odd number, such as a five, seven or nine figure number be used, the middle group of numbers are regarded as a group on their own, with pairs on either side. This may happen, for example, if the files are more numerous or if the number is the same as another number used by the patient, e.g. NHS number or Social Security. An example using a nine-digit number is given in Box 12.3.

Use of colour. The spine and covers of medical records can be of different colours. These colours can be used to indicate the *year* of first attendance at a hospital. In this case records which precede a certain date can be clearly identified and selected for possible culling or retention in a different form such as microfiche.

Colour coding. Colour coding of the notes may be done to aid filing and identify particular notes. For example, a coloured strip of adhesive tape may be added to the spine of notes to identify a particular part of the hospital number. Alternatively, a hard plastic divider may be used which projects from the edge of the notes and can be readily seen when the notes are filed. Mis-filed notes can then be easily spotted, as ones with a colour which does not match the others are more readily noticeable than an incorrect number.

Classification by geography. In a hospital which contains the records of other, peripheral, hospitals, the records which relate to other hospitals may have a different coloured outer cover or other features to identify them, such as a different design or a form colouring or tagging on the spine. The numbering system may start with a letter to indicate which hospital they belong to. By keeping these notes separately, they can be more readily accessed for clinics at the peripheral hospitals.

You need to ensure that on returning clinic bags or other groups of records, records from these hospitals are kept separate from those of the main or other hospitals. On requesting records from the medical records department, it is helpful to medical records staff if you group together requests for records from a particular hospital. You may also need to use a separate booking-out book or a separate section of the general booking-out book to identify these records.

Be especially careful when a patient who normally attends an outlying hospital needs to come in for investigations or for an operation in another or in the main hospital. Multiple sets of case notes may come to light. In this case clear reference to the other notes needs to be made on the outside of each set. For future records, the consultant needs to be informed to ensure relevant documentation is included in both while not duplicating information unnecessarily.

ARCHIVING RECORDS

Generally, records which need to be retained, but are not currently in use, are scanned onto optical discs which are able to hold about 16,000 sets of notes. If the records are then required, printouts of relevant data are made as needed. Backups of optical discs need to be kept in a secure storage place off site.

MICROFILMING

Microfilming is an older technique and is a photographic method, which was used to reduce the size of the records stored. The size of the reduction can vary. If the original was reduced to 1/24 of the original size, the reduction rate is 24 to 1 and described as 24. This was the usual rate for reduction of medical records and could result in a 95% saving in storage space.

It may be necessary to agree a criterion for deciding which medical records should be recorded onto optical discs and whether all or only part of the contents should be included. The equipment necessary to microfilm used to be quite expensive. Most hospitals are now employing more sophisticated methods of storage which involve more advanced information technology methods such as optical disc and in the future, more information will be likely to be stored in electronic form throughout the patient's life.

For microfilming to be carried out, it was necessary to have a range of equipment including cameras. In addition, to assist with the selection and inspection of the images by providing an enlarged view, it was necessary to insert the microfilm into jackets. Special equipment called 'lay up equipment' is used to provide microfiche masters. Duplication equipment will provide the microform.

In order to see the microfilmed records, it is still necessary to have special machines, called readers, which act as projectors, as well as reader-printers. It is also possible to have computerised microfilm indexes using CAR (computer assisted retrieval). This may be worth considering when the rate of retrieval or reference is high.

The confidentiality of these records must be ensured. The resulting records need to be checked before the original paper versions are destroyed.

It is not always easy to read microfilmed notes and they can be of poor quality if derived from sources that have used carbon copies, darkened paper or have been torn or crumpled. Records need to be prepared by ensuring that the patient's name and number are included, that they are in chronological order and that any staples are removed. Each page is then photographed and presented in chronological order on a small card.

It is important that optical discs and microfilmed notes are stored in appropriate conditions and are clearly labelled and catalogued.

When paper records do need to be destroyed, this is often carried out by an external firm which will shred the records. However, it is important that this is carried out under strict supervision.

FORMS

HOSPITAL REFERRAL FORM (BLUE PRL 1) OR REFERRAL LETTER WRITTEN ON COMPUTER

When a GP refers a patient to be seen at a hospital this can be done either on a blue referral form, or on plain paper. The information needed on the referral letter will include the clinical reasons for the referral, but may also include information such as drug sensitivities or allergies. You may find that a method needs to be agreed with the consultant so that this information can be recorded in a suitably prominent position. Other information will form the basis of the patient data set, which can then be included in the PAS (Patient Administration System) and is used for preliminary patient identification. Where GP/Hospital Links are in place, this can be done electronically (see Chapter 8).

GP REQUEST FORMS

GPs may ask the hospital to carry out pathology laboratory reports on a variety of specimens or may request X-rays or other investigations. Often this is carried out electronically through GP/Hospital Links. Fast-track referrals are possible for cancer clinics whereby an appointment is given within 48 hours of receipt of the referral and the patient is seen within 14 days. It is important that data kept on the patient is up to date.

INVESTIGATION REQUEST FORMS

Unfortunately, it is often the case that the doctor's handwriting is not totally clear, so as a medical secretary working in general practice or in hospital you can help ensure the right patient's details relate to the right sample and that the result of the investigation returns to the doctor who requested it.

The consequences of accurate results being sent to the *wrong doctor* who has a patient by the same name could be disastrous, and it is not unknown. Scrupulous care is essential here.

Labels kept in patients' case notes can be useful,

but ensure that a separate label has been used for each piece of the form. This sometimes needs three labels per investigation. A method of ensuring that the results are returned appropriately is to prerecord details such as department code on sample requests. Increased use of bar-coding of lab samples can help eliminate confusion of identification.

If you are helping to prepare for a clinic where all the patients are likely to have the same samples taken, e.g. particular blood tests or cervical cytology, the appropriate forms and labels can be prepared and labelled for each patient. The use of clear, legible writing, usually in capitals, makes everyone's work easier.

Where a particular doctor has exclusive use of a consultation room, many forms can be prepared by ensuring the doctor's code and practice or department code are already written on request forms. This can also be done with sample bottles and containers. It may be that someone else can help with this and that a medical receptionist or nurse or ward clerk may be involved. The result is more efficient collection of data. Samples can otherwise easily be sent to a different doctor who has similar initials and never reach its true destination, which means that the time of the doctor, the patient and the laboratory technician time is wasted, as well as that of others, including yourself, who try in vain to locate the missing information.

Minimising the time that doctors have to spend on clerical work also means that they have more time to spend with the patient.

It is very important that each sample is checked before sending it off.

An input of a little extra time initially can achieve good results.

FORM MED 10 – INPATIENT CERTIFICATE

This can be used by a patient who is currently attending or who has attended hospital as an inpatient. It needs to be completed and signed by an authorised member of the hospital staff. This form can be used to support a claim for statutory sick pay or to continue a claim for state benefits. To start a claim for state benefit, patients need to use form SC1 (Rev) if self-employed, unemployed or non-employed, or Form SSP1 (E) or SSP1 (T) if they are an employer.

PRIVATE PATIENTS

In the case of private patients who have undergone treatment, whether as an outpatient or as an inpatient, the appropriate forms from their insurance companies will need to be completed, if applicable. The consultant may need to refer to the patient's notes for completion of these forms and it may be necessary to hold them back for this purpose.

REGISTRATION OF BIRTH

Following the birth of a baby in hospital, notification is sent to the local Register Office. In the case of a birth being in the community, the midwife will notify the Register Office. The parent should register the birth within 6 weeks and will be given a birth certificate. The parent will also be given a pink registration form (FP58) which should be given to the GP on registering the baby there, and not pasted into the baby book as some parents do.

DEATH CERTIFICATE

This will be issued if a death occurs in hospital. It is very important to record full details, including telephone number of next of kin, so that they may be notified promptly should a death occur. It may also be of particular importance if the person who died had offered to be an organ donor as decisions may need to be made within a short space of time.

Following a death, if a *coroner* is involved the coroner will send Part A of a form to the Register Office. If a post-mortem is necessary, the coroner will send Part B to the Register Office. The next of kin is advised to go to the Register Office to register the death.

When a body is to be *cremated* one doctor needs to sign Part B of the documentation. This can be either the deceased's registered GP or hospital doctor. Part C is completed by another doctor, either a hospital doctor or one who is from a different practice. Each doctor must see the body and they must not be related to each other.

ROAD TRAFFIC ACCIDENTS

When a road traffic accident (RTA) has occurred, the hospital can request reimbursement of emergency treatment costs. The fee is payable by those using the vehicle at the time of the accident and liability for payment is unconnected with any question of responsibility or liability for the accident itself. Usually these costs can be met by the relevant insurance company, but they may be settled by the individuals themselves. This is covered under the Road Traffic Act 1995 Section 158. Records of patients involved in RTAs are sometimes filed separately and may have separate numbers. It is important to note when emergency treatment has related to an RTA.

GP/HOSPITAL/CONSULTANT LINKS

Although a letter requesting referral may be sent in printed form between the GP and hospital, requests for referral may now be sent electronically direct to the hospital where GP/Hospital Links are in place. The letter to the GP following an outpatient appointment or following inpatient treatment can also be sent electronically which, in addition to similar transfer of pathology laboratory data, can speed up considerably the process of information transfer as a whole.

AUDIT

Audit should be an ongoing process. The purpose of audit may be to monitor and review current performance. It may be connected with research into new methods or new drugs or equipment. It may also be used to assess either quantitatively or qualitatively certain aspects in greater depth than had previously been carried out. Related to audit is the clinical coding, which can be used to identify cases of particular interest.

Some forms of audit may be carried out from data already collected and available electronically. This can assist analysis of the data from a point at source.

In order to carry out a particular audit, ways of collecting the data efficiently should be considered at the outset and electronic methods will often provide the best solution if a suitable method can be found. Audit trails are standardly provided electronically. For retrospective studies where such data is not easily accessible, the patient's notes may need to be accessed.

As a secretary, you may need to request particular notes from the records department for audit purposes. It may be important also to retain particular notes of patients involved in an audit study, particularly if it is part of a clinical trial. These notes should be stored in a specific area and a list of them kept up to date and visible. This can prevent the need for someone to go through all the notes in their search for one particular set. If the patient has been admitted or is seen as an outpatient for an investigation, operation or treatment, a discharge form is completed which includes dates of admission and discharge and the codes for the diagnosis and procedures such as OPCS/ICD 10 Codes given (see Chapter 8).

It may also be important to ensure that any rotating junior medical staff have been able to complete their part of the study before they may move on to another department or leave the hospital. It is important that a method of monitoring audit notes is maintained, so that data can be collected as soon as appropriate and so that the records can be released back to the medical records department as soon as possible.

RESEARCH

On occasion, research may be carried out for specific reasons into particular areas. This requires the approval of the Local Ethics Committee. For example, an orthopaedic surgeon may wish to study the effectiveness of different surgical procedures, for research purposes. Another research study could be into the incidence of postoperative infection and consideration of which form of treatment for a specific infection is most effective. Or it may be a study of the efficiency of different forms of prostheses in different categories of patients – how soon do different prostheses need to be replaced and why. In addition, and of increasing importance nowadays, many current forms of audit attempt to discover what are the quality of life benefits and the cost implications of different treatments.

LINKS TO MEDICAL RECORDS OFFICERS

A typical line of accountability can be seen in Figure 12.1.

ACCOUNTABILITY

An established line of responsibility and accountability should be decided so that each member of staff knows to whom they are accountable. In addi-

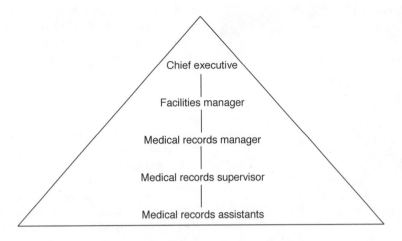

Figure 12.1 A typical line of accountability in the medical records department

tion, they should be aware of whose work they should be overseeing and monitoring.

The job description of individual members of the medical records department may vary considerably. The medical records assistants may be responsible for working in the medical records department and may stay there while outpatient clinics take place. In other situations the role may involve reception of patients during the clinic. Sometimes staff are based in the clinic most of the time and only visit the medical records department to 'pull' (locate and take) records for use during the clinic.

Each member of staff should have a job description, but it is important to remember that this needs to be updated regularly. Any changes in the role need to be agreed and made clear. When new members of staff begin work, they should be able to clarify any areas about which they are unsure of their role. Such areas may come to light particularly during the first week, but other areas may not be encountered until later on. By providing a method of checking that the nature of the work is explained fully and clearly, problems may be avoided in the future.

TRAINING

Staff in a medical records department often receive only one day's general induction training. In addition, some training may be given on PAS systems.

It is important that thorough plans should be made for both induction and ongoing training of staff so that they are fully aware of what their jobs entail and of the importance of working to a high standard. This may involve an investment of time and money and extra staff need to be available to cover for those involved in training.

Needs analysis of the training needs of staff in the department should be made and a plan of training objectives set out. Ongoing monitoring and reassessing of training needs should be carried out and an evaluation of training sessions made, so that staff are kept up to date about changes which may affect them or the work of other related departments.

When training of other staff in the hospital or Trust is being considered it is important for them to be aware of the work of the medical records department so that there is an overall appreciation of how

Reflection Point 6

What advice would you give a new member of staff? Imagine they have started in your department. What are the most important points and what areas should be emphasised in their job outlines with reference to hospital medical records?

Box 12.4 The Caldicott Principles

Some of the general principles of Caldicott are:

Principle 1 – Justify the purpose(s)
Every proposed use or transfer of patient-identifiable information within or from an organisation should be clearly defined and scrutinised, with continuing uses regularly reviewed by an appropriate guardian.

Principle 2 – Don't use patient-identifiable information unless it is absolutely necessary
Patient-identifiable information items should not be used unless there is no alternative.

Principle 3 – Use the minimum necessary patient-identifiable information
Where use of patient-identifiable information is considered to be essential, each individual item of information should be justified with the aim of reducing identifiability.

Principle 4 – Access to patient-identifiable information should be on a strict need to know basis
Only those individuals who need access to patient-identifiable information should have access to it, and they should only have access to the information items that they need to see.

Principle 5 – Everyone should be aware of their responsibilities
Action should be taken to ensure that those handling patient-identifiable information – both clinical and non-clinical staff – are aware of their responsibilities and obligations to respect patient confidentiality.

Principle 6 – Understand and comply with the law
Every use of patient-identifiable information must be lawful. Someone in each organisation should be responsible for ensuring that the organisation complies with legal requirements.

More information and a summary of the recommendations identified from the Caldicott report can be found at www.doh.gov.uk.

each other's work interrelates, particularly with regard to the resulting effect on the availability of notes. These staff may include nurses, doctors, ward clerks as well as others working outside the department.

There is a particular need to consider the training needs of staff who may be devolved to clinical directorates. This is because following devolution, they may not be included in training courses which had previously been provided centrally.

Temporary staff, if untrained, may be unused to the medical environment and may be in particular need of guidance. It may be important to ensure that they have a particular person to whom they can refer, if they are experiencing difficulties. You may be asked to help new members of staff in this way.

You may be involved in preparing job descriptions or notes on how the work is done. As well as including information on how a record should be kept of where the notes are and how they should be filed, it is important to remember to include guidance on the importance of records being accurate and on the nature of confidentiality. By doing this, you can help others become aware of how the records should be kept.

CONCLUSION

As a result of working through this chapter you will now:

- be aware of the issues concerning ownership of and the length of time that health records should be kept, and know of the means of accessing health records
- be aware of the different methods of compilation and storage of health records in the hospital environment
- have an outline of the most important forms used in hospital
- be able to update information concerning service agreements for patient care
- be able to describe the role of audit and to identify how and why it is important to record information accurately
- be able to describe how you may need to oversee the needs of other staff.

Most importantly, it is hoped that throughout the book as well as at the end of this chapter you will build an awareness of the significance of accuracy

Exercises

- Find out how your local hospital stores its medical records; which system is it using now? Are they happy with the way it works? And do they have any plans to change the system in the future?

- Monitor the access to records procedures which are currently used. Are they working well? Are records already being kept on computer? Record access both by patients and by other bodies?

- Work in a small group. Each choose 5 six-digit numbers. All write down the complete list of numbers and as a group decide how these would be filed by terminal digit filing.

- Visit your local reference library and ask to view newspaper articles which are kept on microfilm. What do you think are the advantages and disadvantages of this method? Compare this system of storage with data held on optical discs.

- Ask a laboratory technician if all samples are clearly, legibly and appropriately labelled! What suggestions can you make to help ensure a high level of accuracy?

- Imagine how the following patients may wish their medical notes to be held – a patient who is famous, a prisoner, a person separated from a violent partner, a patient with a history of psychiatric illness. Which data do you think they would consider sensitive? Think of other conditions when information may be particularly sensitive.

- Consider your own medical records – for which purposes would you be happy for them to be used. Would you want the data to be identifiable or would you prefer it to be anonymised.

- Find out more about the Caldicott Principles. To what extent are they being implemented locally? Why may they be difficult to implement? Choose one of the principles and consider how it could be implemented more fully. Make suggestions as to how this could be done.

in your work and the importance of confidentiality. In addition, it is important to remember that you are dealing with people who may not be able to communicate their needs and feelings clearly and who deserve respect and understanding as well as efficiency in the way in which you work with them, so that patient care throughout the health care service is at an optimum.

Finally, it should be noted that a number of changes are currently taking place within the NHS and the new GP and hospital contracts are due for implementation shortly. There are plans to use collated data on every patient through elements of the ICRS into NHS SPINE to provide access to multiple local systems with interoperability. The nature and use of medical records is likely to change considerably in the future and is likely to develop far more fully into electronic forms. Whether a totally integrated ICRS will develop is yet to be seen.

ACKNOWLEDGEMENTS

Bristol Royal Infirmary Trust, Royal United Hospital Trust, Bath

Useful websites

Agency for Healthcare Research and Quality
 www.ahrq.gov.uk
Caldicott report www.doh.gov.uk
1998 Data Protection Act simplified prepared by Medical Protection Society www.mps.org.uk
Electronic Record Development and Implementation Programme – Evaluations
 www.nhsia.nhs.uk/erdip/pages/evaluation

Health Connect www.health.gov.au/healthonline/connect.htm
Health Data Management
 www.healthdatamanagement.com
Health Information Quality www.hiquality.org.uk
Institute for Clinical Systems Improvement www.icsi.org
Medical Records Institute www.medrecinst.com
National Patient Safety Agency www.npsa.org.uk

Further reading

Audit Commission 1995 Setting the records straight. A study of hospital medical records. HMSO, London

DoH 1995 National Health Service Charges to overseas visitors. Patient's guide. Annex 6, Appendix 2, January. DOH, London

DoH 1994 Being heard. The report of a review committee on NHS complaints procedures. DO16/BH/2M HSSH JO6 3055, June. DOH, London

General Medical Council 1995 Duties of a doctor. GMC, London

Hauffman EK Health information management, 10th edn. American Health Information Management Association, Physician Record, Illinois

Markwell D 1995 Computerised patient records in general practice – guidelines for good practice. Produced for NHS Executive Performance Management Directorate Clinical Information Consultancy 24.03.95

Primary Health Care Specialist Group of the British Computer Society 1996 Proceedings of Annual Conference, Downing College, Cambridge

References

DoH 2002 Delivering 21st century IT support for the NHS. The Stationary Office, London www.doh.gov/ipu/what-new/procstratsummary.pdf

Gregory W 1996 The informability manual. HMSO, London

Chapter 13

Outpatient department

Sara Ladyman

OBJECTIVES

- To describe the systems and procedures that take place in an outpatient department, including the secretary's input, with examples of new patient referral and follow up patient systems, the use of the computerised patient administration system (hereafter referred to as PAS) and the preparation and administration of outpatient clinics

- To outline other aspects which require special consideration, including procedures for fast track urgent referrals, patients who fail to attend appointments, overseas visitors, hospital transport requirements, domiciliary and ward visits

- To highlight throughout the chapter the interdependence of procedures, staff responsibilities and the possible repercussions when there is a breakdown in these communications

- To consider throughout the chapter non-routine situations that may require secretarial input.

INTRODUCTION

This chapter is concerned with the administration of outpatient clinics in a hospital. You may find it helpful to refer to copies of the national and local hospital Patient Charters.

OUTPATIENT CLINICS

The majority of consultants will share a purpose-designed outpatient clinic area within the hospital staffed by outpatient nurses and reception staff with outpatient clinics held weekly at set times. Some consultants may have access to their own designated outpatient clinic area where specialist and delicate equipment can be permanently housed, for example the ophthalmology department.

The majority of patient referrals are from General Practitioners (hereafter referred to as GPs). However referrals may include:

- patient self-referral (for example to a genitourinary medicine clinic)
- consultant referral, following an emergency admission via an Accident and Emergency Department
- consultant referral, following a domiciliary visit
- accident and emergency referral
- GP referral – fast track patients, for example with suspect or proven cancers

Not all clinics have pre-booked appointment systems; genitourinary services may have walk-in clinics. Some departments may keep their own confidential patient records, separate to hospital case notes, which usually remain in the department. This is often the case in the genitourinary medicine and psychiatry departments.

Some clinics are for patients requiring minor surgery or invasive investigations as an outpatient procedure, possibly in ophthalmology, dermatology and gastroenterology departments. Be aware that there may be a manual appointment system running parallel to the computerised PAS system for some of these clinics and you should familiarise yourself with these.

NEW PATIENT REFERRAL SYSTEMS AND PROCEDURES

The majority of new patient referrals are received from general practitioners (GPs), seeking specialist consultation, advice or a specific procedure to be arranged for their patients.

You will need to familiarise yourself with the computerised PAS at the earliest opportunity as it is integral to your day-to-day activity and you will receive formal training in the workplace before you can access this system (See Box 13.1.).

Different staff groups will have password access to different parts of the PAS system, according to their role. The operation of a hospital's PAS system will not be described here, as they differ considerably, as does a medical secretary's level of access and ability to make changes to the system. However, generally you will be able to change demographic data for patients on PAS, but you may or may not be able to make or alter appointments yourself and will have to liaise with the appointments staff.

A new patient referral indicates that a patient is being referred for a particular ailment to a consultant. This will initiate a patient care episode. The new patient care episode is separate to the patient having any other episodes of care running concurrently under one or more other consultants in the hospital. They may also have been re-referred to the same consultant again, with the same or a different illness. This will need to be clarified should there have been a duplication of referral made in error and a current episode of care already exists for the patient. In this instance a check of correspondence in the patient's case notes is often required.

Reflection Point 1

If a patient has been seen at the hospital previously what are the variables which may have changed and require verification and subsequent changes to the Patient Master Index and any case notes in existence?

Figure 13.1 outlines an example of a procedure for processing both new and old outpatient referrals.

The GP referral letter is sent to the hospital and may go directly to the consultant or to a centralised appointments department. See the sample referral letter in Figure 13.2.

Reflection Point 2

Why is this so important?

Box 13.1 A computerised patient administration system (PAS)

A PAS will usually include:

Patient Master Index (PMI) Personal and demographic data on all patients who have attended hospital

Modules linked to PMI Provide management and record keeping functions

Modules include: Outpatient Module
Waiting List Module
Accident and Emergency Module

In addition, the system may also be linked to pathology and x-ray imaging departments, thereby providing access to patient results by medical and nursing staff.

More specifically, the Outpatient Module of PAS provides for the effective management of outpatient clinics. Outpatient Module functions may include:

- maintaining a 'diary' of past and forthcoming clinics, identifying patients booked on to specific clinics and their attendance times
- production of a variety of letters, reports and statistical analyses
- clinic rules specifying the frequency of the clinic, duration, number and type of appointments and instructions when doctors are on leave and a clinic has to cancelled or reduced in size
- screen transactions to enable you to answer queries and to make, cancel or change appointments
- lists of patients booked on to specific clinics that can be printed to:
  - assist patient services departments in collecting the patient case notes required for a clinic
  - assist medical, nursing and reception staff with clinic management
  - gather statistics for Department of Health requirements to collect patient charter standard data such as patient waiting times in clinic.

You may use PAS, Outpatient or Inpatient Modules to:
- answer general queries
- register patients
- generate patient identity labels, front sheets, case note labels
- generate new, follow-up or cancellation and rebooking appointment letters
- amend patient details
- make transactions on patient records, e.g. add attendances, make appointments
- cancel clinics and reschedule appointments
- print statistics and reports
- produce outpatient clinic prints
- add waiting list episodes
- print waiting lists.

It is incumbent upon whoever receives the letter first, the appointments desk staff or the medical secretary, to date stamp the letter upon receipt and arrange for the patient's identifying details and receipt of letter details to be entered onto the PAS Referral Module at the earliest opportunity. This information provides the means to:

- start an audit trail for the accurate tracking of the patient through the new patient referral

system, to provide evidence that the hospital is meeting its contractual specifications and obligations, for example meeting government targets for minimum waiting times for first new patient appointments
- facilitate gathering of statistics for national and local patient charter and quality standards and targets on waiting times for first outpatient appointment times

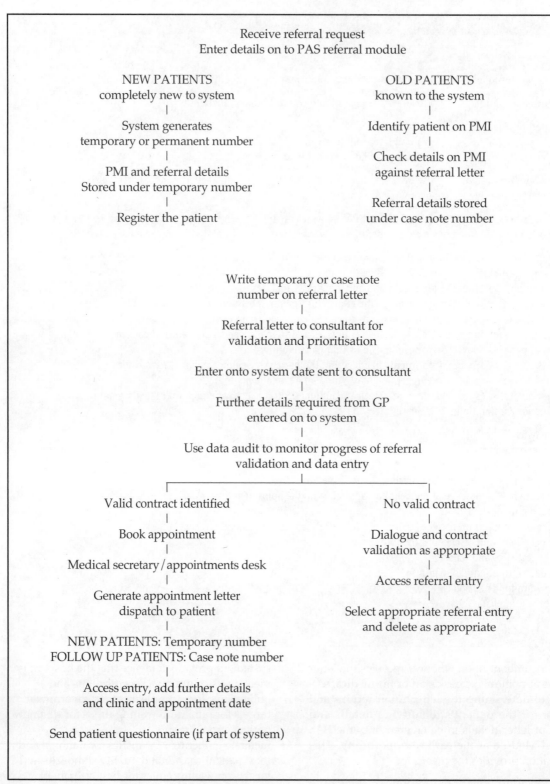

Figure 13.1 Procedure for processing outpatient referrals

Water Mead Practice
1 Meadow Walk
Buckingham
MK18 2HP
Tel 01280 854329
Fax 01280 833441

Dr. R. Mott   Contract I.D.

--

Dr. M. Sread   Practice Code

--

Dr. L. Khan

-- February –

Mr. A. McAllister
Consultant Urologist
General Hospital NHS Trust
Forest Lane
Milton Keynes
MK13 2DF

Dear Mr. McAllister

Mrs. Anne BAYLISS dob 14.04.   **NHS No:**
    Hospital No:
6a Water Mead Gardens, Buckingham MK14 6HP
Tel 356212

Thank you for seeing this lady in your Out-patient Clinic. She has no past history of note apart from bronchitis in childhood. She attended recently with a two-week history of severe pain in the left loin. At that time she had cystitis and I prescribed antibiotics for a urine infection. She returned to the surgery today still complaining of pain in the left loin and she says she still has pain on passing water. I would be grateful if you could see her as soon as possible as I feel she requires further investigation.

Yours sincerely,

Dr. R. Mott

Figure 13.2 Sample referral letter

- ensure timely verification and appropriate changes to be made to patient details at the earliest opportunity, for example GP, patient name and/or address changes
- enable patient's NHS number when known, date of birth, sex, address, and most importantly post code (including a code for patients of no fixed abode), marital status and registered/referring GP/practice and consultant, details which are key to contract validation, to be analysed. By entering the NHS number and date of birth into the Patient Master Index (PMI) on the PAS Referral Module, and then making a further check using their name, it is possible to discover whether the patient is new to the hospital. If among the selection of patients shown it is apparent they have already been allocated a hospital number, there should be a corresponding set of patient case notes or microfiched records in existence.
- A careful check for changes which may have occurred since a previous visit to the hospital include:
- name change
- address change – including postcode
- contact telephone numbers
- General Practice change
- identification of duplicate registrations and case notes for a patient where similar details have resulted in separate registrations, and require an amalgamation of records.

The patient's post code identifies whether the patient can automatically be given a hospital appointment or, where no contract exists, they will need to be treated as an out of area referral (OATS). There will be a procedure to ensure OATS referrals are identified and confirmation that treatment will be funded is made before the patient is offered appointment.

At this point it is important to clarify whether your department has its own procedures for fast track referrals when the GP has identified an urgent appointment is required because a diagnosis of cancer is strongly indicated. National targets require these patients to be seen by a consultant within 14 days of referral. Fast track referral systems may include a specifically designed GP referral proforma containing the patient's identifying details and relevant history, scan and Ca125 blood results. This will be faxed through from the surgery and shoud be brought to the attention of the consultant at the earliest opportunity.

A temporary hospital number (pre-registration number) may be allocated to a patient who has never been seen at the hospital. This will change to a permanent hospital number once the patient has attended their first appointment. The pre-registration or existing hospital number must be written on the referral letter.

The referral letters are given to the consultant or nominated doctor who will validate the referral by deciding whether or not it is appropriate for them to see the patient and allocate patients to the appropriate clinics they hold, which may include outreach clinics held off-site. They will also prioritise the referral letter by indicating a specific time scale to be seen or indicate whether they are to be given an 'urgent', 'soon' or 'routine' appointment. For the latter it is important to be familiar with the consultant's criteria as to how many weeks constitute a maximum wait. It is also important to alert the consultant when a longer wait may be required so appropriate action can be taken. Each clinic will have a reference code on the PAS and appointments are made in the outpatient module.

Reflection Point 3

Although the word 'routine' is used, there is nothing routine about an appointment, for example, to attend a breast clinic. We should therefore be continually aware that each appointment will highlight for patients their own particular concerns about a disease, and possibly their own life process.

In addition to new patients having their appointment dates prioritised clinically, it is important to remember that new patient clinic appointment slots are generally allocated a longer time with the doctor than a patient returning for further consultations.

Reflection Point 4

Why is it important to ensure the new patient is given a new patient appointment slot and not a follow-up patient slot in error?

General Hospital NHS Trust
Forest Lane
Milton Keynes MK13 2DF
Appointments: 01908 465887/547986

6a Water Mead Gardens
Buckingham
MK14 6HP

DATE   – February --
HOSPITAL NUMBER   NP (Pre-registration No. ZA334466)

Dear Mrs. Bayliss

An appointment has been made for you to attend MR. McALLISTER'S NEW PATIENT CLINIC, C6, on – FEBRUARY —.

Please report to Registration Desk TWO on the FOURTH FLOOR OUTPATIENT CLINIC at 2.00 P.M. If you have been handed a referral letter by your doctor please bring it with you. We hope that this date and time is convenient for you. If you cannot come please let us know as soon as you can.

If you have not been to this Hospital before, or if the details printed are wrong, please fill in the Patient Questionnaire and send it to us now. If you have any query regarding this appointment, please have your hospital number (if you have one) or this letter available for reference.

Yours sincerely,

June Davies
Appointments Manager

(Enc. Schematic Map of Hospital with public transport services indicated)

Figure 13.3 Example of proforma appointment letter and patient questionnaire

PATIENT QUESTIONNAIRE

Hospital Number   NP (Pre-registration No. ZA334466)
Surname   Title
First Names
Date of Birth   Sex

Civil State   Single   Divorced
                         Married   Separated
                         Widowed   Other

Current Address
Postcode
Telephone (home)
Telephone (work)

Name of GP (own doctor)
Address

NHS Number   Have you lived in United
                                              Kingdom for past 12 months
                                              YES / NO

Surname at Birth
Other surnames

Town and Country of Birth
Religion
Ethnic origin (This is needed because people of different ethnic origins may have specific health
needs. Please tick the box which best describes your history, values and culture.)
Occupation
Industry or Name of School

Occupation of Spouse
Industry

Name of Next of Kin
Relationship
Address
Telephone

CLINIC   APPOINTMENT   DATE

Figure 13.3 Continued

The important reasons for having special 'new patient' appointments are:

- to allow sufficient time for history gathering, patient examination, tests to be carried out and for further tests to be organised
- to allow the consultant, nominated deputy and other members of the medical team to see an appropriate mix of new and follow up patients.

When sending appointments it is also important to consider whether the patient will require ambulance transportation because there are restrictions on early appointment times. Also, to deal sensitively with appointments for patients who are known to have certain infections, for example methicillin resistant staphylococcus aureus (MRSA). In this instance, the outpatient nurses will need to be alerted as a special consulting room may have to be identified, and arrangements made for it to be cleaned before other patients use it thereafter, hence an appointment at the end of clinic may be more appropriate.

Once the referral letter has been validated by the consultant the appointment can be booked and a computer-generated letter dispatched to the patient. Part of this letter may constitute a patient questionnaire to gather further patient data to be entered on PAS. This data, known as the minimum data set, is a Department of Health requirement, but data may also be collected for statistical purposes to ensure the hospital is responding to the needs of its local population. Analyse the information provided and information requested in the example proforma letter and patient questionnaire shown in Figure 13.3.

The appropriate clinic code, date and time of appointment should be recorded on the referral letter and it may be your responsibility or that of the appointments staff to keep the referral letters readily accessible in a bring-forward system ready for clinic preparation. Note that the practice in some hospitals is to make up a set of new patient case notes, file the referral letter inside and then file the case notes within the medical records department library until clinic preparation.

The procedures and systems associated with the running of a busy outpatient clinic quickly become routine. However, it is important to remember that all enquiries regarding appointments should be vetted before any information is given about clinic attendance. Even the disclosure that a patient is on the PAS system is confidential and every care should be taken to validate callers and the reasons why information has been requested.

CLINIC PREPARATION FOR NEW PATIENTS

Medical secretaries, appointments desk, medical records or clinic reception staff may be involved in preparing case notes for new patient clinics. The principles remain the same and Figure 13.4 outlines the procedure that takes place.

A list of patients to attend the new patient clinic can be printed from the PAS Outpatient Module and this will be printed several days prior to the new patient clinic being held (Figure 13.5).

Outpatient clinics can be organised differently, with a mixture of new patient appointment slots and slots for patients who have already been seen by the consultant who are returning for follow-up appointments. A consultant physician may have different clinics for specific medical conditions, for example a general medical outpatient clinic and a separate diabetic outpatient clinic. It is important for you to familiarise yourself with the types of appointment and clinics available for patients seen in the department.

Reflection Point 5

What are the ramifications of the referral letter being unavailable for the clinic attendance and how can this be swiftly rectified?

It is essential the referral letter is available for the clinic attendance, otherwise the consultant may not agree to see the patient until the referral letter providing clinical information about the patient is available. Whilst it is usually possible to obtain a fax copy of the referral from the surgery or to take dictation over the telephone this will cause delays in the smooth running of the outpatient clinic, cause unnecessary distress for the patient kept waiting and adversely affect Patient Charter outpatient waiting time statistics (Figure 13.4, Figure 13.5).

Print clinic lists of patients
|
Pull GP referral letters and patient questionnaires
|
Access PMI details using pre-registration or case note numbers
|
Link pre-registered case note number to a new hospital case note number
to be activated at clinic attendance
|
Make up patient case notes if not already done
|
Pull existing case notes for patients and file referral letter inside
|
Pull any test results arranged prior to appointment

Figure 13.4 Procedure for processing new patient outpatient clinics

NEW PATIENT PULLING LIST

CLINIC Mr. A. McAllister   SPECIALTY Urology   Clinic Code C6
DATE: DATE LIST PULLED: CLINIC DATE:

TIME	NO.	NAME/ ADDRESS	DOB / HOSPITAL NO.	GP LETTER	PREVIOUS X-RAYS	ROUTINE/SOON/ URGENT
2.00	ZA334466	BAYLISS Anne 6a Water Mead Gardens Buckingham	14.04.-	L	N	R
2.15		HUGHES Keith 39 Brown Rd Buckingham	12.10.-GH386432	L	N	R
2.30	ZA498723	PIPER June 12 Westcroft Lne Gawcott	06.09.-	L	N	R
2.45		PATEL Myra 6 Bierton Road, Bishopstoke	31.03.-GH279432	L	Y	S
3.00	ZA857322	JONES Peter	27.01.-	Bringing letter	N	S
3.15		LAMBERT Clare	GH328954	CANCELLED APPT.		
3.30	URGENT SLOT					
3.45	URGENT SLOT					

Figure 13.5 New patient pulling list

(a) Immediately prior to and during an outpatient clinic

Copies of referral letters obtained as applicable
|
Copies of clinic list printed from PAS and distributed to consultation rooms.
Cancellations and late bookings may need to be added manually
|
Patient reports to reception desk
|
Receptionist confirms patient arrival on PAS. Checks PMI data with patient
|
Referral details transferred to case note number system and new patient number confirmed
|
Endorse details on printed clinic list

(b) At the end of and following the outpatient clinic

Identify patient
|
Enter attendance details on to PAS outpatient attendance module from the attendance form (completed by doctor)
|
PATIENT ATTENDED
|
Temporary number deleted.
Allocated a hospital number (if not already allocated one)
|
Add outcome details to outpatient module
i.e.
follow-up appointment
booked/or not booked
or patient discharged back to GP's care
(decided by clinician)

PATIENT DID NOT ATTEND (DNA)
|
Referral details remain on temporary number
|
New appointment booked/or not booked
(decided by clinician dependent on locally agreed procedure)

Figure 13.6 Outpatient clinic procedures

PROCEDURE FOR NEW PATIENT CLINICS

In the new patient clinic the patient will be clinically examined and this may result in:

- the patient being discharged back to the GP with appropriate advice, thus bringing the episode of care to a close
- diagnostic tests being performed or ordered with a follow-up appointment pending outcome of results
- an emergency admission to hospital, being placed on a waiting list or being allocated a date for an operation using a partial or fully booked system (see Chapter 14 Admissions and Discharges)
- an internal hospital referral for an appointment with another specialist
- a follow-up appointment to return to the clinic for review.

The nurses or receptionist will record waiting time data on an attendance form and the doctors will indicate any follow-up arrangements. This is handed to the receptionist or appointment desk staff to update PAS and to allocate the patient their follow-up appointment as required. The medical secretary however may be required subsequently to make or change a follow-up themselves or with the assistance of the appointments staff using a cancellation and rebooking letter, taking into account any hospital ambulance transport and other arrangements. Outpatient nurses sometimes assume the administrative role during an outpatient clinic where a receptionist or medical secretary is not present. You are not usually expected to be present in the clinic area but should be readily available whilst the clinic is in session to assist with queries which may arise. See Figure 13.6 for procedures relating to the outpatient clinic.

During an outpatient clinic patients may have various tests carried out. Blood samples may be taken by nursing staff, and the appropriate information completed on the request forms, before despatch to the laboratory, or the patient may be sent to a department during clinic for investigations, for example the X-ray department. Box 13.2 indicates the different departments the patient may be required to attend prior to, during or after an outpatient clinic attendance.

The consultant and members of the medical team are responsible for ensuring the GP is kept informed of their findings and this is usually in the form of a letter which may include a preliminary diagnosis,

Reflection Point 6

What are the problems if the request form accompanying a specimen is missing, or a request form taken by the patient to x-ray is incorrect or incomplete? How can this be avoided?

prognosis, drugs or other treatment prescribed for the patient.

Doctors usually dictate this correspondence using handheld dictaphones during clinic. It will probably be your responsibility to ensure there are sufficient dictaphones, audio cassettes and replacement batteries available for the clinic. If you have access to an additional handset this can be labelled and only used for urgent letters so these can be easily identified and transcribed promptly after clinic.

Dictated mini audio cassettes in particular can be easily misplaced. Encourage medical staff to seal the dictated audio cassette in an envelope, with their name and the date of the clinic recorded on the outside and secure it to the dictated clinic notes.

The beginning or end of outpatient clinics is also a time when medical staff may be available to prioritise referral letters, respond to queries, sign correspondence and check incoming results. The medical secretary may find this helpful for day-to-day administration, though it is important to have all relevant information prepared beforehand, including case notes relevant to incoming correspondence.

PROCEDURE AT THE END OF AN OUTPATIENT CLINIC

You should familiarise yourself with the system used at the end of the clinic, ensuring the patient case notes, dictated audio cassettes and dictaphones, etc., are returned to your office.

GPs require current written confirmation of all outpatient attendance to keep abreast of their patients' care and any changes in medication prescribed. Whilst the referral system is rooted in medical ethics and etiquette, the production of prompt written feedback to the GP also forms part of contract specification and is a requirement of the Patient Charter.

Box 13.2 Departments a patient may be required to attend as a result of an outpatient appointment

Imaging department
All clinical specialties have access to imaging services, with the majority of outpatients being examined on demand. Where appointments are required for special examinations, the waiting time may be as little as a week. Equipment may include:
- magnetic resonance imaging machines
- CT (computed tomography) scanners
- Ultrasound equipment.

Haematology department
In addition to clinical advice and interpretation of results, the range of investigations available may include: full blood count, ESR (erythrocyte sedimentation rate), blood film and differential, monospot, sickle cell screening test, serum B12, red folate, platelet function studies, blood grouping and antibody screens. Routine specimens are processed during weekday office hours and Saturday. The department will be computerised and reports may be available on PAS VDUs within minutes of completion and accessible by doctors, nurses and secretaries.

Chemical pathology
The department will offer a comprehensive range of services. The range of tests will include urea and electrolytes (U&Es) and liver function tests (LFTs).

Histopathology
A full range of histopathological and cytological services will be available, including:
- routine histological processing and diagnosis from frozen sections – immunocytochemistry
- electron microscopy
- routine cervical smear diagnosis
- non-gynaecological cytology and fine needle aspirates.

Microbiology
A range of diagnostic services will be available, including:
- bacteriology, virology, parasitology, mycology
- public health and environmental microbiology.
It will also be closely involved with all aspects of infection control and will work closely with the infection control nursing officers.
Routine specimens are processed during weekday office hours and reports can be accessed on PAS VDUs.

Nuclear medicine
Investigations carried out routinely may include:
- the study of organ function
- evaluation of ischaemic heart disease
- the detection of cancer and its spread
- differential diagnosis and assessment of dementia
- the monitoring of renal function, transplant
- diagnosis of acute bleeding
- screening of infection and inflammation
- acute embolic lung disease.
The majority of services are available on an outpatient basis, most requiring only a single visit to the department. Radionuclide therapy is carried out for benign and malignant thyroid diseases.

Physiotherapy
See Chapter 11 on personnel.

When the clinic finishes, responsibility for the case notes and accompanying dictated audio cassettes transfers from the clinic staff to the medical secretary.

The case notes will have been tracked to the clinic. It is in the medical secretary's interests to have a system for recording case notes subsequently found in the office. This usually takes the form of a computerised tracking system on PAS and the use of barcoded case notes. A tracking system, however, is only as good as the users. Ensure that all medical staff and staff using the office are familiar with the system you use. Whilst it may appear laborious, tracking case notes can pay dividends when they have been tracked into a specific area or onwards to another department, rather than searching through case notes in your own and adjoining doctors' offices.

The pattern of your working week will be governed by the number, days and type of outpatient clinics which run. It is therefore essential to familiarise yourself with your consultant's timetable at the earliest opportunity so that you can prioritise your main weekly activities in order to accommodate the other duties expected of you.

Reflection Point 7

You have been away for 3 days. What are the implications if the outpatient clinic typing falls behind?

OUTPATIENT CLINIC LETTERS

Letters dictated for patients attending their first clinic visit will usually be longer than those for patients re-attending as follow-up patients because the consultant will include the history of the patient's condition. Therefore whilst the number of letters to be transcribed for a new patient clinic may be fewer, they may take as long, if not longer, than typing letters from a follow-up patient clinic where many more patients have been seen.

It is usual to transcribe outpatient correspondence in chronological order, using the clinic date as a guide, and generally the consultant's tape is typed first. You will be required to follow the hospital and departmental house style for correspondence. Your font size should never be under 11 because of illegibility when case notes are micro-

Box 13.3 Details required in an outpatient clinic letter

- A reference, including the doctor's and typist's initials and the patient's case note number
- Clinic date and the date transcribed by secretary
- The name and address of the referrer, and their reference (hospital number) if available
- The name, date of birth, address of the patient
- Patient telephone number and GP details if referring patient elsewhere for investigation or treatment
- The name and designation of the doctor dictating the letter
- Details when letters are to be copied to other parties for information

fiched. Each letter should contain the information shown in Box 13.3.

A check should be made against the most recent correspondence on file and the labels on the case notes to ensure the information, including patient details, extracted from the case notes is the most current for each letter typed. If in doubt a check on PAS can be made, as this should be the most current record. Redundant and inaccurate patient labels must be destroyed.

The doctor will have made handwritten notes about the patient in the case notes and these, together with test result forms, previous correspondence and clinic entries, provide an invaluable aid to accurate transcription from audio cassette. You should make a habit of spell-checking and proof-reading all correspondence as part of the process of preparation of correspondence for signature. Doctors may only visit the department at a certain time during the week so an important opportunity is lost to dispatch letters promptly to the GP if alterations have to be made and the letter has to await the doctor's signature once more.

Reflection Point 8

You should track the case notes back to the medical records department as soon as they are no longer required.

Why is this a good policy to adopt?

A copy of the dictated letter must always be filed in the case notes and this must be amended or replaced if any changes have been made to the GP's copy as this must be an accurate record. Each department will have its own policy regarding additional copies of correspondence to be stored on disk or on file.

It is good policy to track case notes back to the medical records department at the earliest opportunity because:

- the medical records department is the first port of call for anyone trying to access case notes
- there is a direct correlation between the number of case notes held in the office and the number of queries and interruptions from staff searching for them, thereby increasing the workload
- there is generally limited office space to store case notes
- when case notes are needed outside working hours, for example in the accident and emergency department, searches in outlying offices may be impractical

Reflection Point 9

What are the legitimate reasons for case notes staying in the office?

Legitimate reasons for case notes being in your office include:

- awaiting transcription of outstanding correspondence
- a doctor's specific request, for example audit and research patients
- awaiting test results and for the doctor to respond to these
- a query to be resolved
- arranging an admission for surgery
- patients for whom a return visit is imminent.

As a rule, once letters have been typed, case notes should be tracked back to the medical records department and despatched according to departmental procedure.

FOLLOW-UP OUTPATIENT CLINIC APPOINTMENTS

The medical records staff or the clinic receptionist will generally prepare the follow-up outpatient clinics, although this may be the responsibility of a medical secretary. You must ensure that any filing of correspondence or results held in your office are in the case notes ready for the patient's visit.

The medical secretary's relationship with the receptionist or medical records staff preparing case notes for outpatient clinics is of paramount importance. It requires cooperation and understanding to accommodate the different needs of the individuals involved. For example, the secretary may need a patient's case notes to resolve a query or to type a letter, at the same times as they are also needed for another clinic.

Reflection Point 10

A clinic receptionist telephones you to ask for a set of case notes required for a clinic in 2 days. You need them to type a clinic letter. How will you resolve this situation?

THE FOLLOW-UP OUTPATIENT CLINIC

Figure 13.7 outlines the procedures for a follow-up clinic. The patient will attend a follow-up outpatient clinic:

- to receive test results following their initial visit to the new patient clinic
- to have further investigative procedures, or be given a date or put on a waiting list for surgery
- for reassessment of the initial problem
- to receive a diagnosis post-surgery
- to have surgical wounds examined, dressed or sutures removed
- for regular check-up
- to have a final check-up before discharge back to the GP's care, thereby ending this episode of care
- *ad hoc* at the request of the GP or patient, because of concerns, and these will usually have been vetted by the consultant or doctor on the team beforehand

Occasionally patients may arrive without an appointment. You should familiarise yourself with the consultant's policy regarding this and the procedure for obtaining case notes, test results, etc., should the consultant agree to see the patient. It may be that each case has to be taken on its own

A clinic list for the follow-up clinic will be generated from PAS
including most recent tracking of case notes
(similar to the new patient list, Figure 13.4)

|

An initial search for case notes will be made
in the medical records department

|

PAS case note to locate case notes not in medical records
or manual tracer cards may be in use and form a vital clue
as to case note location as will the PAS tracking system

|

Medical secretaries will be contacted for case notes
tracked out to them
Case notes to be released as soon as possible

|

Case notes are prepared for the doctor, i.e. all outstanding test
results, X-rays, etc. are entered into case notes so the doctor has all
information to hand for return clinic visit

Figure 13.7 Procedure for a follow-up clinic

merit; for example, a patient may arrive as a result of an administrative error on the part of the hospital and have travelled some distance.

As with the new clinic appointment, there may be a clinic receptionist in attendance or the appointments desk staff will be responsible for updating the PAS Outpatient Module as explained previously. You may wish to refer to the ENT attendance form, in Figure 13.8, to identify the possible outcomes for the patient who has attended the follow-up clinic.

Reflection Point 11

• What are the implications of an outpatient clinic overrunning?

• Who will be affected and how?

• Make reference to your copy of the Patient's Charter guidelines. What does this say about outpatient waiting times?

A clinic may overrun for a number of reasons: staff arriving late, absent doctors for whom the necessary clinic reductions have not been made, overriding the maximum number of appointment slots for that clinic, time spent locating missing case notes or results before patients can be seen.

The implications of an outpatient clinic over-running include:
• Ambulance transport arrangements disrupted
• Overcrowding of clinic areas
• Escalation of stress levels for patients and staff
• Subsequent clinics delayed or disrupted
• Patients and staff leaving late, perhaps in darkness during winter months
• Patient and staff commitments are affected, e.g. those caring for others

Keeping patients and staff informed of delays empowers the patient and doctors who can then, within limits, make decisions, for example a patient choosing to cancel and reschedule their appointment, based on the information to hand.

Reflection Point 12

What steps can you take to assist the clinic run to schedule, in particular with regard to doctors' planned leave arrangements, the appointment system, availability of case notes, etc.?

ENT ATTENDANCE FORM

Time Patient arrived in Clinic
Time seen by Nursing Staff
Time seen by Doctor
Time of leaving Clinic

Diagnosis   1   Code:
              2   Code:

Procedures

	TICK		TICK
None		Microtymp	
Antral washout/suction clearance		Biopsies of ulcers	
Reduction of fracture		Removal of salivary calculus	
Cautery of nasal septum		Audioscope	
Aural polypectomy		Nasal polypectomy	
Myringotomy/grommets insert		Drainage of abscess	
Endoscopy of nose or larynx		Other	

Outcome   TICK   Further appointments

DNA   1   C D/W/M/next routine
Cancelled by patient   2   C D/W/M/next routine
Discharge   3   C D/W/M/next routine
Cross Referral
Operation Full or Partial Booking System
W/L Minor Operation   X-rays required   Yes/No
W/L Day Case   Pathology Reports   Yes/No
W/L Inpatient   Audiology   Yes/No
Other

PATIENT TRANSPORT REQUIRED   YES/NO   Authorised

Medical Signatory

Figure 13.8 An example of an attendance form which the receptionist or medical records staff will then transfer to the PAS

The consultant and his/her medical team will once again dictate a clinic letter to be sent to the GP to update them on the patient's care. It is the medical secretary's responsibility to prioritise and type the follow-up clinic letter dictation, preparing letters for signature and despatch. Once the case notes have been finished with, they should once again be tracked back to the medical records department until they are required again.

Patients, for the most part, are unaware of the complexity of outpatient clinic procedures and systems and you should use your discretion to explain to patients the reason for delays or breakdowns in the system whilst offering them a positive solution to the problem within departmental guidelines.

ADDITIONAL INFORMATION REGARDING OUTPATIENT CLINICS

You should familiarise yourself with the departmental policy and procedure regarding the following points.

URGENT REFERRALS

Urgent or fast track referrals may be made by letter, proforma, faxed or initially by telephone (followed up in writing) from GPs or other sources of referral, for example the accident and emergency department. If an urgent appointment is given for an imminent clinic you should ensure that:

- Permission is sought from the consultant, or nominated deputy as required
- Sufficient time for ambulance transport arrangements to be made if required
- The referral letter and necessary records will be available for the clinic – the referral letter may either be given to the patient to bring in a sealed envelope, faxed by the surgery or sent through the mail if time allows.
- The appointment is made on the PAS and letter giving details despatched and the patient contacted by telephone if necessary
- A request is made for a case note number and folder to be generated or for existing case notes to be located and prepared for the clinic
- PAS and the clinic attendance lists are updated with patient details and clinic reception, nursing and medical staff are made aware the patient is attending

Patients who fail to attend their outpatient clinic appointments

The GP will need to be informed in writing of all patients who fail to attend a clinic appointment without giving a reason. These patients are referred to as 'did not attend' (DNAs). The consultant will write a letter to the GP informing them whether a further appointment has been sent to the patient or whether they have been discharged back to the GP's care. See Chapter 6 on Communication for an example letter. It is not usual to inform the GP when a patient has cancelled and re-booked their appointment.

TERTIARY REFERRALS

The referral must be from one named consultant in an NHS provider unit to another named consultant in an NHS provider unit; within the same hospital or to another hospital

OUTPATIENT OVERSEAS VISITORS

The patient questionnaire (Figure 13.3), should identify patients who have not lived in the United Kingdom for the previous 12 months. When this matter comes to the medical secretary's attention they should inform the appropriate manager, probably within the patient services department. A decision has to be made as to whether they are 'liable to pay' for treatment given or whether there are reciprocal agreements with their country of origin. The patient will need to attend an interview with a nominated member of staff who has had the appropriate training.

TRANSPORT

As a rule, transport for new patients has to be booked via the GP surgery as only they can say whether this is needed on medical grounds. Once the patient has attended a first clinic appointment the clinic doctor can authorise subsequent hospital transport for follow-up clinic attendance and the appropriate form (Figure 13.9) will need to be completed each time the patient attends, usually in the clinic. You must familiarise yourself with the procedures for booking hospital transport in order to minimise the risk of missed appointments, or unnecessary delays. It is important to clarify with

TRANSPORT REQUEST

HOSPITAL NUMBER:

TRANSPORT REQUIRED

Patient walking unaided

Carrying chair, can sit in ambulance

Full stretcher case

Is escort medically necessary?

SURNAME:

FIRST NAMES:

DATE OF BIRTH:

CONSULTANT: WARD:

DATE OF JOURNEY

TIME OF APPOINTMENT

APPROX LENGTH OF STAY

NATURE OF ILLNESS

TO BE TAKEN FROM:

TO BE TAKEN TO:

This is to certify that because of his/her medical or physical condition this patient is unable to travel by any forms of public conveyance.

WILL PATIENT WEAR

OUTDOOR CLOTHES?

SIGNATURE OF MEDICAL OFFICER

DATE:

Figure 13.9 A transport request form

patients their level of mobility, for example whether they can travel by car or ambulance, and whether they have a wheelchair.

There may be a manual ambulance booking system running parallel to entries made on PAS. The transport office may need to be notified in writing with booking requests and when patients cancel or change appointments. It is important to ensure transport has been cancelled for any forthcoming appointments when notified of a patient's death, to avoid causing unnecessary distress to relatives.

PATIENTS IN PRISON

Care has to be taken when arranging these appointments and there will be guidelines. Arrangements will include informing the prison medical centre directly of an outpatient appointment and not the patient or their family. Clarification of the prisoner category may be sought and how many prison officers will be in attendance so an appropriate appointment time can be arranged. Inform outpatient nursing staff, and hospital security if necessary, when a prisoner is coming to the hospital.

DOMICILIARY VISIT

A GP may write or telephone to ask if the consultant will make a home visit if a patient is too ill to attend an outpatient clinic. Familiarise yourself with departmental procedure regarding this. The consultant will be able to claim a fee for a domiciliary visit agreed by a GP.

WARD VISIT

You may receive a request for a ward visit from a hospital consultant or a member of his or her team. A verbal request should usually be followed up by a written request. It is important to take down all details regarding the patient and pass these on to the consultant at the earliest opportunity. Details should include the patient's location, anticipated length of stay, and whether they are well enough to be brought to an outpatient clinic when an outpatient clinic is imminent and, in this case, whether or not they are MRSA positive.

CLINIC CANCELLATION OR REDUCTIONS

When doctors are on leave and outpatient clinics are affected, as much notice as possible is required to put a stop on a clinic, to stop further appointments being booked on PAS and, if necessary, to allow sufficient time to cancel and reschedule patient appointments. Usually a minimum of 6 weeks is required. Any change to clinics has to be put in writing and it is usually the outpatient department staff who cancel and reschedule appointments.

Patient appointments outside normal clinic times

The Consultant may wish to see a patient outside normal clinic times in a consulting room or their office because more time is needed to discuss sensitive issues. The medical secretary should alert reception staff that a patient will be attending, arrange for PAS to be updated, contact the patient by telephone, and whenever possible send confirmation in writing of arrangements, ensure case notes and results are available for the visit and there are no interruptions during the consultation.

CONCLUSION

In this chapter we have looked at the practical administrative issues involved in running an outpatient department, demonstrating the variety of tasks required. These illustrate the importance of effective communication between staff. Emphasis is placed on staff understanding their responsibilities, using the minimum confidential patient information necessary to carry out a task and adhering to hospital protocols. This is essential when considering the number of outpatient clinics and appointments being processed. However, there also has to

be a degree of flexibility in extraordinary circumstances and the medical secretary has to exercise common sense as they are often the first point of contact for patients and those involved in patient care. The medical secretary must have an overview of the whole outpatient system and procedures to assist them in solving a patient's problem. They should also have the ability to refer the patient to the appropriate department or staff member when necessary.

Exercises

- A woman telephones and asks why she has not received an appointment yet to see the consultant. What procedure will you follow to resolve this query and what information do you need from the patient to do this efficiently?

- A man telephones and says that his new patient appointment is for 3 months' time and he wants to see the consultant now. What procedure will you follow to resolve this query and what information do you need from the patient to do this efficiently?

- A GP telephones and asks you to make an urgent appointment for a patient to be seen in the next available clinic. What procedure will you follow to resolve this query efficiently? Consider the information you need and whom you need to inform in order to resolve this matter satisfactorily.

Chapter 14

Admissions and discharges

Sara Ladyman

OBJECTIVES

- To explain the differences between routine, urgent and emergency admissions and define terminology used when managing waiting lists

- To examine an example of an admission management system which utilises the computerised patient administration system (known as PAS), including monitoring bed availability

- To examine an example of a discharge management system which utilises PAS, including communication between doctors and the community

- To outline other areas that require special consideration, including day surgery, intensive therapy unit, when a patient dies, clinical audit and the accident and emergency department

- To consider the non-routine occurrences and anomalies which may involve secretarial input to resolve.

INTRODUCTION

This chapter is concerned with the administration of inpatient episodes of care. You will find it helpful to refer to a copy of the Patient's Charter, and where possible a copy of a hospital's waiting list policy. The patient's perception of a hospital's efficiency is often proportionate to the length of time they wait for treatment. Emphasis is increasingly placed on a hospital's ability to maximise the efficiency of their inpatient management systems as part of the *NHS Plan* with waiting list targets being set to keep patient waits for treatment to a minimum. Medical secretaries must therefore have a clear understanding of their role and responsibilities with regard to outpatient clinic management, outlined in Chapter 13, leading to waiting list management for patients who require surgical intervention, covered in this chapter.

Consultant physicians and surgeons are allocated a number of beds on specific wards for the admission of their patients, giving patients access to specialist medical and nursing inpatient care. Once a specialty has filled its allocation of beds, routine admissions are not usually allowed until patients have been discharged.

Consultant surgeons will be allocated specific theatres and times during the week when they can perform operations on patients who require surgical intervention on a day case or inpatient basis. It is essential to utilise all resources effectively, especially when we consider the specialist medical and nursing care, and the involvement of many other staff and departments before, during and after a patient's stay in hospital.

For the purposes of this chapter we will assume that the admissions department carries out the following duties. However, you should note that the medical secretary might be required to deal with some or all of the procedures for admitting patients from the waiting list.

There is usually a bed manager who will be supported by senior nurses and the duty medical team. A team of doctors in a department may also be referred to as a 'firm' of doctors. Each medical team, or firm, will nominate a duty medical/surgical registrar who is responsible for allocating empty beds. Each medical team will also take it in turn to be 'on take'. Each consultant will have additional responsibility for a set number of days for the overall allocation of beds in the hospital. This is particularly relevant in arranging emergency admissions to beds which could be made available or are not currently in use by different medical teams.

A patient's admission to hospital may be routine, urgent or an emergency. Different procedures apply for each, and these will be outlined in this chapter. The computerised outpatient and waiting list system, also described in Chapters 8 and 13, and referred to as PAS (Patient Administration System), facilitates admission and discharge procedures by utilising an inpatient module. This allows staff to add waiting list episodes, to update and amend inpatient data, to generate letters and patient labels, to print reports and to produce inpatient statistics.

ADMISSION FROM A WAITING LIST

A patient is generally added to an active elective waiting list for surgery after an outpatient clinic visit. The patient may be offered a specific date for surgery by the consultant or nominated deputy. Patients are categorised as day cases or inpatients. Day cases are patients who require admission to hospital for treatment and will use a bed during the day, but are not intending to stay overnight. Inpatients are patients who will need a bed for one or more nights following admission, and may have to be admitted one or more days prior to surgery for clinical reasons.

A patient will only be placed on an active waiting list if there is a clinical indication that an operation is necessary and the patient is ready to have the operation if they are offered a date. The operation must then be carried out within an appropriate time scale. Every patient must be given before leaving, or sent in the post, a letter confirming they have been placed on a waiting list. This admission letter will include details of the consultant they are being admitted under, the patient's name, the date the letter was handed or sent to the patient, the date and time of admission, where to report on arrival, arrangements for transport and a named contact for queries relating to the admission. A response from the patient may be required. Details sent or handed to the patient may also include their pre-assessment appointment, instructions for their admission, and information about their planned treatment, which may be in the form of a patient information leaflet.

Patients must not be added to the active elective waiting list unless they have accepted the consultant's advice that surgery is necessary and they are fit and ready to be offered a date for operation from that point onwards. Some patients may need to lose weight prior to surgery, and some patients may be pregnant at the time a decision is made that an operation is necessary. If the patient is unfit, or cannot commit to having the operation, they must either be reviewed in an outpatient clinic, or discharged back to their GP's care and re-referred when they are fit or ready to pursue surgery.

The patient may be offered, and is sometimes given a choice, of dates for their operation at the time of their outpatient clinic visit, that is, when the decision to admit has been made. In these circumstances the patient is referred to as a 'booked admission' and placed on the active elective waiting list. There is a move towards full or partial booking for all patients. Alternatively, however, the patient may be placed on the active elective waiting list without being given a date for surgery and a date for operation will be offered within an appropriate time scale. All patients of equal clinical priority are treated in chronological order, that is on a first-come first-serve basis, and the PAS system is able to produce a printed waiting list in chronological order to assist the doctor in selecting patients for surgery.

In addition to the active elective waiting list there will be a suspended waiting list of patients who are unavailable for admission because they have become unfit for operation, either medically or for social reasons, after they have been added to the active waiting list. These patients will not count as actively waiting for their surgery until they are transferred back on to the active elective waiting list and will not be counted as such when statistics are gathered. These patients must be carefully monitored to ensure they are suspended for the minimum time necessary. They will usually be managed by using personal treatment plans and this documentation will explain why the operation is delayed, include an action plan and a date when the operation is to be carried out. Patients who are unavailable for their operation for social or personal reasons such as work commitments or holidays, and request their admission date is deferred, may also be placed on the suspended list until they are available to have their operation. The reasons for being placed on a suspended list must be clearly documented without keeping unnecessary detail.

Patients who have been removed from a waiting list where subsequently it is clinically recommended the patient is reinstated, will usually be returned to the waiting list using the original date and not the current date of entry on to the waiting list. Clarification should be sought if there is any query regarding this. It is important that all relevant waiting list history is also recorded at the time of reinstatement, for example previous suspensions and patient deferrals of treatment.

There may also be the option of maintaining what is often referred to as a planned waiting list. This waiting list is designed for patients whose operations are planned in stages. The first operation or treatment date will be given and then as subsequent stages are reached further surgery is planned as part of the patient's treatment programme, for example age- or growth-related surgery in children.

Patients who fail to attend for their operation or to attend an operation pre-assessment clinic prior to admission are referred to as a 'did not attend' (DNA) and actions regarding these patients will be looked at later in the chapter.

Throughout the year there will be operating sessions that the consultant and members of their surgical team will be unable to utilise because of annual or study leave and so on. This must be clearly marked in the admission diary and draft operating lists. As soon as this is confirmed the operating list must be offered to other consultants to ensure optimal usage of theatre space. The operating list is then referred to as a 'relet list'. It is essential that ward, theatre and any staff involved in arranging admissions for a particular consultant are made aware of these changes so that staffing levels, operating equipment and other facilities are planned for appropriately.

WAITING LIST PROCEDURES

For a patient to be placed on an elective waiting list it is essential that an admission card, sometimes known as a 'to come in' card (TCI card), is completed fully and accurately (Figure 14.1) by a doctor in the outpatient clinic. This will include confirmation of the patient's address and postcode, day time and mobile telephone numbers and availability to come in at short notice, usually less than 48 hours if a bed becomes available. Relevant additional information which may affect patient availability is also helpful, for example if they are the main carer in their home, or to accommodate transport arrangements. This information then has to be transferred accurately on to the PAS waiting list module. The waiting list card is generally kept in the patient's case notes or in a filing system kept by the admissions department or medical secretary.

ECR & Elective Admission Request Form
Please complete all information in BLOCK CAPITALS and TICK BOXES as appropriate

Hospital No. _____

Surname _____

Forename/s _____

DOB [____ | ____ | ____]

Sex [Male] [Female]

Address _____

POSTCODE _____

D.H.A. _____

Tel No: Work _____ Home _____

Referring Practitioner:

[Reg GP] [Other GP] [Consultant] [Dentist] [A & E] [Other]

(Name & address only required if referral is not by Registered GP)

Name _____

Address _____

_____

POSTCODE:

Registered GP (only required for patients not registered on PAS):

Name _____

Address _____

POSTCODE:

Consultant _____

Specialty/Sub Specialty Code [   ]   New Patient [   ]

Price Band [   ]   Follow-up Patient [   ]

Intended/Estimated No of Episodes   Proposed Date

Inpatient _____

Day Case _____

Provisional Diagnosis _____

Intended Procedure _____

Admin Category: NHS [   ]   Private [   ]   Amenity [   ]   Overseas Visitor Status [   ]

Admission Details

Date Decision to Admit _____

Priority Type
Routine [   ]   Emergency [   ]
Urgent [   ]   Soon [   ]

Patient Available at Short Notice [Yes] [No]

Patient Informed [Yes] [No]

Admission Time _____

Ward _____

Transport Required   None [   ]   Walking [   ]   Chair [   ]
Stretcher [   ]   Escort Req [   ]

Waiting List [   ]

Planned [   ]

Admission Type
Booked [   ]
Deferred [   ]

Deferral Reason _____

Proposed TCI Date _____

Letter of Confirmation [Yes] [No]

Nil By Mouth from: Date _____ Time _____ am/pm

Operation Date [| |]

Dates to Avoid (Annual Leave, etc.) _____

Investigations to be Arranged Prior to Admission: _____

On Admission: _____

Comments on Admission (Medical, etc.) _____

Name of Doctor Completing:
(Please Print) _____

Date of Completion _____

Computer Input By (Initials) _____   Date _____

For CVU Use
Approved: [Yes] [No]   Agreement No. _____

Signed _____   Date _____

Figure 14.1 A 'To Come In' (TCI) request form

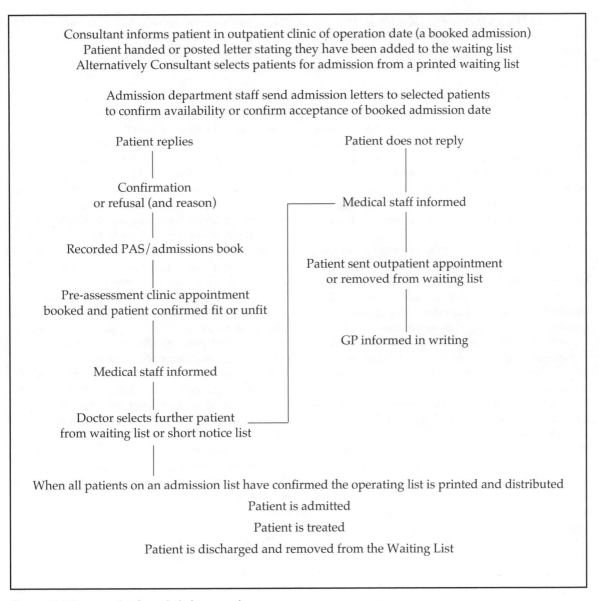

Consultant informs patient in outpatient clinic of operation date (a booked admission)
Patient handed or posted letter stating they have been added to the waiting list
Alternatively Consultant selects patients for admission from a printed waiting list

Admission department staff send admission letters to selected patients
to confirm availability or confirm acceptance of booked admission date

Patient replies   Patient does not reply

Confirmation
or refusal (and reason)   Medical staff informed

Recorded PAS/admissions book

Patient sent outpatient appointment
or removed from waiting list

Pre-assessment clinic appointment
booked and patient confirmed fit or unfit

GP informed in writing

Medical staff informed

Doctor selects further patient
from waiting list or short notice list

When all patients on an admission list have confirmed the operating list is printed and distributed

Patient is admitted

Patient is treated

Patient is discharged and removed from the Waiting List

Figure 14.2 An example of an admission procedure

When the information is transferred to PAS a check is made to confirm that an agreement or contract to treat the patient exists locally. When this is not the case, for example when a patient may live outside the area, agreement must be sought for them to be treated as an out of area treatment (OAT).

Patients are usually required to attend a pre-assessment clinic shortly before their admission date. The pre-assessment nurse and doctor will assess the patient and will make a decision as to whether or not they are fit for their operation. If they are unfit they will be transferred to the suspended waiting list as described previously. The pre-assessment appointment may also be booked at the time of the outpatient clinic visit. This reduces the risk of patients arriving on the admission day and having to have their operation cancelled or deferred because they are medically unfit and thereby underutilising beds and operating lists. It also provides the patient with an opportunity to clarify information or ask further questions that may not have been addressed in the outpatient clinic. A paediatrican will always undertake pre-assessment of children for surgery.

It is usual for a minimum of 3 to 4 weeks' notice of admission to be given, to allow the patient sufficient time to make arrangements, and to enable administrative tasks to be completed. This includes notification and confirmation of availability from the patient for the allocated date and attendance of a pre-assessment clinic or other arrangements as necessary. Occasionally admission departments run a computerised and manual system in tandem though this is becoming less common with the installation of more sophisticated PAS systems. Booked admissions, patients who have been given their date for operation during an outpatient clinic for example, will also need to have arrangements confirmed within this time scale.

A printout from PAS of the waiting list for each consultant will be produced and this will contain details of all patients who will need to be treated before the end of the year in order to be operated upon within the waiting target. The consultant or nominated doctor in the department will plan forthcoming admissions and it may be the secretary's responsibility to ensure that an up to date copy of the list is printed off regularly and available for reference. A record should be kept for patients who have specified they can be admitted should cancellations or spaces become available. A number of 'fire break' operating sessions or slots may be kept free throughout the year. These are utilised in a shorter than normal time scale and filled with emergency and fast track patients requiring surgery, and for rescheduling patients who have had their operations cancelled and must be offered a second date within a prescribed time scale.

An admission procedure similar to the one outlined in Figure 14.2 may be utilised.

Each consultant will implement their own selection criteria for arranging patient admissions based primarily on clinical need. Other factors taken into consideration when allocating an operation date may include obtaining test results, amending treatment plans and referring to the patient case notes as necessary.

An operation diary or preprinted forms may be used by the doctor in conjunction with a current waiting list to draft lists of patients to be contacted for operations in designated theatres on specific dates. These draft operation lists will usually comprise of several patients for different operations, and until patients have confirmed acceptance of the date offered this proposed operating list will be fluid and may change several times before it is finalised. The consultant or nominated doctor will decide the appropriate mix of patients who can be accommodated within the time scale of the theatre session as different procedures take different lengths of time. Other factors such as the experience and grade of doctors operating and whether the patient has any complications or infections will also be taken into account. Patients on the waiting list for the same operation with no medical complications must be offered dates sequentially. Likewise it is the doctor who decides which short notice patients are to be admitted, and they too should be offered short notice availability of operation dates in chronological order.

The medical secretary will find it helpful to refer to a copy of the theatre schedule, usually produced annually, which includes details of operating sessions which have been cancelled, for example around the Christmas holiday period or because of medical audit sessions. Relevant information must be transferred into the admissions diary from the theatre schedule to ensure that patients are not booked onto non-existent or rescheduled operation lists.

The patient must be contacted or handed in clinic a letter stating they have been placed on the waiting list, and an admission letter which includes the proposed date of surgery and instructions, such as advice on food or drink intake prior to admission. It may also include details of a pre-assessment appointment to see a nurse and doctor for a medical check, a reduction or withdrawal of medication, and any tests to be carried out shortly before admission to hospital. (Figure 14.3 is an example of an admission letter.)

There will be a procedure for patients who have not confirmed acceptance of their admission date or did not attend (DNA) their operation date. A check must be made that the patient has not cancelled the offer of surgery or moved address. The consultant or nominated deputy will decide how to proceed in these circumstances. The consultant will write to the GP indicating whether the patient will need to be seen again in an outpatient clinic or referring them back to their GP if the patient DNAs more than once. For urgent admission patients who have DNAd it is essential to make every effort to contact the patient by telephone to agree a further date before sending out confirmation of the operation date in writing.

Regrettably, some patient admission dates have to be cancelled, sometimes on the day of admission. This can cause a great deal of distress and

Dear

We have provisionally booked a bed for you in .... Ward on

.... under the care of ....

On receipt of this letter please telephone the above number to confirm or refuse this booking. Failure to do so may result in the cancellation of the booking.

Please telephone this office between 10.00 a.m. and 11.00 a.m. on the day you are due to come in to check there is a bed available for you as we occasionally have to cancel a planned admission.

Please report to the Front Hall Reception Desk at 11.00 p.m. where you will be directed to the Admission Lounge before going to Ward _____.

We enclose a handbook 'Coming into Hospital' with information on what to bring and routine in the ward. We trust this will be helpful to you.

Yours sincerely,

Admissions Officer

Figure 14.3 Example of an admission letter

inconvenience for patients and their relatives who have mentally prepared themselves for the surgery, made arrangements in the workplace and for caring for others in their absence. Cancellations may be due to the high level of unforeseen emergency admissions, delays in discharges or the closure of beds due to infection. For example, in recent years methicillin resistant Staphyloccocus aureus, known as MRSA, has emerged as a major infection control problem on wards. It is an organism spread relatively easily from person to person and is difficult to eradicate.

Once confirmation of attendance for operation has been received from all the patients on the draft admissions list for a specific operating session the admissions department or medical records staff will be responsible for locating the patient case notes, ready for admission. The case notes will need additional paperwork, including blank inpatient history sheets, consent forms, various charts and patient care documentation for completion by the nurses or doctor on the ward or in the preoperative pre-assessment clinic usually held in outpatient clinic areas. X-rays and outstanding results will also have to be located and filed with the case notes to enable doctors and nurses to complete this patient interview and at this point the decision to admit is confirmed. This minimises the risk of patients being admitted to a bed and then found to be unsuitable for surgery at that time, blocking a bed unnecessarily and resulting in a wasted operating slot. The medical secretary may be contacted regarding case notes and results in their possession and these should be released at the earliest opportunity. The admissions staff or medical secretary may have to add patients to the ward diary, entering the date of admission and date of surgery which may differ when patients have to be admitted earlier for medical reasons.

The admissions list is also circulated to other departments, including the ward, the chaplains and the medical social worker, so that they can make their arrangements accordingly.

Scenario 1

A patient telephones to ask you if he needs to follow any special instructions prior to admission. How would you respond to this query?

THE OPERATING LIST

The medical secretary may have responsibility for the timely production and distribution of the consultant surgeon's operating list; that is, the list of patients who will be operated on in theatres in a particular operating session. In order to prepare for forthcoming operating sessions theatre staff and others will need to refer to the finalised typewritten operating list. The operating list is drawn from information recorded in the admission diary and draft operation lists and should be distributed well in advance of the operating date. The operating list will include the name of the consultant, the name of the doctor performing the operation and their grade, and the name of the anaesthetist who will be present. Patient details will include full name, age, hospital number, ward, operation details, type of anaesthetic required (general, local, spinal block etc.) and highlight any clinical risks (for example if medications will be temporarily suspended). It is important that abbreviations are not used and that

all information is spelled out to ensure the understanding of all staff. The operating list may indicate specific times anticipated for each patient's operation and the doctor will have prioritised the patients in the order of operation. The theatres and anaesthetics department staff will coordinate the operating lists for the various specialisms. The admissions staff or medical secretary may be required to circulate operating lists to staff and departments who work in conjunction with theatres, for example the central sterile supplies department (CSSD), who provide sterile instruments and equipment for each operation, and the haematology department for blood matching. The operation list should include the date it was produced and the name and contact telephone number of the admissions department or medical secretary who produced the operating list, to avoid confusion and to ensure· amended lists, due to unforeseen cancellations and so on, can be identified in chronological order and the most recent list acted upon.

The operating list and admission dates must also be transferred across to the ward diary via the admissions staff in good time to ensure ward staff can plan staffing and patient activity levels, order special equipment and so forth and make arrangements to receive the patients onto the ward.

The case notes will usually be held by the ward or admission lounge staff in preparation for admission by staff responsible for receiving and admitting patients for their surgery. The admission lounge is an area manned by admission clerks who will manage the transition of the patient to the ward rather than the patient reporting directly to a busy ward environment where staff may have conflicting demands on their time. The admissions lounge is usually adjacent to an Accident and Emergency Department so that an emergency team is on hand in the unlikely event of a patient collapsing.

A few days prior to admission the case notes will be made available for the medical and nursing staff on the ward. The majority of wards have a full or part time administrative assistant, known as a ward clerk or ward assistant. The ward clerk may have responsibility for updating the PAS system once the patient has been admitted and allocated a bed on the ward. They may also assist with updating the bed state, ensuring results are checked by a doctor and filed in the case notes, sorting incoming mail, receiving patients and visitors and liaison with other

HOSPITAL NUMBER   243675

4th May --

Mr. K. Davidson,
14 White Cross, Bakers Town
BT21 8SK

Dear Mr. Davidson,

You have been on (Consultant's name) Waiting List since (date added to List).

Sometimes patients change address, have their operation elsewhere or decide they no longer wish to have the operation. We may also be able to offer you a date at short notice if a patient cancels.

Please telephone us on the above number, or complete and return the tear off slip and return in the enclosed stamped addressed envelope.

If you require further information please do not hesitate to contact me between 8.00 am and 6.00 pm Monday to Friday on (direct dial telephone number).

Yours sincerely

Waiting List Officer

Cut off below and return in SAE:
- -
Hospital Number: Patient Name: Address:

Telephone Number: Mobile Telephone Number:

Please amend any of the details above if they are incorrect, and tick the following statements as appropriate:

I still want to have the operation ___

I have had the operation done elsewhere ___

I no longer want to have the operation ___

I am available to come into Hospital at short notice (within 5 days) ___

My holiday dates are:

Signed: Date:

Figure 14.4 An example of a PAS-generated waiting list validation letter

5th May

Dr. B.E. Smith (GP),
10 Blackhorse Road,
Bakers Town
BT22 7QD

Dear Dr. Smith,

RE   KEITH DAVIDSON
DOB   10.12.--

ADDRESS   14 White Cross, Bakers Town
POSTCODE   BT21 8SK

HOSPITAL NUMBER   243675

OPERATION   FASCIECTOMY

Resulting from recent validation of my Waiting List, the patient detailed above has been contacted and has expressed a wish to be removed from my Waiting List. After studying the patient's case I have decided to remove this patient from my List.

If you know of any reason why this patient should be reinstated, please do not hesitate to contact me.

Yours sincerely,

Mr. J. Daniels
Consultant in Plastic Surgery

Figure 14.5 Example of a PAS-generated letter to a GP to assist in validating a waiting list

hospital departments.

Unfortunately operations do have to be cancelled on the day of admission because of a lack of beds which are being occupied by emergency patients, patients awaiting discharge to the community or insufficient operating time. Any patient cancelled for non-medical reasons must be offered a date within 28 days of the original date and, to minimise the risk of the patient being cancelled again, this must be recorded on the waiting list module and in the patient's personal treatment plan.

All patients on a waiting list will be periodically validated to ensure that an operation is still required by the patient, their registration and contact details are still correct, and they will be treated within the appropriate time scale. Validation of the waiting list is essential to ensure patients do not breach the maximum wait for their operation, to optimise bed occupancy and maximise operating theatre usage. Details of the waiting list and expected waiting times are distributed monthly to individual consultants and the admissions management team for action as required. A summary of waiting list waits will also be made available at Trust board meetings and distributed between consultants and sent out to GPs who refer patients to the hospital for treatment.

Statistics are regularly sent to the Department of Health for monitoring and comparative performance data for different hospitals is published to enable hospitals to measure their efficiency in waiting list management against the average.

Whether the medical secretary is directly or indirectly responsible for waiting list management they can help maximise the efficiency of the service by ensuring personal and demographic details of patients are accurate by updating the PAS system and manual records when informed of changes, and making the admissions department staff aware of changes in a patient's situation. (See Figures 14.4 and 14.5 for examples of PAS computer-generated letters to assist in validating waiting lists.)

URGENT ADMISSIONS

As well as providing waiting list management information the admissions department will be responsible for communicating telephone and written enquiries and cancellations as appropriate. In the case of urgent admissions, (as opposed to emergency admissions), it is important that admissions staff clarify with the doctor or nurse whether or not the patient has been advised that an offer of an admission date is imminent. The patient will need to be made aware of the reasons for being admitted urgently by the clinician before these arrangements are made. This is particularly important if the patient is part of a fast track outpatient procedure when the diagnosis is sensitive, for example in cases of suspected or proven cancer. It may be necessary to liaise with the patient through a cancer services support nurse, for example, who will be in contact with the patient. The admissions staff will then update the PAS waiting list module, and the manual systems, immediately the date for surgery offered to the patient has been accepted.

EMERGENCY ADMISSIONS

Same-day admissions can occur when the patient requires admission immediately from the accident and emergency (A&E) department, an outpatient clinic, through a GP or from another hospital. The referring doctor or doctor on call usually contacts the admissions staff with the patient's name, sex,

age, diagnosis and consultant to be admitted under. The admissions staff are responsible for locating a vacant bed, agreeing this with the duty medical registrar or duty surgical registrar (i.e. a member of the medical staff with responsibility for admissions on that particular day). The GP will be contacted if they have been instrumental in arranging a patient's admission.

DAILY INFORMATION ON BED AVAILABILITY

The admissions staff are responsible for collecting information on bed availability to assist in bed management and monitoring. This information is provided by the 'bed state'. The bed state is a continuous record of the status of each bed in the hospital and this is held and updated on the PAS. The status of each bed is defined in four ways (Box 14.1).

Box 14.1 The bed state

- Occupied: a bed which currently has a patient in it
- Booked: a bed, which has a patient, coming into it in the next 24 hours
- Available: a bed which does not have a patient booked in the next 24 hours
- Reserved: a bed which has a patient coming back into it within 48 hours, not a planned admission but perhaps an urgent planned admission

---

The admissions staff will operate a number of different systems to ensure that timely and accurate information is gathered on bed occupancy.

Nursing staff are required to notify the admissions department immediately a bed on the ward becomes available when a discharge of patient has been agreed by the consultant. The PAS system is updated regularly.

Reflection Point 1

In what ways can a medical secretary assist with minimising the stress caused by a potentially traumatic cancellation of a patient's admission date?

BEDSTATE AT 8 a.m. WARD DATE

Bed No.	Hospital No.	Name	Consultant	PATIENTS – IN			PATIENTS – OUT				For Discharge or Transfer Today
				DATE of Admission/Transfer	FROM	DATE Return to Ward	DATE of Discharge/Transfer	TO	DATE of Death	DATE Home on Leave	
1	FW0000	DAVIES CLAIRE NHS	PB	12.3.90	CAS						
2	FW0000	DAVIES CLAIRE NHS	PB	12.3.90	W/LIST						
3	FW0000	DAVIES CLAIRE NHS	PB	12.3.90	CLINIC						
4											
5											
FX											

Figure 14.6 A manual bed state form

The admissions departments staff may ring the wards at set times during the day to check the bed state for accuracy, and for any available beds caused by discharges and deaths. (See Figure 14.6 for an example of a manual bed state form.)

In an acute bed shortage the bed manager, supported by the 'take' firm, will contact all firms and ask that whenever clinically possible patients are considered for discharge or moved to make beds available for the 'take' firm to utilise. There will be a clinical referee to help resolve difficulties. The Emergency Bed Service and Ambulance Service must also be notified of these decisions.

The Emergency Bed Service provides a central information service for GPs and hospital doctors on the availability of beds in surrounding hospitals and ambulances to divert to hospitals with available beds.

BED MANAGEMENT AND MONITORING INFORMATION

There will be a bed allocation team who will be concerned mainly with retrospective monitoring of bed management and planning services. Statistics generated from PAS, including hospital initiated cancellations and patients remaining in A&E for 24 hours or more (i.e. patients who should be moved to an appropriate ward within 48 hours of admission, before routine cases are admitted) will be utilised. They will address issues of bed blocking where patients are kept in hospital unnecessarily without clinical need. There may be a number of reasons for this. Usually it is because there are insufficient or unavailable resources to accommodate the patient in the community. For example, lack of an available space in a care home to take a patient who has Alzheimer's may lead to a bed being blocked and unavailable for forthcoming admissions.

CONFIDENTIALITY

If a caller asks which ward a patient is on, it may be because they wish to send a card or flowers. It is possible, however, that someone who has knowledge of the wards and the types of operations or treatments provided there may deduce the reasons, rightly or wrongly, for a patient being on that ward without you specifying this. For example, Ward 10 may be specifically for

the care of patients who are HIV positive and have associated illnesses. Care must therefore be taken when giving any information to callers and a check made beforehand that the patient is happy for any information to be given out. PAS may have a privacy facility for recording a patient's wishes in this respect.

DAY SURGERY UNIT

The unit will usually provide facilities for adult patients and children who can safely be admitted for surgical, therapeutic, diagnostic or endoscopic procedures and sent home on the same day. Specialties using a day surgery facility may include general surgery (e.g. inguinal hernia repair), ophthalmology (e.g. cataract extraction), orthopaedic surgery (e.g. arthroscopy), ear, nose and throat (ENT) surgery, urology and plastic surgery. They will have their own operating theatres and team of staff. Figure 14.7 shows an example of a letter to patients being admitted for day surgery.

There may be overnight hostel accommodation available for patients when travelling time would otherwise make it difficult for them to attend for treatment. Medical secretaries must familiarise themselves with the procedures involved for admitting patients to day surgery and the follow up procedures such as the production of proforma discharge letters and the typing of discharge summaries as required.

It should be noted that some surgical procedures might also take place in the outpatient department, for example in dental, ophthalmology and dermatology specialisms. The medical secretary must be aware of any special requirements for recording these cases on PAS.

INTENSIVE THERAPY UNIT (ITU)/INTENSIVE CARE UNIT

There will be intensive care beds and high dependency care beds for the specialist care and treatment of critically ill patients by a team of staff who generally possess a critical care qualification. ITUs will generally provide waiting areas and accommodation for next of kin. Patients may, for example, have sustained major trauma, require treatment for burns, sepsis or multi-organ failure,

Dear

Your doctor has recommended that you have an ENDOSCOPY. This is a telescope examination of your oesophagus (gullet), stomach and duodenum. The examination is performed as a single procedure using a flexible lighted instrument and is carried out in the Unit by a specially trained doctor. It will help discover the cause of your symptoms or clarify any abnormality seen on X-ray.

Do not eat or drink anything from midnight before your examination. Medication should also be omitted unless you are a diabetic or on medication for a heart condition. If this is the case please contact the department for instructions.

Please report to the Day Surgery Unit (sign posted throughout the Hospital). There you will be asked to change into a gown. You may bring your own dressing gown if you wish. Please bring your slippers.

A doctor will take a brief history from you and a small needle will be inserted into your arm or hand. From the DSU you will be transferred to the Endoscopy Unit on a special trolley. Here you will be given something to make you very drowsy. When you are totally relaxed the doctor will pass a tube over the back of your throat and down into your gullet. This will not interfere with your breathing and is not painful. The examination lasts about ten minutes and a nurse will remain with you throughout. Once the examination is over you will be returned to the DSU to sleep off the effects of the injection. There is a waiting area if your escort wishes to wait for you.

Please Note: It is essential that you are collected and escorted home by a friend or relative. YOU MUST NOT DRIVE YOURSELF HOME. If there is a problem with a companion taking you home please contact this Department immediately.

Please note the date and time of your appointment:

DATE: .... TIME: ....

Useful information following Endoscopy:

1 Advised not to smoke or take alcohol for 24 hours.
2 You should not drive or operate machinery for 48 hours following Endoscopy.
3 Contact your own doctor two weeks after your Endoscopy for result of examination.
4 Rest for remainder of the day and you should be able to return to work next day.
5 Occasionally some patients experience a slightly sore throat. This will subside without medication.

Yours sincerely,

Day Surgery Unit Manager

Figure 14.7 Example of a letter to a patient for day surgery

Scenario 2

A patient telephones you and asks you where she is placed on the waiting list and when she can expect to be called for admission. What action should you take and what information can you provide? What variables outside the hospital or your own control may influence the time a patient may spend on the waiting list?

require coronary care or require a period of care in ITU following major surgery before transferring back to a ward.

COMPULSORY ADMISSIONS

It should be noted that whilst the aim is always to advise voluntary admission wherever possible, patients can be detained in hospital under the Mental Health Acts in order for their mental state to be assessed and, if necessary, treated, or transferred to an appropriate psychiatric unit. There will be a duty psychiatrist and duty psychiatric social worker on call and available to assist in these cases (see Chapter 3).

DISCHARGES

All hospitals will have a discharge policy outlining all matters that must be attended to before the patient leaves the hospital following treatment. This will include, as appropriate:

- advice from doctors and nurses on the ward to patients on how best to look after themselves and what to expect following surgery and appropriate information sheets, for example on pain management
- production by the doctor of a proforma style letter to post or to be handed by the patient to their GP containing information about treatment and recommendations about future medical care and hospital follow-up is required
- any medications the patient is discharged with, dressings which will need changing, stitches removing and so on by the practice nurse, or an appointment to return to the ward

- medical certificate
- arrangements regarding special pension or benefits, with which a hospital social worker may assist
- other arrangements, such as social services, meals on wheels, home help, day care, nursing aids, nursing care (for example Macmillan nurses)
- date and time of next outpatient clinic appointment, if required
- community nursing staff visit date
- return of valuables
- arrangements for getting home, including hospital transport (patients may be transferred to another ward, hospital, to a nursing or residential home and arrangements will need to be made accordingly)
- date of discharge entered on to the PAS
- case notes forwarded to the medical secretary for dictation by the doctor of a discharge summary to the GP if required, using the PAS case note tracking system
- X-rays returned to the X-ray department film stores.

The medical social work department will liaise closely with the ward, the primary health care team and the community services regarding the patient's discharge to ensure continuity of care.

To reduce the number of forms in circulation at discharge a self-carbonated discharge letter form may be used as follows (see Figure 14.8).

- the form, completed legibly and clearly by a doctor, can be sent to the pharmacy department in order for drugs on discharge to be prescribed
- the top copy is sent to the GP on the day of discharge (or given to the patient to deliver)
- the second copy is filed in the patient's case notes
- the third copy is sent to the clinical coding department
- the fourth copy is for pharmacy records.

Once the consultant has made the decision to discharge the patient they may be transferred on the day of discharge to a discharge lounge. A registered nurse supervises the patients and facilitates the smooth transition from acute care to home in a relaxed and managed environment. The patient is relieved of the perception that there is pressure on the ward to release the bed as soon as possible. There are categories of patients who will

DISCHARGE LETTER

Hospital No.:

Surname:

First Names:

Date of Birth: Sex:

HOSPITAL: CONTACT TEL No.

Date:

Address:

Dear Dr. ....

Your patient, who was admitted on .... to Ward ....

was discharged

under the care of .... was/will be transferred on .... to ....

died

DIAGNOSIS (firm (F) or provisional (P)) operations, problems and unexplained abnormal findings

INPATIENT SUMMARY AND RECOMMENDATIONS FOR FURTHER MANAGEMENT

	Notifiable diseases only Date notified	ICD coding

HISTOLOGICAL DIAGNOSIS KNOWN/NOT KNOWN. DETAILS

PATIENT WILL/WILL NOT BE SEEN IN OUTPATIENTS. DATE

Drugs taken home and supply provided	Dose	Frequency	Duration necessary	Supply given wks/days	Drugs taken home and supply provided	Dose	Frequency	Duration necessary	Supply given wks/days

DRUGS TO AVOID AND REASONS (including drug sensitivities)

INFORMATION GIVEN TO PATIENT	Information given to Relative or Friend
Diagnosis	
Prognosis	
Resumption of work	
Other	

SERVICES ARRANGED BY THE HOSPITAL (please tick appropriate box if service has been arranged)

MEALS ON WHEELS   ☐ HOME HELP   ☐ HOME NURSE   ☐

GERIATRIC/HEALTH VISITOR   ☐ PART III ACCOMMODATION   ☐

OTHER (please state)   ☐

Cons.

Yours sincerely,

A fuller summary will/will not be sent

S. Reg.

Copy handed to patient/posted to GP

Please print name

Reg.

H.O.

Figure 14.8 A discharge letter

CONSULTANT		GP: Dr
ADMISSION DATE: / /		PATIENT NAME:
DISCHARGE DATE: / /		HOSPITAL NUMBER: DOB:
WARD: HOSPITAL:		ADDRESS:
CONTACT TEL NO.:		POSTCODE:

PRIMARY DIAGNOSIS	MAIN PROCEDURE:	DATE
2.	OTHER PROCEDURES:	
3.		
4.		

CLINICAL COMMENTS

A further summary will be sent

RECOMMENDATIONS FOR FURTHER MANAGEMENT (HOSPITAL, GP)	SERVICES ARRANGED BY HOSPITAL
Date and time of Outpatient Appointment if made: Transport arranged?: Y/N	

DRUGS TO TAKE HOME	☐ Tick if no drugs required	☐ Tick if child resistant closure not required		Pharmacist Check	
Drugs – Approved Name	Route	Dose	Frequency	Duration necessary	Pharmacy

DRUGS TO AVOID AND REASONS (including drug sensitivities):

Signature:	Grade:
Print Name:	Date:

not be transferred to the discharge lounge and these include patients who may be confused, unconscious and other patients awaiting transfer to another hospital, or those who are unable to stand and may be bedridden.

The doctor may dictate a fuller discharge summary to be typed and sent to the GP after a patient has been discharged and the medical secretary will need to keep abreast of patients being admitted and discharged so that there is prompt dictation and transcription of these summaries, irrespective of whether or not they play a more active role in waiting list management.

PROCEDURES WHEN A PATIENT DIES

When a patient dies in hospital the ward sister usually contacts the nearest relative or personal representative of the deceased. The hospital chaplain will be available and the body will be taken to the hospital mortuary until arrangements are made to have the deceased taken to, for example, a Chapel of Rest outside the hospital.

Patient death administration is processed by staff in the patient affairs office who are generally part of the hospital administration department, together with the doctor concerned with the patient's care. There will usually be a private room available for staff to speak with the relatives of the deceased at this very distressing time.

Doctors should inform the patient's GP as soon as possible either by telephone or letter that his/her patient has died.

The doctor responsible for the patient should complete the following paperwork.

Death certificate. Unless the case is to be referred to the coroner, this should be issued as soon after the death as possible, to prevent further distress to the next of kin of the patient.

The doctor should ensure that all sections of the form are complete and that he/she prints his/her name at the end of the certificate. A register will be kept of all death certificates issued.

The form is sent to the Registrar for Births and Deaths, unless the case is referred to the coroner

The Town Hall Registrar will not accept a certificate if the cause of death is abbreviated or if there is no definite cause of death. Terms such as 'probably' and 'unknown' are unacceptable.

Where there is doubt as to the cause of death or

> ### Box 14.2 Circumstances necessitating an autopsy
>
> - Patients who have been in hospital for less than 24 hours
> - Patients whose death may be related to drugs, poison or industrial disease
> - Accidental death/recent fall/fracture
> - Suspicious death/circumstances
> - During a surgical operation/while under anaesthetic
> - Death is sudden, unexplainable, for example sudden infant death

death by natural causes has to be confirmed, the coroner will authorise an autopsy. This may be followed by an inquest. Box 14.2 gives circumstances which may necessitate these procedures.

The coroner will send the death certificate to the Registrar of Births and Deaths once a satisfactory conclusion has been reached.

The medical team may also request a post-mortem, with specific consent of the relatives, to:

- study the effects of treatment, involving the retention of tissue for laboratory study
- remove tissue for the treatment of other patients and for medical education and research.

Post-mortem form. If the medical team feel it is appropriate to request a post-mortem, the patient's relatives must give their permission and a consent form must be completed and a histopathology form submitted by the doctor requesting the post-mortem.

Medical audit form.

Cremation form. Where appropriate.

A 'free from infection' certificate. If the body is to be transported to another country, this form has to be completed, stating that the body will cause no hazard if transported in a sealed coffin.

Staff in the patient affairs office will also be responsible for ensuring that the correct patient details are forwarded to the patient services department. This ensures the cancellation of any known appointments, waiting list entries, and admissions or transport arrangements on PAS. Case notes should be amended accordingly when they eventually return to the medical records department and are generally stored separately and subsequently microfiched. The PAS must be updated as quickly as possible, at least within 48 hours of being notified of a patient's death. Patient affairs staff are responsible for returning a patient's belongings to the relatives and liaising with the mortuary staff.

Failure to collect and provide accurate information of this very sensitive nature may result in the wrong patient appearing on the PAS as being deceased, which may have serious ramifications. Consider a patient not attending (DNA) an appointment for an X-ray to be taken prior to admission, and you are aware that the patient is very elderly. The first check should be with PAS to see whether it indicates that the patient has been admitted as an emergency or has died, before an attempt is made to contact the patient to ascertain why they missed the appointment and to arrange another as required. A telephone call to the patient's surgery may also be an appropriate step in some circumstances before contacting the patient. Failure to update PAS

Reflection Point 2

When a patient has been discharged the case notes are sent to the medical secretary at the earliest opportunity in order for a fuller discharge summary to be dictated by a nominated member of the medical team and subsequently typed by the secretary for dispatch to the GP. (See Fig. 14.9, Excerpt from an inpatient discharge summary.)

Reflection Point 3

Analyse the information which has been recorded in the discharge summary and reflect on the reasons why this information has to be provided before proceeding with the chapter.

and other computerised systems may result in a deceased patient's relative receiving 'did not attend' or further appointment letters, or an ambulance calling to collect a patient for an outpatient appointment , all of which will cause distress.

MEDICAL (CLINICAL) CODING

Medical coding involves the abstraction of clinical information from case notes or discharge summaries and the conversion of that information into an alpha-numeric structure so that without additions or personal identifiers, the codes can provide a comprehensive reflection of morbidity and a description of diagnoses and procedures for individual patients. This diagnostic and procedural information can be put into a comparative form which can then be analysed for statistical purposes.

There are two coding systems in use.

The International Classification of Diseases and Health Related Problems (ICD) is periodically updated and published by the World Health Organization. It is an international standard through which all clinical activity relating to inpatient diagnoses is measured. It is intended to provide a comprehensive list of codes to classify all known diseases and injuries (see Chapter 8). Hospitals produce contract minimum data sets (that is, the demographic, social and clinical information gathered on PAS) which are coded, and regular central returns made from hospitals to the Department of Health. This information provides users of NHS data with better clinical, social and epidemiological information to improve the planning and running of health services at district, national (e.g. National Audit Office) and international levels (e.g. World Health Organization). Statistics are used to aid decision-making and to target health promotion in particular areas of the country, for example where there is a higher incidence than the national average for heart disease.

The Office of Population Censuses and Surveys (OPCS) statistics are revised periodically and provide a further national standard through which all operative procedures are coded in respect of inpatient and day case activity. That is, operations, procedures and their complications will have an identifying code. Revisions of the codes in order to accommodate changes in medical treatments are made as they become available.

Each medical firm will have a medical or clinical coding officer whose responsibility it is to ensure that coding from each firm is timely, accurate and complete for each inpatient episode. Data is entered onto the PAS and facilitates the production of reports and statistics.

Accurate and timely clinical coding (Box 14.3) is

PATIENT'S GP	Dr M. Shah
ADDRESS	14 Bridge Street, Shackleton, Herts.
HOSPITAL NO	264 299
SPECIALISM	GENERAL SURGERY
CONSULTANT	PETER JONES
SURNAME	STANLEY
FIRST NAME	QUEENIE
SEX	F
DOB	04.06.
PATIENT'S ADDRESS	
POSTCODE	
ADMITTED	01.05.
DISCHARGED	10.05.

History
80-year-old lady living in sheltered accommodation. Referred by her General Practitioner.

Past Medical History
Congestive cardiac failure and episodic angina. Also suffers from folate deficiency anaemia.

On Examination
Referred to us as an emergency with bleeding per rectum. Sigmoidoscopy indicated a malignant tumour of the rectum. Biopsy was reported as rectal carcinoma.

Diagnosis on Admission
Admitted for resection of rectal carcinoma.

Procedure
Abdominoperineal resection with colostomy.

Postoperative
Uneventful postoperative course.

Discharged after 10 days.

Drug therapy on Discharge
Nil

Final Diagnoses

		ICD codes
Primary	Cancer of rectum	000.0
Secondary	Folate deficiency anaemia	000.0
	Angina	000.0
	Adenocarcinoma	M000/0

Procedure

	OPCS Codes
Abdominoperineal resection	H00.0

Figure 14.9 Excerpt taken from an inpatient discharge summary

Box 14.3 Minimum requirements for accurate, timely and complete coding coding

- Summaries should be legible
- Patient identification details should include the following:
  - registration/hospital number
  - surname and forename
  - address and postcode
  - date of birth, gender and marital status
- Consultant and specialty
- Date of admission and discharge
- Ward
- Medical diagnoses should include:
  - principal diagnosis
  - subsidiary diagnoses
  - external cause of condition, if appropriate
  - histology results
- Any operation or procedure undertaken with dates
- Any complications arising

Box 14.4 How statistics are used

Local use of statistics
- Number of patients seen by consultant by site and in bed occupancy days
- Analysis of referral patterns
- Activity for different operations

National and international use of statistics
- Assessing health needs of the country
- Epidemiology
- Public health
- Population registers

Successful billing

Contracting information, for example the production of activity reports, are used by providers and purchasers to facilitate planning and to support the contract negotiation process.

Reflection Point 4

The medical or clinical coding clerk relies on the information provided in the discharge letter and discharge summary to code the patient's inpatient episode. A patient with a series of admissions would have several code allocations per admission. With reference to Figure 14.9, the discharge summary, how many of the requirements needed for accurate, timely and complete coding can you identify?

DEPARTMENTAL MEDICAL (CLINICAL) AUDIT

In addition to medical coding being entered on to the PAS, computerised departmental audit systems have been introduced to provide medical staff with an opportunity to collect detailed information on every inpatient seen within a firm. Each consultant will set their own audit aims.

Whilst firms conform to a single standard in the area of diagnostic and procedural coding, they can also access other coding systems, for example Read codes. This is one example of a comprehensive, hierarchically arranged classification and medical thesaurus of terms used in each medical specialism and structured for use in computers, and cross referenced to the ICD. Read and other systems are intended to support the work of doctors with day-to-day patient care and are not designed specifically for wider research purposes or as a statistical tool outside of the department. The role of departmental audit is viewed as complementary to the collection of statistics described above The local audit systems enable doctors to add their own specialist codes to assist them in setting their own standards. They can then measure their local practice, in relation to diagnoses, operation and procedure outcomes, for their own patients, against national and international standards and work towards improving or maintaining these as necessary.

one way of ensuring that medical information is of a high enough quality to reflect accurately the health care practice patterns of doctors and other health care practitioners. As well as ensuring the GP has up-to-date information about the patient's hospital episode, as with patient clinic letters, hospitals can be penalised when discharge summaries are not sent or delayed and this has a direct cost implication for the hospital.

The original function of medical coding was to provide epidemiological data for statistical analysis, by using agreed national and international codes. This information is increasingly used to assist in costing patient care by grouping together comparative costs for treatments.

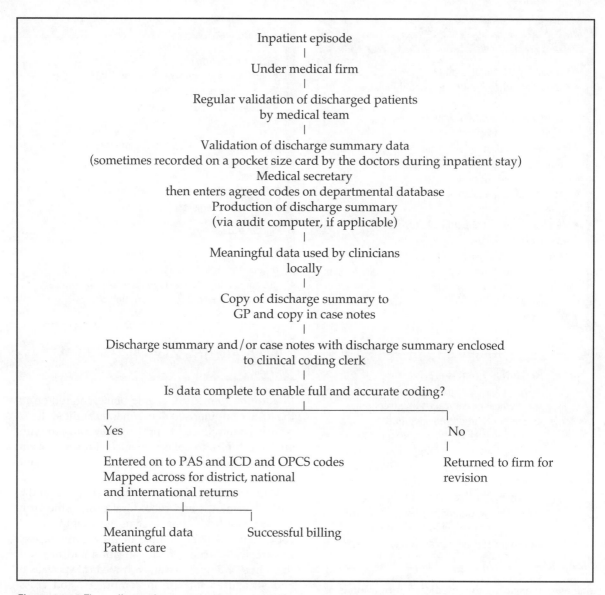

Figure 14.10 The coding cycle

It should be noted that departmental audit data collected on a local system is of a highly sensitive and confidential nature, as it reflects the performance and activity of individual doctors within a team and is therefore not generally made more widely available. The success of internal audit to a large extent relies upon the confidence of medical staff that this information will be used positively to assist in improving departmental standards of patient care.

The departmental computerised audit system may also generate GP letters and summaries. Read and other coding systems can be 'mapped up', i.e.

converted to, ICD and OPCS computer programs on the PAS, which in turn can be mapped up to other hospital computer systems, including those for finance, though in the latter to maintain patient confidentiality patient identifying details will have been removed.

Firms will usually hold regular validation meetings to approve data to be entered on to the departmental database and to ensure audit data is meaningful. Both the medical secretary and the coding clerk may participate in these meetings. Figure 14.10 illustrates the coding cycle. Box 14.4 summarises the use of statistics at different levels.

ACCIDENT AND EMERGENCY DEPARTMENT

The accident and emergency (A&E) department falls outside the usual formality of contracted services between general practice and hospitals, at least for the first 24 hours of a patient's care. Therefore, treatment is available to anyone who presents themselves to the A&E department.

The A&E department provides 24-hour emergency care to a wide cross-section of patients 365 days a year. Its role is to provide clinical assessment and emergency treatment and a referral system back to the patient's GP or to hospital specialist as appropriate. A&E departments will have their own module on PAS and usually keep their own patient records, though they may request hospital case notes, if they are in existence, to assist in treating the patient.

Designated A&Es will also provide a major incident service for their surrounding area and may keep major incident flying squad stores. There will always be a consultant and/or senior registrar 'on call' in A&E and they must usually be informed in the event of the following:

- death in the young (under 40)
- deaths where violence may have occurred
- seriously ill children/non-accidental injury – known or suspected
- significant burns to children and adults
- stabbings/shootings/rape/serious assault
- episodes with major press or police involvement.

Generally there will be an adjacent fracture clinic consulting area. There may also be clinics held for plastics/minor burns, soft tissue, rheumatology and a weekend dental clinic.

The majority of patients attending A&E are ambulant. There will be a 24-hour reception area where staff take details from patients and register them on the A&E module on PAS. Patients are issued with a hospital number and a casualty and incident number. A screen in the PAS module will allow the hospital staff to record a free text summary of the patient's condition. This can be provided by the patient, their relative or the paramedic involved in the case as appropriate.

Patients will then be seen by the 'triage' nurse (triage meaning the order of treatment of the patients being based on clinical urgency). The triage nurse will assess each patient upon their arrival, obtain a further history, take baseline observations as required (e.g. blood pressure), carry out first aid and prioritise the more urgent cases and the patient's access to the A&E doctors.

Patients arriving by ambulance will be taken straight to the treatment room, or if appropriate, to the crash room, where the crash team will administer emergency treatment. The ambulance personnel will pass on as much information as possible to the A&E reception staff so that the patient can be registered on PAS.

Reflection Point 5

The Patient's Charter standard for A&E is 90% patients should be seen within 5 minutes of arrival.

All patients who ask to see a doctor must see a doctor. The casualty doctor will complete casualty records, detailing further history, investigations, diagnosis (as far as possible) and will initiate treatment, discharge the patient back to the GP, refer to a hospital specialist for an outpatient attendance, or admit the patient for inpatient care. Patients who are not admitted remain the responsibility of the A&E department, so follow-up arrangements must be made as appropriate. There may also be dedicated A&E beds for stays of 24 hours.

The casualty officer, who is a doctor, will liaise with the duty registrar of the medical firm 'on take' to find an available bed. Hospital case notes are made up if none already exist and the patient then becomes the responsibility of the firm of the consultant who is 'on take' when they are admitted to the ward. The consultant's secretary will be responsible for typing the discharge summary to the GP when the patient subsequently leaves the hospital.

The department will have a number of treatment cubicles, X-ray equipment in designated rooms, a fully equipped theatre for urgent surgery and minor procedures, a plaster room, and may have designated paediatric cubicles and a paediatric waiting area as well as a relatives' room. There may be doctors' 'on call' rooms nearby, a radiation decontamination unit and isolation suite.

Other staff within the department may include:

- porters, with 24-hour cover
- liaison sisters, with special responsibilities for the elderly, those with alcohol and drug problems

Dear Dr

Re

The above patient attended the A&E Department of this Hospital on

.... at ....

The presenting complaint was LACERATION TO JUST ABOVE WRIST, LEFT ARM.

Diagnosis: LACERATION LEFT WRIST.

Treatment: DRESSING/BANDAGE/SLING.

SUTURING/STERISTRIP.

The patient has been discharged back to your care.

Yours sincerely,

Consultant
Accident and Emergency Department

Figure 14.11 Example of an A&E attendance letter

'I am a registered medical practitioner currently employed as a senior house officer in the A&E Department of St Mary's Hospital.

The patient, Joshua Smith, was brought by ambulance to the A&E Department of this Hospital at 2000 hours on 6th June -- following an alleged assault.

I examined him and found him to be suffering from the following injuries: a 2 cm laceration x 1 cm deep on the right cheek of the face and superficial abrasions to the right hand. The patient's wounds were cleaned and sutured under local anaesthetic with a total of 5 sutures. The patient was discharged from the Department at 2200 hours. He was advised to have his sutures removed in four days....'

Figure 14.12 Example of a doctor's statement for a police officer

- paediatric liaison nurse
- pharmacy, for dispensing a small stock of antibiotics and painkillers
- duty radiographer for taking X-rays.

As the A&E departmental secretary, you may be required to enter the information from the casualty card onto PAS using free text and generate the letter to the GP (Figure 14.11), updating them on the patient's care and follow up. A referral letter to the outpatient department for further care may be required or a letter for the patient to return to a specialist clinic held in A&E for review or re-dressing.

The medical secretary may also become involved with the typing of statements for the police, Criminal Injuries Compensation Board reports and solicitors' medical reports and statements. Patient confidentiality is paramount, and it is essential that permission in writing from the patient is obtained as well as permission from the A&E doctor. Requests for patient names, addresses and information by the police should always be referred to senior casualty staff or the duty administrator. It must be remembered, however, that the police play a major supporting role in casualty situations, for example in locating next of kin, and they have to supply a report to their superiors when they are first on the scene of an accident and so on. The doctor will usually dictate a statement providing factual information for the police. See Figure 14.12 for an example of a doctor's statement for a police officer.

CONCLUSION

In this chapter we have looked at the practical administrative issues in running inpatient services including those prior to admission, during an inpatient stay, at discharge and following discharge. By demonstrating the variety of tasks and procedures which must be carried out, the importance of effective communication between all staff groups involved is highlighted. Emphasis should be placed on staff adhering to systems and procedures, as this is essential when we consider the number of patients who require inpatient care. It is important for medical secretaries to have an overview of the whole system to enable them to resolve queries, or to refer patients to the appropriate department or staff member. The medical secretary is often the first point of contact for patients, their relatives and staff in a patient's care.

Exercises

It is a Monday morning. You have just been informed the operating list has to be cancelled for that Thursday morning because the operating theatre your consultant uses has had to be closed for infection control. You have four patients to be admitted on the Wednesday for major or minor surgical procedures. They are to be operated on the Thursday. You manage the waiting list and sent letters out to the patients some weeks earlier giving them their TCI 'to come in' dates and all the patients have confirmed acceptance of these dates and have attended their pre-assessment appointments. How will you contact the patients? How do you think this may affect the patients and how may they react to this news? What and how will you explain to them what has happened? What follow up administrative procedures and arrangements will need to take place? Are there any other issues this situation may raise?

You are the medical secretary in the accident and emergency department. You receive a telephone call from the police. They say that a man by the name of Paul Johnson, date of birth 10.12.62, has been brought into hospital following a fight. He had allegedly been stabbed. (Paul Johnson is a local celebrity – being a member of a first division football team.) They want to know whether or not they can come in to see him. They would also like a statement from the doctor who is seeing him about his medical condition. How would you deal with this query? What issues does it raise?

SECTION 4

The secretary in general practice

Chapter 15

General practice and primary care

Barbara Jones

CHAPTER CONTENTS

OBJECTIVES

- To provide a brief history of general practice
- To describe the role of the GP in primary care and health promotion
- To identify the personnel working within primary health care
- To give a brief overview of areas used in health centres
- To stress the importance of standards within premises, maintenance and security.

INTRODUCTION

This section deals with general practice within the National Health Service and the wide-ranging areas of primary care. The present direction of health care focuses on general practice, allowing and encouraging GPs to take a major part in the standard of primary health care of their practice population and to take an active part in the motivation of the primary health care team.

Before you begin to study this chapter, you may find it useful to obtain a copy of a practice leaflet.

BRIEF HISTORY

The National Health Service (NHS) as we know it today came into being with the introduction of the NHS Act in 1946. Prior to that, the National Health

Insurance Scheme had been instituted in 1911 and all employed and self-employed people were obliged to pay contributions that entitled them to receive free medical care from a general practitioner. The introduction of the NHS Act extended this obligation to the whole population – 'A free Health Service for all'. There have been several changes made over the years and Acts of Parliament have been issued in order to carry out these changes. The NHS Act of 1977 requires that the Secretary of State continues to monitor and promote improvements in the health of the nation, not only in the diagnosis and treatment of illness but also through prevention measures. The NHS (General Medical Services) Regulations 1992 set out the terms and services which gave a framework within which all general practitioners worked and listed specific duties to be carried out. Payments made to general practitioners for this work were paid in accordance with the *Statement of Fees and Allowances,* most often referred to as the 'Red Book'. With the introduction of the new GP contract and PMS appointments, the use of the GMS Terms of Service and 'Red Book' will be radically altered. All doctors who wish to practise in the UK must, by law, be registered with the General Medical Council.

The introduction of fundholding in 1991 allowed some practices to purchase directly from hospitals the health care needed for their patients. They held their own budgets for various areas of health and were free to purchase from whichever 'provider' (hospital or Trust) they felt would supply the best service and value for money, for their patients.

The government has now abolished the 'internal market' within the NHS and based patient care on need and not on the practice's fund availability. Primary Care Groups (PCGs) and Primary Care Trusts (PCTs) have been set up since 1999, replacing fundholding. These consist of groups of practices within an area developing and managing the needs of patient care within that area and so delivering a service which is relevant and effective.

This new system abolishes the implication of a two-tier system of health care, whereby the best service was apparently available only to those who had budgets and money available within those budgets to pay for treatment. It has also introduced Clinical Governance, which involves every member of the primary health care team, and patients, encouraging best practice and observation of national standards, continually working for improvement in personal development and health care standards, and moni-

> **Box 15.1 Terms of service for doctors in general practice (DoH)**
>
> - Provision of services to patients – covering health checks and advice, diagnosis and treatment of the patient.
> - Obligations to the Primary Health Care Trust (PHCT) – to inform them of their hours of availability, regulations governing the employment of deputies and their ability to practise.
> - Acceptance of fees – rules and regulations governing the NHS fees payable for General Medical Services (GMS).
> - Practice leaflet – information about the personnel and services available and keeping this up to date.
> - Prescriptions and referrals – obligations to prescribe and refer patients for treatment.
> - Annual Reports – to provide Annual Reports for the PHCT on the activity and progress of the practice workload and employees.

toring services through the Commission for Health Improvement (CHI) and National Service Frameworks (NSFs).

THE ROLE OF THE GP IN PRIMARY CARE AND HEALTH PROMOTION

Most GPs practise within the National Health Service. They are not employed by the NHS but work under contract as *independent contractors* for the PCTs in their area. Details of their obligations as a GP working as part of the health service are laid out in the Department of Health *Terms of Service for Doctors in General Practice* (Box 15.1).

Registered GPs have a list of patients who have chosen to be treated by them and for whom they are responsible. Should a GP accept a new patient or remove a patient from his or her list, the relevant Health Authority must be informed immediately so that accurate details of the list size and the patients the doctor is responsible for are maintained.

The *Terms of Service for Doctors in General Practice* cover the wide-ranging areas of health care a doctor needs to provide and specific duties doctors must carry out. Besides treating patients who attend surgery, prescribing medication and making necessary home visits, they also have to carry out an active health promotion role within their practices. They are obliged to give advice on the patient's health status in the following areas:

- Obesity/exercise/smoking/alcohol and drugs – offering appropriate services to identify, control or reduce the risk of disease by giving advice on suitable lifestyle changes
- Over 75-year-old health checks – offering and providing health checks for elderly patients
- New patient health checks – providing health checks for new patients in order to give a basic insight into their health status
- Vaccination and immunisation – offering and providing the necessary vaccinations against measles, rubella, pertussis, Hib, polio, diphtheria and tetanus
- National screening – taking part in the national cervical cytology screening, and screening for diabetes, asthma and chronic/ischaemic heart disease as required by the government.

These priorities may change as information is collected and analysed highlighting other areas that need to be targeted. The government is constantly reviewing health promotion targets in order to address the wider influences on health such as the environment and poverty. Cytology and immunisation and health promotion targets are linked to income for the practice and the medical secretary's role in collecting accurate information and managing clinics is very important (see Chapter 16).

Reflection Point 1

How do practices encourage patients to participate in health screening?

PERSONNEL WORKING WITHIN PRIMARY HEALTH CARE

The personnel you will find working in primary care may vary depending on the size and type of surgery you work in. In a small *single-handed* practice, although having the district nurse, health visitor and midwife working with them, any additional services may have to be referred to the local hospitals. A larger, *group practice*, of two of two or more doctors working together to look after patients registered with them, would have bigger premises and the resources to hold several in-house services for patients, including chiropody and physiotherapy facilities.

This section provides a brief description of the people you may work with in general practice.

MEDICAL STAFF

Obviously these are the main core of general practice and patients will consult with them for medical advice and diagnosis of their symptoms. From this consultation they may be referred for specialist treatment at hospital or to one of the in-house services available to the patients, should the doctor feel this necessary.

Working arrangements will vary from practice to practice but depending on whether the doctor is employed on a full-time or part-time basis the number of hours he or she is available for surgeries and patient care will be set in a regular pattern. Rotas will be in place to cover weekend on-call work, out of hours call out and holiday cover.

Often in a group practice when a doctor is off for holiday, sickness or study leave there is flexibility in the surgery rota to allow the other doctors in the practice to cover the surgeries or a *locum doctor* is employed.

THE LOCUM DOCTOR

Locums are fully qualified doctors who have also completed 12 months in general practice as 'trainees', which gives them the qualification to work in general practice.

Often they are looking for permanent work as full partners within a partnership of doctors but carry out temporary work until they find a suitable position. *Partnerships* are groups of doctors who work together from one main surgery (plus small branch surgeries in some rural or large practices) to care for patients. As they are working as a small business and have overheads and responsibilities relating to this, *partnership agreements* which bind them legally to fulfil their part of the commitments of the practice are necessary. Carrying out locum work provides a valuable insight into the surgeries in the area and how they are run.

Locums can provide their services for one session only or longer periods if required and are paid by the hour or session at BMA rates. The GP remains contractually responsible for the services given by a locum to their patients, unless the locum is on the PCT's medical list.

GENERAL PRACTICE REGISTRARS

These are fully qualified doctors who are carrying out training to become general practitioners. They have to complete 12 months' training under the guidance of an approved GP trainer before they can apply to be general practitioners in their own right. Very often they have considerable hospital experience in medical fields other than general practice.

RETAINER DOCTORS

These are doctors, generally female, who work a reduced commitment of up to two sessions per week on the government-sponsored retainer scheme. This scheme allows women with family responsibilities to keep up to date and use their medical skills until they are able to increase their commitments to general practice.

ASSISTANTS

These are qualified doctors, like GPs, but they are employed directly by the GPs on a salaried basis. They often work part-time for just two or three sessions per week. They have the final clinical responsibility for the patients they treat but do not have a say in the running of the practice as they are not full partners.

ON-CALL AGENCY DOCTORS

There are agencies that work locally and nationally to provide on-call cover services. Surgeries are able to book doctors from the agency for short notice emergency rota cover.

Out of hours cover for night visits for patients is often covered by a cooperative of doctors in an area. A rota sharing the on-call nights is distributed and each surgery carries out its part in the rota. Whoever is on duty will see or speak to all the patients who request night visits irrespective of which surgery they are registered with.

THE PRACTICE NURSE

The practice nurse assists the doctor in delivering medical care to the patients. They hold health promotion clinics on topics including asthma, diabetes, family planning, holiday vaccine, heart disease and stroke clinics, besides carrying out basic nursing procedures such as dressing wounds, taking blood pressure, cholesterol and blood tests, giving injections and carrying out registration health checks. The practice nurse also has to keep up to date with training and additional courses. The intention is that the practice nurse can take all routine medical work from the doctor, freeing him or her to concentrate on more complex work and diagnosis. The practice nurse's training enables her or him to inform the doctor and highlight any concerns regarding patients. The role is gradually changing and expanding. The government is promoting the development of nurse practitioners who may become even more important in general practice as they will be allowed to diagnose and prescribe certain groups of medicines and undertake chronic disease management. Practice nurses will also work on applying and structuring health promotion protocols and guidelines.

HEALTH CARE ASSISTANTS

Health care assistants carry out the more basic nursing tasks such as taking blood samples, blood pressure checks, health checks on patients aged over 5 years, data entry on the computer, clinical stock control/ordering and generally helping to free the Practice Nurse to carry out more complex duties such as triaging appointments or holding minor illness clinics.

PHLEBOTOMIST

Phlebotomists are trained only to take blood samples from patients. They are not qualified to carry our any other nursing tasks but again help to reduce the Practice Nurse's workload.

ANCILLARY STAFF

Practice manager

Most practices today employ a practice manager to supervise and implement the smooth running of the practice. They take the workload from the senior partners and allow them to concentrate on patient care. The practice manager will be responsible for all staff personnel matters and the selection and training of administration staff.

They will meet with the partners and discuss prac-

Box 15.2 Job description for a medical secretary

JOB TITLE: *SECRETARY*

MAIN PURPOSE OF THE POST: *To provide a wide range of duties including secretarial, clerical and computer input to facilitate the administration work required to provide an efficient medical service to the patients.*

RESPONSIBLE TO: *Practice manager.*

MAJOR DUTIES AND RESPONSIBILITIES
1. Secretarial duties.
2. Clerical duties.
3. Computer duties.
4. Monitor of stationery stock levels.
5. Any other delegated duties considered appropriate to the post.

SPECIFIC TASKS

1. Secretarial duties
   - All hospital referrals (5 partners, retainer doctor, locum doctors).
   - Typing miscellaneous letters.
   - Hospital enquiries – results, appointments, etc.
   - Deal with enquiries/requests from solicitors, consultants and hospitals relating to patients.

2. Clerical duties
   - Sorting insurance reports, DSS forms, filling in tracer card to obtain records ready for the doctor.
   - Monitoring all inadequate/abnormal smears and sending appropriate letters to patients.
   - Sorting the morning post and allocate to the correct partner.
   - Selecting appropriate mail for the computer operator.

3. Computer duties
   - Entering date of receipt of insurance reports, etc.
   - Using the Medical System word processor to record referral letters.
   - Using the Medical System word processor to produce smear repeat letters.

4. Monitor of stationery stock levels
   - On a regular basis monitor general usage and request requirements for stationery orders.
   - Liaise with the practice manager for order/purchase of requirements.

tice policies and systems, manage the practice accounts and staff payroll, liaise with the PCT on behalf of the practice and organise primary health care team meetings. They will also ensure that procedures are in place to maximise the practice income from item of service claims and check all quarterly payments from the PCT for accuracy. They will be responsible for the execution of health and safety procedures within the practice and the implementation of the practice complaints procedure.

Office manager/administrator

Sometimes the practice manager has the help of an office manager or administrator who will monitor and control the work carried out with item of service claims and the basic smooth running of the administration side of general practice. This is often a role taken over by the senior receptionist or medical secretary. Depending on the type of practice you work in, if you are able to develop your skills and knowledge to cover all aspects of general practice work, then a career progression towards management is appropriate.

Business manager

The Business Manager will manage the practice accounts and negotiate contracts on behalf of the practice, or in conjunction with the partners, for any enhanced services the surgery is able to provide. They will prepare reports, figures, statistics and accounts. In some practices the Business Manager and the Practice Manager are the same person. Although fundholding was phased out under changes within the NHS, budgetary control remains an important function within general practice.

Computer staff

Most surgeries employ data input clerks to ensure all health promotion details are entered on the computer. They may carry out only these duties or also be involved in medical audits and development of the full use of the computer system, setting up templates for the accurate and appropriate capture of information on the health status of patients within the practice and the 'at risk' groups such as Coronary Heart Disease (CHD), asthma, diabetes etc. Efficient collection of data adds to the income of the practice. See also Chapter 16 for more information.

Receptionists

Most receptionists are employed on a part-time basis. Their duties cover not only basic reception desk duties and first-line patient contact but also filing, processing repeat prescriptions, giving out test results to patients once they have been checked by the doctor (the doctor usually contacts the patient where results are abnormal or indicate that an appointment should be made for the patient to discuss the result), booking ambulance transport, X-rays, appointments, home visits, pulling records for surgeries and countless other tasks which are essential parts of the job. Often there is a full-time senior receptionist who has a supervisory role in addition to reception duties and ensures the smooth running of reception and efficient processing of item of service claims.

Medical secretary

Depending on the type of surgery you are working in, your duties may vary from basic audio typing of referral letters and booking hospital appointments to working with the doctors and nursing staff to implement the surgery cervical recall system, medical audits, taking minutes of primary health care meetings, and developing the practice computer system to maximise its use.

In a single-handed doctor practice you would probably be carrying out reception, secretarial and, if the practice is a dispensing one, dispensing duties which would give you an excellent foundation of experience to develop your career.

In a larger practice there would be more staff available to specialise in different areas of administration. As a medical secretary you could be working with the practice manager on improving inefficient work processes, improving working conditions and ensuring the smooth running of the practice. Box 15.2 provides a sample job description.

Other primary health care team members

The primary health care team consists not just of the general practice staff but of all the additional medical disciplines that work together to provide a complete and caring service to the patient. They are all qualified in their own fields of work and are attached to the practice. They are not employed directly by the practice but through the PCT or through the contract set up with the Trust who employs them.

District nurses carry out their work with housebound patients who need clinical assistance to cope with their illness. Their work may also cover running clinics, for example a diabetic clinic, which monitor the disease and give lifestyle advice to patients.

Health visitors are well known for involvement with child care development but this is only one area of their work. They can be involved with health clinics, parenthood classes, 'Look After Yourself' lifestyle clinics and links with the elderly – not just the baby clinic and childhood immunisation programme. Patients do not have to be referred to the health visitor by the doctor, they can refer themselves. Suitably qualified health visitors can also prescribe some basic medication relevant to their patients' requirements.

Midwives carry out visits to patients before and after the birth of their babies, hold antenatal clinics including relaxation and child care instruction within the surgery to monitor the pregnancies and, as part of the 'named-nurse' continuing care policy, are pres-

Box 15.3 Reasons for contacting the social services department

1. *Fostering and adoption of children* – the GP will be involved in giving medical opinions about the adopters, fosterers and the children if they are registered with the practice.
2. *Accommodation for the elderly* – Should it become increasingly difficult for an elderly patient to look after themselves, or close relatives of the elderly patient are unable to cope with looking after them, the doctor may contact the social services for their help in arranging full-time care for the patient, or various in-house help or aids such as additional stair rails, equipment to help the patient bathe easily, cooker adaptations, meals on wheels and home helps.
3. *Respite care* – Some relatives who care for elderly patients in their own homes can have short periods when the patient can go into nursing home care for respite care. This gives the carer a few weeks 'holiday' and eases the strain of caring for an invalid or sick relative.
4. *Accommodation for patients* – Poor housing conditions often aggravate some health problems and the GP may recommend better housing as a clinical priority for these patients.

ent for the birth of the baby whether the delivery is at home or in the hospital. They visit the mother for a specified length of time after the birth to ensure that mother and baby are well and there are no problems.

Physiotherapists work in-house supplying a rapid-access physiotherapy service for patients and can also continue the treatment at the hospital should more complex equipment be required to treat the patient.

Chiropodists/Podiatrists work in-house or at health centres or hospitals usually looking after the foot care of diabetic patients or the elderly, children with foot problems, pregnant women and disabled patients.

Counsellors work for the practice on a sessional basis, counselling patients referred to them by the doctor. By employing a counsellor the practice can benefit in many ways. Practices have counsellors to help people deal with their personal problems and counselling of this nature cannot be carried out in a normal surgery appointment time. The counsellor is trained to lis-

ten to patients and to help them come to terms with personal problems in a positive way. The prescribing of antidepressants and tranquillisers can be greatly reduced when patients are able to cope with their problems. Patients have to be referred by the GP to the surgery counsellor. Patients can self-refer to a private counsellor and would pay any fees for this service.

Community psychiatric nurses are named nurses attached to the surgery and they use their skills and training to treat more complex mental problems than the counsellor. They often carry out rehabilitation work with patients discharged from psychiatric units to live in the community and with drug addicts, working closely with the GP.

Social workers are attached to the practice and they are the link doctor's contact when patients need additional care or services beyond medical assistance. You may have to contact the social services department for a variety of reasons (Box 15.3).

Macmillan nurses are nurses especially concerned with the care of cancer patients and are often linked with hospices in the locality.

Alternative medicine practitioners may practise aromatherapist, acupuncture, homeopathy, or reflexology. These services are not commonplace and you will find that most practices do not hold them in-house and in these cases patients would have to pay privately for consultations.

It is important that you get to know the members of the primary health care team and all the practice staff as you will be working with them as part of the team. Knowledge of each role and the part they play within the organisation helps strengthen your ability to work as an efficient and valued team member.

Reflection Point 2

Make a note of all the professionals you come into contact with at work or on your GP placement. How does the practice encourage a feeling of team participation?

ENSURING GOOD SERVICE

All general practices today have to have a *practice charter* listing items and standards the practice provides to its patients and the basic expectations the surgery has of its patients. Public and patient involvement groups are encouraged in most forward looking surgeries to help promote understanding and good relationships when working through changes or developing services. Patient satisfaction questionnaires are important and necessary in this area too (Figure 15.1).

A *complaints procedure* is another requirement and there are standard information packs with guidelines to help practices put together their own procedures. Samples of these are given in Figures 15.2-15.6. Patients' Forums and PALS (see Chapter 2) ensure patient and public involvement in the NHS Strategy now being developed to promote good relationships between doctor and patient throughout the NHS, and to look at clinical governance from the patient's perspective.

Reflection Point 3

Are these notices available in languages other than English? Consider the local population using the practice. Is this and other sources of information clear and accessible to everyone?

OVERVIEW OF AREAS IN HEALTH CENTRES

The basic layout required in health centres includes a reception desk, patients' waiting area and a consultation room for the doctor. Not many years ago this was the norm. Today, with all the additional services doctors are obliged to provide and the services they want to provide for their patients 'in-house', much larger accommodation is required. Not only does the waiting room provide a seating area with magazines for patients and various health leaflets, you may also find areas set aside specifically with children in mind with several choices of toys and games. The in-house services supplied speed up the delivery of treatment and you will find rooms for practice nurses, counsellors, physiotherapists, chiropodists, midwives, alternative medicine practitioners and some surgeries supply an area office for district nurses and health visitors to use as a base. These additional in-house clinics allow the patient to be treated quickly, close to home, so providing better health care. There are usually additional offices for the practice manager and secretarial and computer sup-

port staff, and a library or common room where team meetings, training sessions and study can take place.

THE IMPORTANCE OF PREMISES PRESENTATION

As previously mentioned, the premises of today's surgeries are much larger and kept to a higher standard. From the patient's point of view it is important that the waiting room is pleasant in appearance, clean and well organised with useful, informative leaflets and information to hand – and of course a good supply of recent magazines. Any notice boards should be well maintained with posters neatly and clearly laid out – not pinned up in a cluttered and disorganised manner so that patients cannot read them clearly. A badly laid out information notice board is worse than useless to patients or the surgery attempting to inform them.

Some surgeries may have piped music in the waiting room, which is pleasant to listen to and relaxing for the patient, or perhaps a television screen with video presentations of health information.

A play area or corner for young children with simple toys and children's books is usually available, but again this should be kept tidy and all toys should be in a clean condition and washed regularly. Care needs to be taken in this area with regard to age suitability, hygiene and space required.

Reflection Point 4

List the toys you think are suitable and unsuitable.

Seating should be in good condition and not torn and dirty. First impressions are very important and simple measures of regular maintenance in these areas will keep your surgery welcoming and efficient.

Reflection Point 5

If you were planning to redecorate and replace items in your surgery, what would be the most important points to take into consideration?

Our responsibilities

1. You will be treated sympathetically and politely by Practice Staff.
2. Your privacy and confidentiality will be respected at all times.
3. We will do everything possible to ensure that our systems for providing a health care service to you are reliable and effective.
4. Patients are at liberty to see any of the partners irrespective of the doctor they are registered with.
5. You will have a right to information about your own health, treatment and its likely outcome.
6. You will be offered a Health Check on joining the Practice and given information and advice on maintaining good health and avoiding illness.
7. All patients of 75 years and over will be offered an annual health check.
8. Urgent emergency cases will be seen the same day in the surgery.
9. You will be seen within 30 minutes of your appointment time unless some unforeseen emergency delays the doctor. In such a case the receptionist will keep you informed.

Your responsibilities

1. To be polite to doctors and staff.
2. To give the practice adequate notice if you wish to cancel an appointment.
3. To request home visits before 11.00 a.m. and only if they are medically necessary and you are too ill to attend the surgery.
4. To give at least 24 hours' notice for a request for a repeat prescription. These should be collected within one month.
5. When you are notified that a repeat prescription is due for a review you should make an appointment to see the doctor before your next request.
6. If you need to speak to a preferred named doctor you must wait until after booked surgery appointments.
7. No smoking on the premises.
8. To inform the surgery straight away if you change your address.

Figure 15.1 A practice charter. (Reproduced by permission of Elms Medical Centre, Chester)

THE ELMS MEDICAL CENTRE

Complaints Protocol

1. All complaints concerning the practice should be referred immediately to the Practice Manager.

2. The Practice Manager will reply to/contact the complainant within two working days and investigate the complaint.

3. All details of the investigation will be recorded.

4. Once the investigation is complete the Practice Manager will report back to the Practice.

5. The Practice Manager together with the partnership will decide how best to report back to the complainant.

6. An explanation will be sent to the complainant within ten working days. (If this is not possible, the Practice Manager will contact the complainant to explain the delay and set a revised time scale for the conclusion of the procedure.)

7. If, following the practice's explanation, the complainant remains dissatisfied, they will be informed of their rights to pursue the complaint via the Primary Care Trust (PCT).

   The PCT number is 01244 650300

   (Freephone Number 0800 132996)

Figure 15.2 A complaints protocol. (Figures 15.2–15.6 reproduced by permission of Elms Medical Centre, Chester)

Cleanliness in the surgery is obviously very important. Surgery cleaners or contract cleaners should ensure that treatment rooms are thoroughly cleaned to avoid any possibility of infection being spread from unhygienic standards. The waiting room areas, reception and toilets should be cleaned daily and all rubbish placed outside in appropriate containers ready for collection. All treatment room and consultation room clinical waste is classed as *hazardous waste* and should be placed in yellow waste collection bags ready for collection with the yellow sharps polythene box containers that hold used syringes. These are collected separately by an authorised contractor and are incinerated, for they are governed by the Control of Substances Hazardous to Health Regulations 1989 (see Chapter 17).

STATIONERY STOCK ITEMS

The doctors' surgeries should be well stocked with relevant forms and information that are used regularly and the medical secretary should check these stocks weekly and ensure they are restocked and arranged tidily. The doctor does not want to have to search for regularly used forms in the middle of a consultation.

General stationery stocks should be monitored and a list of stock requirements given to the practice manager for reordering; often this is the responsibility of the secretary. Postage costs and postage stamps will be recorded and a record kept.

Reflection Point 6

What other stocks should be checked?

SECURITY

A great deal of equipment and confidential information is held in surgeries so security is of prime importance. Not only the commitment every employee makes to confidentiality of patient details and information but the need to safeguard the building that houses this information is of prime importance. You may be asked to sign a notice of confidentiality, as shown in Figure 15.7. Burglar alarms and security lighting are additions to robust locks and sometimes, depending on the area the

---

THE ELMS MEDICAL CENTRE

Notice to Patients

In this Practice we operate a Practice Complaints Procedure as part of the N.H.S. system for dealing with complaints.

Our aim is to provide you with a high standard of care and we will try to deal swiftly with any problems that may occur.

Our Practice Manager or Senior Receptionist can give you further information.

Figure 15.3 A notice to patients about the practice complaints procedure

premises are in, and insurance requirements, metal shutters are installed.

Personal safety is obviously important. Although very few patients are aggressive or disruptive to the general running of the surgery, there are a small number that have to be carefully managed. The experienced receptionist will cope relatively easily with these patients and it would be an advantage to spend part of your induction period to the practice in reception observing these skills. Keeping calm, not taking any verbal abuse personally, quietly but positively dealing with the situation will often keep the agitated and abusive patient under control – at least until the practice manager or a doctor is available. (See also Chapter 5.)

Violent patients are a similar concern and obviously your safety and the safety of other patients in the waiting room are of paramount importance. Some surgeries have alarm buttons to press when staff are in threatening situations. For uncontrollable patients calls should be made directly to the police

This leaflet explains how you can share your views or concerns about any aspect of the service you receive from us.

If you would like more information about this you can telephone The Complaints Manager on FREEPHONE 0800 132996

If you prefer you can write to

The Chief Executive
South Cheshire Primary Care Trust
FREEPOST (no stamp required)
1829 Building
Countess of Chester Health Park
Liverpool Road
Chester CH2 1YZ

The Elms Medical Centre

*Your views –
good or bad –
are always welcome.*

Our simple procedure can resolve concerns quickly and confidentially by giving you an opportunity to express your views – good or bad.

The person responsible for dealing with your comments and complaints is the Practice Manager.

If you have discussed an issue with her and are still unhappy we respect your right to make a complaint.

We have forms available for you to fill in with details of your complaint.

Your complaint should be made as soon as possible, ideally within a matter of days, so that we can investigate accurately while things are still fresh in everyone's mind.

If, for some reason this is not possible you should let us have details of your complaint:

- within 6 months of the incident

OR

- within 6 months of discovering that you have a problem, provided this is within 12 months of the incident.

We will send you a written acknowledgement within two working days of receiving your complaint and will do all we can to complete our investigation within ten working days.

We will then write to you again with an explanation or suggest a meeting with those involved.

If you are still dissatisfied or perhaps you don't want to raise the problem directly with us, you have the right to raise the matter with South Cheshire Primary Care Trust.

Figure 15.4 Excerpt from a leaflet explaining the complaints procedure

COMPLAINTS FORM

Complainant Details

Surname _____ Forenames _____

Address_____

_____

_____

_____

Telephone_____ Date of Birth_____

Patient's Details (where different from above):

Surname _____ Forenames _____

Address_____

_____

_____

_____

Details of Complaint
(including date(s) of events and persons involved)

_____

_____

_____

_____

_____

_____

(Continued on next page)

Date: _____ Complainant's Signature: _____

Where the complainant is not the patient:

I authorise the complaint set out above to be made on my behalf (name) _____
and I agree that the practice may disclose to (name) _____
(only in so far as is necessary to answer the complaint) any confidential information about me which I
provided to them.

Patient's Signature: _____ Date: _____

Figure 15.5 A complaints form

COMPLAINT ACTION SHEET

Complainant Details

Surname _____ Forenames _____

Name of Patient (if different)_____

Consent required: YES / NO   Date of Birth: _____

Contact Telephone Number: _____

First Contact made by: Telephone _____ Letter _____ Personal Contact_____

Date of Incident: _____   Complaint Received: _____

Received by: _____

Summary of Complaint:

_____
_____
_____
_____
_____
_____

Action Taken:

_____
_____

DETAILS OF RESPONSE

By (name): _____

First Contact made by: Telephone _____ Letter _____ Personal Contact _____

Date:

_____
_____
_____
_____
_____
_____

Outcome: SATISFIED / DISSATISFIED

If dissatisfied has the complainant been informed of PCT contacts   YES ☐   NO ☐

Figure 15.6 A complaint action sheet

CONFIDENTIALITY

In the course of your duties you may have access to confidential material about patients or other health service business. On no account must information relating to identifiable patients be divulged to anyone other than authorised persons.

Failure to observe these rules will be regarded by your employers as serious misconduct which could result in serious disciplinary action being taken against you, including dismissal.

Signed _____

Date _____

Figure 15.7 A notice of confidentiality

station to have them removed from the premises. Very often doctors will refuse to treat patients who are violent or abusive to staff and will have them removed from the list if incidents occur repeatedly. The Health Authority or various private training companies hold courses in dealing with this type of patient.

Reflection Point 7

Find out if there is any training available in your surgery.

COMPUTERS

Computers and medical equipment need to be security code marked and computer file servers should be enclosed in security casing and secured to the floor.

BUILDING MAINTENANCE

GPs by law have a duty to ensure the safety of anyone who enters the surgery and may be liable if there is an accident. Therefore it is extremely important to keep the building and all equipment in good repair. All maintenance to the fabric of the building, equipment and security systems is organised by the practice manager. Yearly maintenance checks are made on equipment and the building security system and any repairs are carried out immediately.

CONCLUSION

This chapter has provided an overview of general practice and the people who work there, and the roles and functions they fulfil. It has also provided an introduction to your role as a medical secretary within general practice. The most important thing to remember is that in general practice you are part of a team that ensures the effective running of the practice. Do take the opportunity to find out as much as possible about the practices you have been involved with either as a medical secretary or as a patient.

Exercises

- Compare different practice leaflets if available. Try to think of them from the perspective of the patient. Are they helpful? Could they be improved?

- Find out more about other personnel involved. Talk to them about what they do.

- All practices are different. While on work placements compare notes on the variety of provision and collect material to help you build a full picture of your surgery's methods of ensuring good service.

Further reading

Lilley R 2003 The new GP contract: How to make the most of it. Radcliffe Medical Press, Abingdon

National Health Service 1996 Practice-based complaints procedures. HMSO, London

Quinn NE, Simon P 1996 The GP receptionists handbook. Baillière Tindall, London

Chapter 16

The working practice

Barbara Jones

OBJECTIVES

- To provide a broad outline of the numerous tasks carried out daily in general practice

- To explain the uses of computer systems in general practice

- To give an overview of procedures carried out in general practice and associated claims

- To emphasise the importance of accurate storing and retrieval of information

- To give a brief description of the various rotas and protocols used to ensure good practice.

INTRODUCTION

This chapter explains how general practice works and the medical secretary's role in assuring the smooth running of the practice. There are a vast range of tasks performed in general practice and teamwork and accuracy when carrying out your part are essential.

GENERAL PRACTICE TODAY

High standards are needed in today's general practice. Not only are there high levels of skills and services available for patients, patients themselves have high expectations of health care professionals and are far more demanding of the services they receive.

With the introduction of Primary Care Trusts, closer links with surgeries, hospitals and othe health care agencies, including the voluntary sector, help to develop services appropriate for the needs of the area or localities.

PRACTICE CHARTER

Guidelines for your surgery will be contained in the practice charter and it will state the maximum length of time patients are expected to wait until they are seen. They should be informed if the doctor is delayed and offered another appointment on another day if they cannot wait. Patients need to know what basic standards they can expect from their surgery and the practice charter provides this. In order for the standards to be met there should also be some commitment from the patient and many surgeries have patient's charters to give guidance on the basic expectations the surgery has of its patients. When patients and doctors work together in this way standards and services can be delivered in a positive and effective manner. (See Figure 15.1 in the previous chapter for an example of a practice charter.)

COMPUTERS IN GENERAL PRACTICE

In order to keep pace with the many changes and provide a caring yet efficient service in general practice, use of modern technology is essential (see also Chapter 8). There are several computer medical systems developed especially for use in the doctor's surgery such as Vamp, EMIS, Meditel and Genisyst. These systems provide quick and efficient retrieval of information. Whichever system you are working with, it will be networked throughout the surgery. This allows doctors, reception and the medical secretary access to enter their specific work onto the patients' files at the same time. The computer stores all this information and it can be searched, audited or retrieved at any time within minutes. All the clinical systems have a basic word-processing programme which enables the medical secretary to type referral letters and process bulk recall letters to groups of patients by mail merging quickly and efficiently.

Most practices will also have various software on additional computers which enable them to carry out word processing with advanced capabilities for producing professional posters, newsletters and leaflets. Spreadsheet software is also invaluable for producing activity statistics, rotas, financial forecasts, etc. The practice accounts system and payroll, whether they are specific software packages purchased for the task or in-house spreadsheets, are also quick, easy and accurate in producing the financial records of the practice.

Computer systems in general practice are fast becoming indispensable. All the information required on all aspects of the work carried out in the practice once entered on the computer can be easily retrieved in a variety of ways and statistics can be produced to give a simple picture of the facts you are looking at. Entering patients on the medical database dispenses with the necessity to compile an age/sex register.

The manual age/sex register consisted of writing out two identical index cards containing basic details of patients when they registered. They were then filed into two sections of male and female and one set filed alphabetically and the other in date of birth order.

Once entered on the computer, details from the database can be searched rapidly on many areas, not just name and date of birth. Addresses, families, streets or roads or even postcodes depending on the information you need to match can be obtained with just a few key strokes, not an afternoon or days checking through thousands of cards.

As long as you have adequate back-ups for the daily input of data you need never worry too much should the computer go down or 'crash'.

Details entered on the practice computer can be accessed from any computer in the building as long as it is networked to the main file server. Claims, medical histories, health promotion details and also referral letters can be viewed quickly and easily from anywhere in the building without having to check files, folders or log books in reception, the practice manager's room, or treatment room.

National Service Frameworks (NSFs) have been introduced to provide guide lines and to standard-

Reflection Point 1

What are the security and confidentiality issues concerning the increased use of computers in general practice?

APPLICATION TO GO ON A DOCTOR'S LIST
(Form FP1)

General Information

Applications to go on a doctor's list are filled in and used when the patient wishes to register with the practice but does not have his NHS medical card available.

FILLING IN THE FORM

1. Ensure the form is filled in completely with:
    a) The **patient's Surname, Forename, any previous Surname**.
    b) **Date of birth** and **whether male or female** (this is particularly useful when accepting foreign patients with unusual names).
    c) Their **full permanent address with Postcode**.
    d) Enter **the NHS number**, if known.
    e) Their **previous doctor** and his **address**.
    f) The **patient's previous address, town or country of birth**.

2. *If the patient has been abroad* and is returning to reside in this country *or moved from abroad to live here*, ensure that:
    a) The **date of arrival** is filled in and the **date when the patient left this country**.

3. **Ensure the patient signs the form and dates it.**

4. On the reverse of the form **the parent** of a child applying to go on the doctor's list should **tick the box for child health surveillance**.
    The patient can also indicate whether or not they would like to be an organ donor.

5. On the reverse of the form you should also **ensure the doctor's name, code number and signature with date are entered**.

    It is essential that all new patients over 5 years old **MUST BE OFFERED AN APPOINTMENT** TO SEE THE **PRACTICE NURSE FOR A HEALTH CHECK**.

Figure 16.1 Instructions for filling out Form FP1 (application to go on a doctor's list)

ise information on specific diseases such as diabetes, asthma, heart disease and mental health. The use of computerised systems is essential to provide quality information quickly and easily.

PATHOLOGY TESTS – LABORATORY LINKS TO PRACTICE

Another development that is gaining momentum in general practice is the linking up of hospital computers with the general practice computer to provide fast and efficient service in supplying the results of patients' laboratory tests. Tests are carried out at the pathology laboratory and the results entered on the hospital computer. These are sent down the modem line to the practice 'mail box' at a certain time during the night and the practice computer 'picks up' information placed in its mail box at a set time during the night or early morning. When the computers are switched on in the morning the patient's results are already on computer for the doctor to view and assess.

BASIC REGISTRATION PROCEDURES

When a patient comes to the Reception Desk to register with the Practice they should be asked to fill in a GMS1 (purple form) if they do not have their Medical Card.

Ask them to go to the side of the Reception Desk if reception is busy to fill in the form.

When they have completed the form the receptionist should check that all the details have been filled in correctly.

An appointment can then be made for the patient with the nurse for a registration health check *(or an appointment with the doctor if the patient needs to be seen).*

The GMS1 or Medical Card should then be placed in a doctor's tray ready for the doctor's signature. (Applications should be signed daily.)

The Senior Receptionist will make out the Provisional Record folders with the necessary basic continuation sheets for each new application and the folder will be filed with the Provisional Records awaiting full records from the Support Services.

Once the applications have been signed by the doctor they should be forwarded to the Administration Office to be processed on the GP Link computer.

When the full notes arrive at the surgery from the Support Services they will be cleared as received on the computer if using GP Links and forwarded to be summarised and sent out to the branches.

The provisional notes at the branch will be matched and added to the full notes and the complete file will then be stored in the main records filing system.

The empty Provisional Folder can then be re-used for another patient.

Keeping provisional files separately not only prevents duplication of files and applications but it is a good check on any outstanding medical records.

The Senior Receptionist should check each week if any Provisional Files are over six weeks old. If there are any, a list should be drawn up with the patient's name, date of birth, address and date of registration and forwarded to the Practice Manager who will arrange contact with the Support Services requesting the notes.

Figure 16.2 Instructions relating to basic registration procedures

Procedure for Completing a Temporary Resident/
Immediately Necessary/Emergency Treatment Form

1. Obtain relevant details to complete the form (over the telephone or at the desk).

2. Make the appointment entering TR by the name of the patient in the Appointment Book.

3. **Write the date and time of the appointment at the top of the form.**

4. **Place the form at the front desk** – to await the appointment.
    (This will prevent any TR forms being lost/duplicated or incomplete forms being sent to the doctor for signing and notes can be kept on those who did not attend.)

5. When the patient arrives for the appointment carry out the following:
    a) Quickly **check the form** to ensure we have all the necessary information filled in.
    b) **Give the form to the patient** to confirm that all the details entered are correct.
    c) When satisfied the form has been completed correctly give the patient the form and **ask them to take a seat and hand it to the doctor/nurse when they are called in**.

6. Once the patient has been seen the doctor/nurse will then fill in the consultation details. The doctor will sign and date the form and it should be placed with the records and returned to reception at the end of surgery. **N.B. (Practice Nurse appointments will only have consultation details and should be placed in a doctor's tray for the doctor to sign once they have been seen and have been returned to reception with the other surgery records.)**

7. Staff filing records should remove any TR forms and place them in the TR box, and file them alphabetically.

8. The Senior Receptionist will check them weekly and return all TRs that have expired to the Administration office to be checked and forwarded to the Support Services.

Figure 16.3 Instructions for completing a temporary resident form

---

Deceased Patient Protocol

When the surgery is informed that a patient has died at home:

1.   **Pass the message on to the Doctor** together with the patient's Medical Record.

2.   **Write** the **name of** the **patient** on the **Notice Board** in reception.

3.   **Doctor** will **inform the District Nurse** if it was a terminally ill patient.

4.   **Secretary** will **inform** the **hospital** by telephoning.

5.   Ensure the **cause of death** is **entered** in the **Medical Record** and on the computer.

Figure 16.4 A deceased patient protocol

The government hopes to develop these links even further, so that hospitals and surgeries can send referral letters via links and actually book appointments for patients at the hospital on the same day they visit surgery. Information links with other providers would certainly cut down on the amount of paper that is passed via surgery delivery services informing practices of courses, item of service updates, and the mass of information that is churned out weekly in order to keep communications between providers up to date. Once these advances have been perfected the benefits of computer networks can be fully appreciated.

REGISTERING NEW PATIENTS

The use of the computer in processing registrations and claims forms is another area where time and efficiency has been applied. Managed well, this system has been a great success for improved accuracy of claims and prompt payment.

The medical computer system is used in all aspects of general practice. If we begin at the beginning, the first contact a patient makes at a surgery to register is logged on the computer. The details from this medical card, form GMS4 or a purple registration form GMS1, are checked through with the patient to ensure all entries are completed. There is a section on the back of the GMS1 form which allows patients to give consent for their inclusion on the Organ Donor Register. The details are then entered on the computer system and sent through a modem line via GP Links to the NHS Support Services and are acknowledged within

48 hours. Once acknowledged, the patient is included on the list of the practice and the doctor begins receiving a payment each quarter for supplying medical services.

Once the patient is accepted onto the list, the Support Service requests the medical records from the patient's previous doctor and usually within 4 to 6 weeks the full medical notes are with the practice. If the doctor requires the records immediately the Support Services will request them from the previous doctor or if they are moving into the area from another Health Care Trust they will contact them to obtain the records urgently.

Patients registering with the practice must be living within the practice boundary. The doctors define their practice area in the practice leaflet and patients living outside this should not be registered. When patients register with the doctor they are usually asked to make an appointment with the practice nurse for a registration health check. This allows the practice to obtain information from patients on their medical history and details of any medicines they are presently taking. Details from the health check are valuable ways of obtaining the health promotion data which is requested each year.

Basic instructions on how to register patients and when to fill in the various claims forms are usually available in all practices (Figures 16.1-16.3). These help staff learn new procedures and are invaluable when new staff or college students begin work in the practice. Although the forms and regulations governing them are the same you will find that each practice has its own way of implementing them.

Reflection Point 2

Patients don't have to give a reason when they change doctors. Should doctors have to give a reason when they remove patients from their practice list?

PATIENTS LEAVING THE PRACTICE

When patients leave the practice the Support Services requests the patient's records and it is the practice's duty to return these records immediately. The patient's new doctor may require urgent access to the medical history; therefore it is a responsibility that must be fulfilled. Medical records are the property of the National Health Service and therefore belong to the government. The doctors are responsible for them during the time the patient is registered with the practice and strict confidentiality rules must be adhered to by practice staff.

CHANGING DOCTORS

Patients have a right to change doctor without giving a reason and therefore they can move from practice to practice if they are not satisfied with the service they are receiving. In cases like this their medical records will be requested via GP Links if you are computerised or from a computer printout sheet called the FP22.

DECEASED PATIENTS

If a patient dies the Registrar of Births and Deaths notifies the Support Services and they will then remove the patient from your list and request the return of the medical records. More internal work within the practice has to be carried out when a patient dies as they may be on a consultant's list at the hospital or on a practice recall list (Figure 16.4). If this is the case the hospital has to be contacted so that no future appointments will be sent to the patient's home. It can be very distressing for relatives if this happens. It is usually the medical secretary's job to contact the hospital and inform the necessary department of the death.

FORM FP69

This is a green card which is issued to the surgery when an item of mail has been sent from the Support Services to the patient and been returned by the Post Office as not living at that address anymore. The Support Services then put a tag on the patient's computer details, and produce and send the green card to the practice. If it is not returned with the patient's new address, or confirmation of the address already on the system within six months the patient is taken off the list. The records are returned and stored at the Support Services until the patient registers elsewhere in the same area or the United Kingdom and then the notes are passed on to the new doctor.

REMOVAL OF A PATIENT FROM THE PRACTICE LIST

A doctor can remove a patient from his or her list without giving a reason but it is good practice to give the patient a letter explaining the reasons for their removal. This may be because the patient has moved outside the practice boundary or because there has been an irretrievable breakdown in the relationship between the doctor and patient. Patients who behave badly at the surgery by being violent or abusive to staff, or make inappropriate demands upon the practice by making frequent request for home visits for minor issues, can be removed from the list at the doctor's request.

APPOINTMENT SYSTEMS

Each doctor, nurse or in-house specialist will have their own schedule of surgeries. Doctors will normally have two surgeries per day – morning and afternoon/evening. Consultation times may vary from doctor to doctor, with one allowing 10 minutes per consultation and another 7 minutes, another only 5 minutes, another less but with a block every few patients to allow for 'catch up' time. Check the appointment system where you are and analyse how it is worked out and what types of things have been taken into consideration when setting it up.

Consultation statistics can be compiled easily from computerised appointment systems but practices usually have an adequate manual system in place to monitor the workload and home visits made by the doctors (Figure 16.5).

The various clinics held in the practice, e.g. diabetic, asthma, antenatal, child health, minor surgery, will all be set in a regular pattern and the correct length of time allowed for each type of consultation.

The community midwife will hold her clinics to monitor the progress of the mother and developing baby and gradually build a relationship with the mother-to-be to give her confidence to discuss any problems or worries. Should the mother wish to have a home delivery then this relationship is paramount. The shared-care system of midwife, doctor, health visitor and members of the primary health care team all working together for the benefit of the patient is highlighted in the antenatal and child health clinics, where several disciplines of medical care are pulled together.

Child health clinics run by the health visitor in conjunction with a doctor from the surgery monitor child development and immunisation status. These clinics are usually noisy, relaxed and welcoming. Mothers with babies and toddlers attend to have the baby weighed and discuss with the health visitor any queries they may have about feeding or concerns about their child. As their baby grows regular development checks on height/length, weight, hearing and eyesight, movements, etc., are carried out by the doctor at various ages, usually 6 weeks, 4 months and 3 years. If the child does not seem to be developing to the standard levels required, the doctor can refer the child to a relevant hospital consultant for appropriate treatment or diagnosis at an early stage.

The practice nurse will be responsible for holding clinics in the surgery with direct access to the doctor if any urgent treatment is required. The nurse's rotas may be set for different types of clinics, e.g. asthma, well woman, or a general clinic is held which covers all areas and in which opportunistic screening or monitoring is carried out. As various checks and procedures take different lengths of time, basic timetables have to be made available for the receptionist when booking appointments and written instructions should also be in place (Figures 16.6 and 16.7). This avoids overbooking appointments and allows a greater understanding of the procedures being carried out. Some surgeries have introduced nurse triage of urgent appointments and home visits. The expertise of a qualified triage nurse helps to alleviate the increasing demands on doctor time and inappropriate home visits. She is qualified to discuss medical prob-

Reflection Point 3

A patient is demanding an immediate appointment – consider ways of coping with this demand and a full appointments schedule.

lems and, following strict protocols, give basic medical advice, or book the patient into an urgent appointment. Some nurses, district nurses and health visitors are also qualified to prescribe specific medication.

You should speak to the practice nurse in your surgery and find out how tests and checks are carried out and how the way you carry out your job could help improve the system or communications.

ADVANCE BOOKING OF APPOINTMENTS

Surgeries will all have their own set ruling on advance bookings. Some have no limit, others only allow booking one month ahead, some only next day appointments. Often there is a high percentage of non-attenders in the surgeries which book ahead. Perhaps this is a reason for next day only appointments. Doctor time wasted when patients do not turn up is very annoying, especially when receptionists are having to tell other patients there are no appointments available. The education of patients in this area would be a great advantage for the busy practice.

Advance appointments are usually made for courses of immunisations, recalls for cytology screening, blood pressure monitoring, specific review requests by the doctor. Minor surgery clinics usually have a waiting list and advance bookings are needed here. When a person is to have a minor operation in the surgery, no matter how small, he or she should sign a basic consent form agreeing to the procedure to be carried out. In some cases, for example elderly patients, it is wise to inform patients that they may like to have someone with them or arrange transport home after the surgery.

There is also the 'Open Surgery' where no appointments are made and patients turn up and sit and wait and take it in turn to see the doctor. In this case, systems have to be in place to provide a smooth and orderly running of the session to avoid patients jumping the queue and causing disruption. Medical records have to be retrieved quickly as patients arrive

APRIL	Doctor	Branch A	Branch B	Branch C	Home Visits	Total Consultations
	DR A	62	280	91	49	482
	DR B	194	259	183	65	701
	DR C	122	219	129	46	516
	DR D	112	72	165	47	396
	DR E	97	192	65	21	375
	DR F	193	212	102	49	556
		780	1234	735	277	3026

MAY	Doctor	Branch A	Branch B	Branch C	Home Visits	Total Consultations
	DR A	194	188	189	40	611
	DR B	191	217	81	55	544
	DR C	150	303	99	60	612
	DR D	151	140	175	54	520
	DR E	107	180	42	45	374
	DR F	163	91	89	21	364
		956	1119	675	275	3025

JUN	Doctor	Branch A	Branch B	Branch C	Home Visits	Total Consultations
	DR A	310	176	97	47	630
	DR B	179	179	123	56	537
	DR C	217	201	104	45	567
	DR D	108	131	175	41	455
	DR E	258	261	136	53	708
	DR F	150	149	42	38	379
		1222	1097	677	280	3276

JUL	Doctor	Branch A	Branch B	Branch C	Home Visits	Total Consultations
	DR A	214	174	99	44	531
	DR B	180	189	191	67	627
	DR C	110	334	121	46	611
	DR D	96	55	37	27	215
	DR E	191	209	175	52	627
	DR F	220	251	91	55	617
		1011	1212	714	291	3228

AUG	Doctor	Branch A	Branch B	Branch C	Home Visits	Total Consultations
	DR A	175	197	79	50	501
	DR B	159	168	106	42	475
	DR C	122	261	72	55	510
	DR D	147	95	97	47	386
	DR E	91	140	137	45	413
	DR F	166	120	75	37	398
		860	981	566	276	2683

SEPT	Doctor	Branch A	Branch B	Branch C	Home Visits	Total Consultations
	DR A	189	265	53	47	554
	DR B	181	196	185	53	615
	DR C	123	152	126	42	443
	DR D	103	249	117	32	501
	DR E	157	114	149	39	459
	DR F	152	177	46	34	409
		905	1153	676	247	2981

Figure 16.5 Consultation statistics

Home Visit Totals

Doctor	Apr	May	Jun	Jul	Aug	Sep	Oct	Nov	Dec	Jan	Feb	Mar	Year Total
DR A	49	40	47	44	50	47	43	0	0	0	0	0	320
DR B	65	55	56	67	42	53	56	0	0	0	0	0	394
DR C	46	60	45	46	55	42	61	0	0	0	0	0	355
DR D	47	54	41	27	47	32	53	0	0	0	0	0	301
DR E	21	45	53	52	45	39	39	0	0	0	0	0	294
DR F	49	21	38	55	37	34	67	0	0	0	0	0	301
Total	277	275	280	291	276	247	319	0	0	0	0	0	1965

Doctor Consultation Totals

	Apr	May	Jun	Jul	Aug	Sept	Oct	Nov	Dec	Jan	Feb	Mar	Total
Dr A	482	611	630	531	501	554	0	0	0	0	0	0	3309
Dr B	701	544	537	627	475	615	0	0	0	0	0	0	3499
Dr C	516	612	567	611	510	443	0	0	0	0	0	0	3259
Dr D	396	520	455	215	386	501	0	0	0	0	0	0	2473
Dr E	375	374	708	627	413	459	0	0	0	0	0	0	2956
Dr F	556	364	379	617	398	409	0	0	0	0	0	0	2723
TOTAL	3026	3025	3276	3228	2683	2981	0	0	0	0	0	0	18219

Branch Totals

	X	Y	Z	TOTAL
APRIL	780	1234	735	2749
MAY	956	1119	675	2750
JUNE	1222	1097	677	2996
JULY	1011	1212	714	2937
AUG	860	981	566	2407
SEPT	905	1153	676	2734
OCT	917	1037	720	2674
NOV	0	0	0	0
DEC	0	0	0	0
JAN	0	0	0	0
FEB	0	0	0	0
MARCH	0	0	0	0
TOTAL	6651	7833	4763	19247

Figure 16.5 Consultation statistics (continued)

in order that the doctor will have all the necessary information or recent laboratory tests to hand when seeing the patient.

Receptionists normally book all appointments but the medical secretary may be asked by the doctor to contact the patient and book a suitable appointment with the nurse, a doctor, counsellor, physiotherapist, etc. Ensure you know how to use the system whether it is computerised or manual.

HOME VISITS

Home visits are intended for the elderly, house-bound or very sick patients too ill to come down to surgery. Some people abuse this service and request home visits for trivial reasons – sometimes simply because there have been no free appointments available for that morning. Requests for

---

PRACTICE NURSE APPOINTMENTS

1. **09.00 a.m. Appointments**
   (i)   These are for **3 blood tests only**.
   (ii) Patients for blood tests after fasting may have **water only** from **9.00 p.m.** the previous evening.
   N.B. *Non-fasting blood tests may be done at any time **before 3.00 p.m.** in ordinary sessions.*

2. **Telephone Calls**
   Only urgent calls are to be put through during clinic sessions.
   Non-urgent calls, e.g. Reps or patients requesting advice will be taken between 12.30 p.m.-1.00 p.m. and 5.30 p.m.-6.00 p.m.
   N.B. *Some calls are not appropriate for the Practice Nurse to deal with, e.g. questions about contraception, medication and illness.*

3. **Drug Company Representatives**
   From September **Reps** will be seen by appointment only at **12.30 p.m. on Tuesdays**.

4. **Reasons for Patient Appointments**
   When making appointments please state reason.

Figure 16.6 Instructions for practice nurse appointments

home visits usually have to be made before 11.00 a.m. Staff taking requests for home visits have to be accurate in obtaining and passing on information. The patient's name, address and telephone number if they have one and, should someone else be phoning in for them, that person's details would also be useful in case the doctor wishes to contact them for further details of the sick patient. A brief description of the reason for the call will give the doctor insight into the urgency of the visit and also alert the receptionist. Obviously a patient with a pain in the chest or left side, difficulty breathing, having a fit, collapsing, etc., would ring alarm bells for the receptionist to pass the message immediately to the duty doctor. It is not the receptionist's job to diagnose the severity of the illness – this is solely the doctor's responsibility. Should you take a call of this nature, do not hesitate to pass it on to a doctor or in his absence the nurse for further medical advice. The receptionist should get the patient's medical records out ready for the doctor and ensure the correct address is on the record. Sometimes

Reflection Point 4

Discuss the most professional and tactful ways of finding out the details needed for a home visit.

patients could be staying with friends or relatives while they are ill or perhaps could have moved and not informed the practice. Always check these details as delays in finding the patient's home in urgent requests could be fatal.

Patients should always be asked if they can get down to surgery, as doctors can see more patients in the surgery in the time that it takes travelling out and visiting just one patient. Sometimes requests are made for home visits for very minor symptoms and each surgery will have its own standard procedure of accepting and filtering these calls.

PRACTICE NURSE CLINICS

CLINIC	TIME	URINE SAMPLE	DOCTOR ON PREMISES	NOTES
ASTHMA	Monday 3.00–5.30 p.m.	1st Appointment	YES	NEW PATIENTS – 30 minute appointments (i.e. 1st Appointment) Patients may be seen at other times by Jenny. Patient must bring inhalers, etc., with them.
BABY IMMUNISATIONS	Tuesday 2.00–3.30 p.m.	NO	YES	**NB. Not carried out if baby unwell.** Appointments may be made during ordinary sessions if unable to attend clinic.
BLOOD TESTS				**3 only at 9.00 a.m. (none Wednesday)**
Fasting Blood Tests	9.00 a.m.	NO	NO	For Fasting Blood Tests – Patients are allowed only water for 12 hours before the test is taken.
Non-fasting	Before 3.00 p.m.	NO	NO	For Non-fasting Blood Tests appointments can be made anytime before 3.00 p.m.
CORONARY HEART DISEASE SCREENING	Wednesday 3.00–5.15 p.m.	YES	NO	30 minute appointments. ECG appointments can be made during CHD Clinics (30 minute appointments).
DRESSINGS	Anytime	NO	YES	
EAR SYRINGING	Anytime	NO	YES	ONLY patients who have been referred by the doctor or have had their ears syringed before can make an appointment. Drops (e.g. Olive Oil or Sodium Bicarbonate) to be used in ear twice a day for four days before appointment.
ECG	CHD Clinic or 11.45 a.m.	NO	NO	30 minute appointment.
HOLIDAY IMMUNISATIONS	Anytime	NO	YES	APPOINTMENT to be made to discuss requirements and start immunisation programme.
INJECTIONS	Anytime	NO	YES	ZOLADEX, MYOCRISIN, B12, SUSTANON given by nurse. **NB. NOT the contraceptive injection.**
NEW PATIENT HEALTH SCREEN	Anytime	YES	NO	15 minute appointment.
OVER 75 YEAR CHECK	Anytime	YES	NO	30 minute appointment.
REMOVAL OF SUTURES	Anytime	NO	YES	
SMEAR ONLY	Anytime			Repeat smears – 15 minute appointments.
DIABETIC CLINIC	*Tuesday 9.30–10.30 a.m.*	*YES*	*YES*	***Carried out by District Nurse***

NB. The Well Woman Clinic has now been cancelled. Patients requiring smears can make appointments at any time with the nurse using a 15 minute appointment.

Figure 16.7 A timetable for practice nurse clinics

REPEAT PRESCRIBING

The use of the computer with repeat prescribing is again invaluable. Computers record all processed requests for medication and can be set to limit the number of prescriptions issued in order that the doctor can monitor the progress of the drug. If this has been done or the practice has a protocol then most patients on repeat medication will have to see their doctor within a set time for review. Good practice dictates that regular monitoring of repeat prescribing is a necessity. Most practices will have a protocol to cover this which will include setting limits on the computer to indicate when a patient needs to see the doctor before another repeat can be issued (Figure 16.8).

Computerised scripts also give a quick method of checking if a patient is over-using a certain drug and it can be brought to the attention of the doctor immediately. Often there is a simple reason for it but if a patient is over-using a prescribed drug it could be doing more harm than good and the doctor needs to assess the situation.

When repeat prescriptions have been run off they also produce an attached side slip of paper listing all the medications the patient has on repeat. The patient then selects the items he or she requires and returns the slip to the practice a few days before the medication runs out. The receptionist then processes the request and the doctor signs it. The script is then placed ready for collection at the surgery or, as is increasingly popular, a named chemist of the patient's choice can collect it. Often these chemists provide a delivery service, which is ideal for housebound or elderly patients.

Reflection Point 5

What guidelines do you have in place for monitoring repeat prescribing? What advantages do prescribing protocols give the practice?

CONTROLLED DRUGS

These are drugs which cannot be included in a repeat prescribing list but have to be handwritten by the doctor. They include drugs used by addicts and they have to be issued on a special prescription which gives the chemist authority to dispense the drug on a daily basis (see Chapter 18).

DRUG AUDITS

Information from the repeat prescribing can give insight into the prescribing patterns of doctors and highlight areas where expensive drugs are being used inappropriately. A practice formulary will help standardise this but very often the formulary is an ongoing process. Regular searches on the computer for specific drug usage and meetings to discuss the drug budget can help control the amount of spending in this area.

PROCESSING CLAIMS

Data on contraceptive care, minor surgery, vaccination and immunisation, temporary residence, registration health checks and maternity services can all be claimed quickly and efficiently via GP Links. Manual paper systems are far more time consuming for staff and computers are the most efficient and effective way of collecting data.

As a medical secretary you may be responsible for entering and collating some of the data for patient medical summaries, cytology, childhood immunisations etc. This involves accurate record-keeping of women eligible for cervical cytology screening, informing the Support Services of all women who have had hysterectomies, who are pregnant and are unable to attend for their screening until after the birth, or who are having some type of treatment which prevents them having their smear test at that time. The Support Services, once notified, will then take them off the target list until the agreed time. A search on the computer of all those females who have not had their smear test and a mail merge of their addresses with a standard letter should be a job suited to the medical secretary. Keeping details of the immunisation status of children under 5 years and sending out appointment letters for them to attend the baby clinics for their immunisations when they are due may be a combined task for reception and secretary. However it is processed in your practice, inaccurate records of the cytology and immunisation registers can lose the practice a great deal of money. Computerisation of these details gives quick and accurate information, helping you to keep ahead of the necessary target levels.

Repeat Prescribing Protocol

This protocol sets out the procedures used for dealing with requests for repeat prescriptions at the main surgery and branch surgeries in order to provide a rapid, accurate and safely monitored service to the patient.

Authorisation

Repeat prescriptions are computer-generated. The items are put on the computer only with doctor authorisation and the following standards apply.

No controlled drugs are included.

Drugs with an abuse potential are only included at the doctor's discretion.

The number of prescriptions to be issued is authorised by the doctor, entered on the computer and the computer will then indicate 'expired' once this number is reached. Any additional requests made after this can only be processed after obtaining authorisation from the doctor to update the computer to allow further issues of repeat prescriptions.

This information will also show up on computer generated surgery lists which are used for all surgeries. Drugs can be added or omitted by the doctor writing the drug dose and quantity on the surgery list.

There is a liaison slip which is attached to the manual record when hospital requests for drugs are made via discharge letters or clinic letters. The doctor fills in the information he requires on the computer prescription. This is on approved FP10 computer forms and comes complete with counterfoil which lists numerically the drugs which can be repeated.

Requesting a Repeat Prescription

Ideally, the patient will present the counterfoil from his previous prescription to the reception staff with the requested items endorsed. They will accept it and inform the patient that the repeat prescription will be available in 24 hours.

In the case of postal requests a stamped self-addressed envelope is required in order to return the prescription by post.

The patient may request prescriptions to be collected from the branch surgeries. A daily processing of prescriptions at the branch surgery ensures they are available for collection.

Telephone Requests

We encourage the patient not to telephone for repeat prescriptions yet sometimes this is unavoidable. Telephone requests are accepted between 11.00 a.m. and 12.00 noon in the morning and from 2.00 p.m. to 3.00 p.m. in the afternoon. These should be emergency calls only and patients are told the prescription will be ready after 2.00 p.m. the following day.

Figure 16.8 A repeat prescribing protocol

Generating a Prescription

The repeat prescription requests are entered into the computer and one member of staff and one terminal are dedicated to this task in the mornings. (Urgent requests during the afternoon are processed by the receptionist on duty.)

All patients who are on repeat medication have a repeat prescription request limit on their computer file. Each request is entered on the computer and attention is drawn to the number of repeats that have been issued.

Once the number allowed has been reached the computer indicates that authorisation has 'expired'. This alerts the receptionist to gain further authorisation from the doctor before further repeats are issued.

The receptionist enters all the requests for prescriptions received that morning into the computer and once completed the computer will print out a batch of all of the morning's requests. This is usually completed by 12.00 noon.

The prescriptions are then separated for the individual doctors and are presented for signing.

By 1.00 p.m. each day the process is completed by the reception staff. The prescriptions are sorted for posting to the patient or collection.

Generic Prescriptions

When the doctor changes a patient's prescription from a brand named drug to the generic equivalent a short letter is attached to the prescription explaining the change to the patient.

This avoids causing the patient concern when they collect the prescription from the chemist.

Exclusions

The computer will not print out a prescription if it has expired and will only prescribe the amount of drug authorised.

Any amendment has to be made by the doctor of the patient and the patient may be required to make an appointment for a review of his medication.

Non-Computer Generated Repeat Prescriptions

Under certain circumstances patients request repeat prescriptions which they have had previously but they are used infrequently or for other reasons are not on the computer repeat prescribing system, e.g.

> Hayfever tablets
> Paracetamol for infants
> Preparations for head lice.

Under these circumstances the staff will accept the request but inform the patient that it cannot be issued until after surgery when the doctor will authorise the prescription whilst he is signing the computer printed repeats.

FEES PAID DIRECTLY TO DOCTORS

INSURANCE MEDICAL REPORTS

These are requests by insurance companies for medical reports on patients. A full medical is not usually required but a standard form is supplied to obtain the necessary information for the report on the patient's health status. A patient's consent sheet or section will always be included with these requests as a report should not be processed without it. If the patient signature on a consent form is not included with the paperwork you should contact the company requesting the patient's consent and hold the application on file until it is received. Copies of these reports should be kept on file for 6 months. A patient has the right to see the report before it is sent off to the company. A place on the application form indicates this by selecting the option to see the report. If this is the case you must hold back the report for 28 days to allow the patient to contact the surgery to make an appointment with the secretary or practice manager to see the report. Once the report has been seen it can be sent off. If the patient has not contacted the surgery within 28 days the report can be sent off. The income to the practice varies depending on the amount of information required. If a full medical is needed then the fee payable is greater. The BMA provides guidelines on appropriate and acceptable levels of charges for the doctor's work.

Sometimes a company will request a full medical and report on a person who is not registered with the practice. This is usual as some companies prefer to have an independent doctor's opinion and it may be part of your duties to contact the person and arrange a suitable time when the doctor can carry out the examination.

PRIVATE SICK NOTES

Sometimes patients require a private sick note for their employer or for a sickness insurance policy. A fee is charged for this and is payable by the patient.

TRAVEL INSURANCE FORMS

Patients travelling abroad for their holidays often take out travel insurance. If they should have to claim on these policies for medical reasons they require medical evidence to support their claim. A fee is claimable from the patient or the insurance company, whoever is requesting the details.

DEATH CERTIFICATES

After a patient has died the doctor attending the patient issues a death certificate and seals it in the envelope provided ready for collection at the reception desk by a member of the deceased's family. A fee is charged for this.

CREMATION FEES

If the deceased is to be cremated the undertaker will ask the doctor to complete Form B of the cremation forms. The doctor completing Form B asks a second doctor to complete Form C. These doctors must not be in partnership or related and they will receive the appropriate fee from the undertaker.

CORRESPONDENCE AND PAPERWORK IN GENERAL PRACTICE

Letters, advertising circulars, forms, laboratory tests are part of the incoming mail that has to be dealt with in the practice and it is important that the mail is forwarded to the correct person or section to process it. Practices will all have their own system of processing the mail in the most efficient way and you should familiarise yourself with the responsibilities of the members of the practice team so that you can play your part in directing the mail to the correct person. Figure 16.9 gives an example of the types of incoming mail and how it is processed in one surgery. Processing doctor referral letters for patients has to be carried out as soon as possible once you receive the tape or details. Delays or missed referrals could delay appointments with consultants or prevent the patient receiving necessary treatment. A system should be set up to control the efficient processing of this. In Figure 16.10 an example of a system is shown. All dictation tapes are numbered and when returned to the secretary they are logged in. Any urgent letters included on the tape are noted in the comments section and if there are any private referrals they are noted. The secretary who is typing the tape enters her initials and once completed enters the date. This sim-

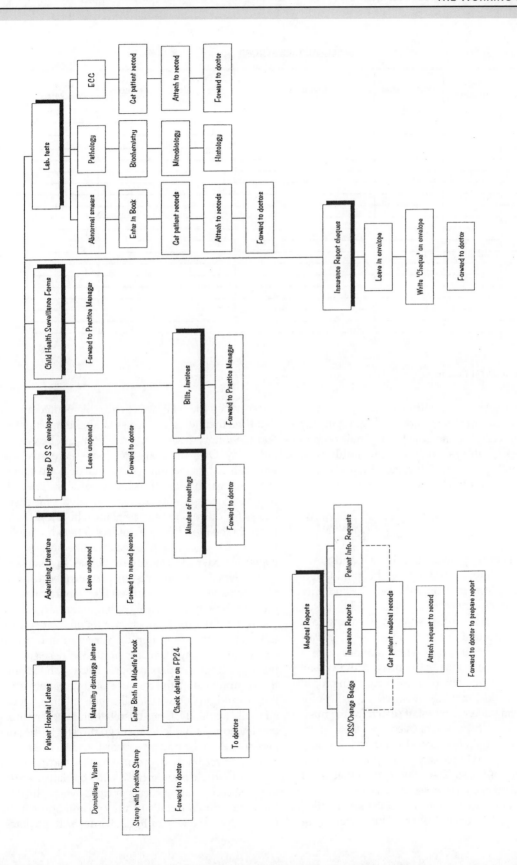

Figure 16.9 Types of mail

REFERRAL TAPE RECORD

Date Received	Tape Number	Doctor Initial	Comments	Private Referrals Included	Secretary	Date Completed

Figure 16.10 Referral tape record

ple record ensures strict rotation of the tapes so that none get missed or mislaid and also highlights any delays from receipt of the tape to the final completion. Causes of delays, such as staff holidays or sickness, can be accounted for and suitable action taken to provide additional secretarial cover.

FILING

One job in general practice that is vast and never ending is the filing. Each day more hospital letters and laboratory tests come into the practice and once seen by the doctor need to be filed quickly in the patient's medical record. It is a never ending task but a most important one that should never be carried out casually or in a haphazard manner.

If clinical correspondence is filed in the wrong patient's record, time will be wasted searching for it, and there will be annoying embarrassing delays for the doctor and patient while staff search for the missing item. Should a copy be requested from the hospital or laboratory it could take days to find and this does not give a very good impression of the professionalism and efficiency of the staff. A filing system that is not accurate and up to date is worse than useless.

In general practice the patients' notes will be filed in small 'Lloyd George' folders. These were pro-

duced when the NHS was first implemented and at that time there was less access to all the consultants' and laboratory tests and X-rays that can be carried out today. Over the years they have served the system well but increasingly some practices are changing over to the larger A4 size folders. They do require more space for storage but give a far easier access for doctors to see at a glance the latest test or letter. In the Lloyd George folders, letters have to be folded, cut or shrunk to a smaller size on a photocopier in order to fit neatly in the file. In some surgeries, letters and test results are scanned directly into the patient's computerised file. Laboratory tests are sent directly from the hospital to the surgery via computer links and as doctors enter all their consultations onto the computer, the surgery can function easily without paper records or notes. These surgeries may shred the paper copies once scanned into the computer and the amount of time taken scanning would probably match the time no longer needed to file manually. Once hospitals and surgery links are developed fully letters will go directly to the surgery to link to the patient's record, and vice versa.

Whichever method you use, letters and tests are always filed chronologically with the latest at the top. The continuation sheets or cards where the doctor writes down details of the consultation can be filed in the same way or in date order with the latest

DOCTOR COMBINED ROTA

APRIL

	1 Tues	2 Wed	3 Thurs	4 Fri	5 Sat	6 Sun	7 Mon	8 Tues	9 Wed	10 Thurs	11 Fri	12 Sat	13 Sun	14 Mon	15 Tues	16 Wed	17 Thurs	18 Fri	19 Sat	20 Sun	21 Mon	22 Tues	23 Wed	24 Thurs	25 Fri	26 Sat	27 Sun	28 Mon	29 Tues	30 Wed
Day Time	HGJ	JRW	TMB	HGJ			TMB	DJO	JRW	HGJ	TMB			DJO	HGJ	TMB	HGJ					DJO	JRW	TMB	JRW			JRW	HGJ	TMB
Out of Hours				DJO 2									TMB 1	HGJ				DJO 12-1		TMB 8-12										
Nights		JRW					TMB							HGJ/JRW						SELL			3rd O							
Holidays													JRW	JRW	JRW	JRW						HGJ	HGJ	HGJ	HGJ			DJO	DJO	DJO

MAY

	1 Thurs	2 Fri	3 Sat	4 Sun	5 Mon	6 Tues	7 Wed	8 Thurs	9 Fri	10 Sat	11 Sun	12 Mon	13 Tues	14 Wed	15 Thurs	16 Fri	17 Sat	18 Sun	19 Mon	20 Tues	21 Wed	22 Thurs	23 Fri	24 Sat	25 Sun	26 Mon	27 Tues	28 Wed	29 Thurs	30 Fri	31 Sat
Day Time	HGJ	TMB				DJO	JRW	TMB	HGJ			DJO	HGJ	JRW	TMB	DJO			HGJ	JRW	DJO	TMB	HGJ			JRW	TMB	HGJ	JRW		HGJ
Out of Hours		JRW 1		HGJ 5-10															DJO												HGJ 1
Nights		TMB																				TMB									
Holidays	DJO	DJO																								DJO	DJO	DJO	DJO	DJO	

JUNE

	1 Sun	2 Mon	3 Tues	4 Wed	5 Thurs	6 Fri	7 Sat	8 Sun	9 Mon	10 Tues	11 Wed	12 Thurs	13 Fri	14 Sat	15 Sun	16 Mon	17 Tues	18 Wed	19 Thurs	20 Fri	21 Sat	22 Sun	23 Mon	24 Tues	25 Wed	26 Thurs	27 Fri	28 Sat	29 Sun	30 Mon
Day Time		JRW	TMB	HGJ	JRW				TMB	JRW	TMB	HGJ	JRW			TMB	JRW	HGJ	TMB	HGJ			DJO	JRW	DJO	HGJ	DJO			DJO
Out of Hours							HGJ 1																							
Nights																HGJ			JRW											
Holidays		DJO	DJO	DJO	DJO	DJO			DJO	DJO	DJO	DJO	DJO			DJO	DJO	DJO	DJO	DJO			TMB	TMB	TMB	TMB	TMB			

Figure 16.11 An on duty rota

at the back. This will depend on the doctor's preference in your surgery.

PRACTICE ROTAS

Practice rotas are essential for the smooth running of the practice. They are an effective method of communication to ensure that the participants and attached staff know where clinics are being held and the staff who will be manning them, where and when doctors will be holding surgeries and when they are away. There are many types of rota and you will come across several different variations and layouts of rota in your working life. It may be a rota that includes you or simply one for your reference to enable you to carry out your work in an efficient way by knowing the exact whereabouts of doctors and staff.

DOCTOR ROTAS

Every doctor in any surgery will work by rotas or take part in some sort of rota. It may be purely as part of an out of hours service for patients in the case of a single-handed doctor but their surgeries and various clinics will be worked on a weekly or monthly basis. Several rotas may be in use at one time in larger surgeries, such as the daily surgery rota, the on-call rota and the out of hours rota (Figures 16.11 and 16.12). These may also include or combine holiday rotas when doctors take it in turns to have certain school or bank holidays off. If the main surgery has branch surgeries, these will also have to be included and considered in the doctor and staff rotas. If the partners have opted out of out of hours cover there would only be the daytime on-call and holiday rotas to process.

STAFF ROTAS

Staff rotas for morning and afternoon shifts, Saturday morning surgeries and holiday cover will also be in existence. All surgeries and the many types of clinic sessions are usually worked out on a weekly basis and hence are also part of the rota system. A great deal of 'good will' goes on in general practice when it comes to emergency cover if staff are taken ill suddenly, or the doctors decide to hold an additional surgery over bank holidays. For good planning and avoiding the day-to-day stress of ensuring cover, rotas are an essential tool in the smooth running and effectiveness of the practice. Figure 16.13 provides an example.

As a medical secretary it may be one of your responsibilities to update and circulate the rotas. If it

ON CALL ROTA
APRIL

Date	Day	Day Time	Out of Hours	Nights
1	Tuesday	HGJ		
2	Wednesday	JRW		JRW
3	Thursday	TMB		
4	Friday	HGJ		
5	Saturday		HGJa.m./DJO 2	
6	Sunday			
7	Monday	TMB		TMB
8	Tuesday	DJO		
9	Wednesday	JRW		
10	Thursday	HGJ		
11	Friday	TMB		
12	Saturday			
13	Sunday		TMB 1	
14	Monday	DJO	HGJ	
15	Tuesday	HGJ		
16	Wednesday	TMB		
17	Thursday	HGJ		HGJ/JRW
18	Friday		DJO 12-5	
19	Saturday			
20	Sunday			
21	Monday		TMB 8 – 12	
22	Tuesday	DJO		Co-op
23	Wednesday	JRW		
24	Thursday	TMB		
25	Friday	JRW		
26	Saturday			3rd on
27	Sunday			
28	Monday	JRW		
29	Tuesday	HGJ		
30	Wednesday	TMB		

Holidays

JRW	14TH - 18TH
HGJ	21ST - 25TH
DJO	28TH - 30TH

Figure 16.12 An on call rota

January

	Dec 30	31	Jan 1	2	3	4	6	7	8	9	10	11	13	14	15	16	17	18	20	21	22	23	24	25	27	28	29	30	31	Feb 1
	M	T	W	T	F	S	M	T	W	T	F	S	M	T	W	T	F	S	M	T	W	T	F	S	M	T	W	T	F	S
Veronica	d	d	d	d	d	o	d	d	d	d	d	o	d	d	d	d	d	o	d	d	d	d	d	o	d	d	d	d	d	o
Helen	pm	am	am	o	pm	o	pm	am	am	am	o	o	pm	am	am	am	o	o	pm	am	am	am	o	o	am	o	pm	pm	pm	o
Lisa	am	am	o	pm	pm	am	pm	am	am	o	pm	o	pm	am	am	o	pm	o	pm	am	am	o	pm	o	pm	o	pm	pm	am	o
Sylvia	am	o	pm	pm	am	o	am	o	pm	pm	am	o	am	o	pm	pm	am	o	am	o	pm	pm	am	o	o	pm	am	am	am	o
Judith	o	pm	pm	am	am	o	am	o	pm	pm	am	o	am	am	o	pm	pm	o	am	am	o	pm	pm	o	pm	pm	am	am	o	o
Joyce	pm	pm	am	am	am	o	o	pm	pm	am	am	o	am	o	pm	pm	am	o	pm	am	am	am	am	o	pm	am	am	am	pm	o

February

	Feb 3	4	5	6	7	8	10	11	12	13	14	15	17	18	19	20	21	22	24	25	26	27	28	Mar 1	3	4	5	6	7	8
	M	T	W	T	F	S	M	T	W	T	F	S	M	T	W	T	F	S	M	T	W	T	F	S	M	T	W	T	F	S
Veronica	d	d	d	d	d	o	d	d	d	d	d	o	d	d	d	d	d	o	d	d	d	d	d	o	d	d	d	d	d	o
Helen	pm	am	am	o	pm	o	pm	am	am	am	o	o	pm	am	am	am	o	o	pm	am	am	am	o	o	am	o	pm	pm	pm	am
Lisa	am	am	o	pm	pm	am	pm	am	am	o	pm	o	pm	am	am	o	pm	o	pm	am	am	o	pm	o	pm	o	pm	pm	am	o
Sylvia	am	o	pm	pm	am	o	am	o	pm	pm	am	o	am	o	pm	pm	am	o	am	o	pm	pm	am	o	o	pm	am	am	am	o
Judith	o	pm	pm	am	am	o	am	am	o	pm	pm	o	o	pm	pm	am	am	o	am	am	o	pm	pm	o	pm	pm	am	am	o	o
Joyce	pm	pm	am	am	am	o	o	pm	pm	am	am	o	pm	am	am	am	am	o	pm	am	am	am	am	am	pm	am	am	am	pm	o

March / April

	Mar 10	11	12	13	14	15	17	18	19	20	21	22	24	25	26	27	28	29	31	Apr 1	2	3	4	5	7	8	9	10	11	12
	M	T	W	T	F	S	M	T	W	T	F	S	M	T	W	T	F	S	M	T	W	T	F	S	M	T	W	T	F	S
Veronica	d	d	d	d	d	o	d	d	d	d	d	o	d	d	d	d	d	o	d	d	d	d	d	o	d	d	d	d	d	o
Helen	pm	am	am	o	pm	o	pm	am	am	am	o	o	pm	am	am	am	o	o	am	o	pm	pm	pm	o	am	o	pm	pm	pm	am
Lisa	am	am	o	pm	pm	am	pm	am	am	o	pm	o	pm	am	am	o	pm	o	pm	pm	am	am	am	o	pm	am	am	am	am	o
Sylvia	am	o	pm	pm	am	o	am	o	pm	pm	am	o	am	o	pm	pm	am	o	o	pm	am	am	am	o	o	pm	am	am	am	o
Judith	o	pm	pm	am	am	o	am	am	o	pm	pm	o	am	am	o	pm	pm	o	am	am	o	pm	pm	o	pm	pm	am	am	o	o
Joyce	pm	pm	am	am	am	o	o	pm	pm	am	am	o	pm	am	am	am	am	am	pm	am	am	am	am	am	pm	am	am	am	pm	o

Key: 'd' = DAYS; 'am' = MORNINGS (from 8.15 a.m. to 1.00 p.m.; Saturday 8.30 a.m. to 12 noon); 'pm' = AFTERNOONS (from 1.15 p.m. to 6.00 p.m.).

Figure 16.13 Reception staff rota

is, then accuracy and full knowledge of the surgery and advance notification of cancellations or holiday bookings will be vital.

CONCLUSION

From the contents of this chapter you can see that there are many areas to general practice. You may not have to know every detail of all the forms and procedures but a good general knowledge of all these aspects is essential. Knowing who deals with what, when people are available, where people are, etc., enables you to pass on doctor, patient, hospital queries to the right person quickly and efficiently. This will eliminate delays and give a good impression of the

working efficiency of the surgery. It will also show you as a confident, capable and caring secretary.

Exercises

An up-to-date procedure folder or book is a useful reference tool. Would you be able to work with the practice staff in producing one? What problems might you encounter?

List the rotas used at your practice. Are they helpful or confusing? Could you improve communications by implementing a set rota?

Further reading

Jones T 1996 The structure of the NHS. Publishing Initiatives, Thetford

Pickersgill D 1992 The law and general practice. Radcliffe, Oxford

Quinn NE, Simon P 1996 The GP's receptionist's handbook. Baillière Tindall, London

Salisbury C, Sawyer T 1998 Handbook of practice nursing, 2nd edn. Churchill Livingstone, Edinburgh

Chapter 17

Clinical considerations

Stephanie J Green

OBJECTIVES

- To promote an awareness of health and safety issues in general practice
- To describe procedures for infection control and disposal of waste
- To provide an understanding of sterilisation procedures
- To highlight the importance of safe handling of specimens
- To provide an outline of tests and investigations in common use.

INTRODUCTION

This chapter is intended to make the medical secretary aware of their responsibilities within the general practice and of various important practical issues in relation to the clinical environment. It will refer in a more applied way to issues mentioned in previous chapters, especially Chapters 3 and 10. As medical secretaries work as one of the team within the general practice environment, an understanding of the issues covered in this chapter is most important.

General practices need to provide safe and healthy working conditions with everyone able to work together in an informed and therefore confident manner. They should all know where problem areas might be and how they can be overcome safely and satisfactorily. When working in a medical environment in whatever capacity, it is important that the following issues are addressed by each member of the team. Whatever our role, none of us can work alone here.

In Chapters 3 and 10 reference has been made to health and safety legislation at work. In this chapter, we will look at the specific application to general practice, not forgetting that the responsibilities lie with both the employee and employer, as in any other workplace.

HEALTH AND SAFETY

The aim of the Health and Safety at Work Act 1974 is to ensure the safety, health and welfare of both people at work and those who are not working but may be at risk from those who are – in the case of general practice this will be clients or patients. There are obligations laid down for employers, who should prepare a consultative policy for health and safety in their workplace. There are also requirements for the employee, these are:

- To take due care of themselves and others while at work
- To abide by agreed policies
- To make correct use of protective clothing
- To attend training
- To ensure that safety procedures are observed and maintained.

General practice will have particular concerns which will be addressed in this chapter, but it will do no harm to remember some of the day-to-day issues that are included within the health and safety legislation. These are the provision of eating facilities, heating, lighting and consideration for visitors, whether it is the postman or a patient. There will be more specific medical points to consider here, but there is a legal obligation to produce a safety policy if there are more than five employees – which will inevitably apply to most general practices. In hospitals there are special departments devoted to occupational health and infection control.

ACCIDENTS

The responsibility for the prevention of accidents rests with every member of the workforce. Every member of the team should be safety conscious,

Reflection Point 1

As a medical secretary there will be specific health and safety issues which might affect your work. What do you think they are? What does health and safety legislation have to say about the management of these issues. If you do not know ... FIND OUT! As a clue, one of them might include the optician.

Box 17.1 Procedure for accidents

- Report any accident to the practice manager.
- Maintain an accident book. This should be available for recording any incidents. Each incident should be described fully, signed and dated.
- Serious incidents resulting in permanent damage or death should be reported to the Health and Safety Executive.

from the safe cleaning of floors to the safe disposal of contaminated waste. In general practice the points listed in Box 17.1 should be followed.

CONTROL OF SUBSTANCES HAZARDOUS TO HEALTH – COSHH

These regulations state that any dangerous or hazardous substance which is being used in general practice should be:

- Identified
- Given a description of the precautions which are to be taken and the hazards they might present
- Given a plan of use
- Provided with a contingency plan, should an unplanned occurrence take place.

Likewise, staff who may come into contact with hazardous substances must understand any risks involved and the precautions which must be taken. New staff must be given adequate instruction and supervision.

In a clinical environment such as general practice, there are bound to be substances which could be hazardous to health and safety and in a small workforce these could involve staff other than the practice nurse. These may include:

- Bleaches
- Industrial methylated spirit.

These should be stored in a locked cupboard and separated from other lotions.

INFECTION CONTROL

HAND CARE

One of the most important aspects of controlling infection is basic hand washing. Poor hand washing techniques have been found to be an easy source of cross-infection, as areas of the hands can be missed if this is hastily carried out. The importance of this fact has been the subject of discussion at the highest levels and has resulted in new government directives. Refer to Chapter 10 to remind yourself.

Reflection Point 2

How do you wash your hands? Make a list of the occasions you know you should use thorough hand washing as part of a procedure. Is this just theoretical or do you think you actually carry this out? Now consider the general practice – are there additions to make to your list?

Extra protection for hands needs to be considered. Staff should always cover cuts and abrasions with a waterproof dressing, which should be regularly changed. If you have a problem with chapped skin or dermatitis, gloves should be worn to protect you from infection. There are different types of gloves that may be used:

- The household variety are used for cleaning.
- Non-sterile single use gloves are used for examination and may be made of thin polythene or latex. Single use gloves are manufactured to a Department of Health specification.
- Surgical gloves are of a different specification and withstand sterilisation.

Wearing gloves does not remove the need to wash your hands thoroughly before and after any task or patient contact. This will include cleaning instruments, handling specimens, disinfectants and for cleaning up any form of spillage.

Having considered the importance of hand care, we also need to look at other aspects of basic hygiene. It has been shown that bacteria can multiply on moist soap and fabric towels, so to reduce the risk of cross-infection, anti-bacterial pump action soap dispensers and paper towels should be provided and elbow taps fitted, especially in clinical areas, to reduce hand-to-hand contamination. In surgical areas hand disinfectant solutions, which are often a mixture of chemical disinfectants such as chlorhexidine and alcohol, will be used before invasive procedures are undertaken.

PROTECTIVE CLOTHING

There are occasions when there is a further risk of contamination, including of clothing. For these procedures, disposable plastic aprons, face masks and eye protection may be necessary. All staff need to be familiar with procedures for dealing with body fluids should accidents happen. We may well be aware of the risk that HIV infection poses, but we must not underestimate the risk from other serious infections, such as hepatitis B.

SPILLAGE

If you are required to clear up any spillage of blood or any body fluids, the following points must be observed:

- Wear rubber gloves and apron
- Use disposable towels to absorb the spill
- Use domestic bleach or Milton 10,000ppm to treat the spill and leave for 10 minutes. After 10 minutes, discard the towels into the standard yellow waste bag for disposal.
- Alternatively, chlorine granules may be supplied to cope with these situations – these inactivate any infectious agent; follow the manufacturer's instructions on the container. This may well be the method of choice in general practice.

Spillage on carpets can be a problem – if it has had a protective treatment applied to it, it may be possible to clean it with hot soapy water once the spillage has been cleared. Check with the manufacturer's instructions first. Perhaps this should be a planning consideration in the first place!

Spillage of mercury from a broken sphygmomanometer or thermometer needs very different treatment. This requires special precautions as it can give off toxic fumes. It should be contained within the machine where possible or tipped into an airtight container and covered with water. There are special kits available to cope with mercury spillage and advice might be obtained from a local pharmacist.

INJURY

As part of infection control it is necessary to consider what is best practice in the event of injury (Box 17.2).

IMMUNISATION

Most practices will provide protection for their staff with immunisation against hepatitis B and all staff should make sure that they are up to date with protection against tetanus, polio and tuberculosis.

WORK SURFACES

As already discussed in Chapter 10, general cleaning must be of a high standard. However, in clinical situations, extra care must be taken. Work surfaces and trolleys should be cleaned before and after any procedure. Soap and water or Milton solution is adequate for cleaning glass surfaces or any others used during a sterile procedure.

DISPOSAL OF WASTE

Waste can be divided into

- Clinical waste
- Sharps
- General waste.

CLINICAL WASTE

This is waste such as human tissue, body fluids, contaminated material, swabs and dressings. The Health and Safety Act 1974 and the Environmental Protection Act 1990 state that this type of waste must be disposed of in yellow plastic bags, sealed, labelled with its source and incinerated. In this way

---

Box 17.2 Dealing with injury

Needle stick or sharps injury
- Encourage free bleeding
- Wash with soap and water
- Do not suck the wound
- Report the incident to the practice manager and record in the accident book
- Seek further advice or treatment from the Public health Laboratory

Splash injury in the eyes
- Crying will help to wash substances out
- Wash out using copious amounts of cold water
- Seek further treatment

Blood
- On skin with no cut or abrasion, wash with soap and water
- In mouth, spit out, rinse and spit again. Seek further advice.

---

clinical waste is readily recognised nationwide. Primary Care Trusts will have a contract with a specialist waste disposal firm to operate a service which will provide bags and ties and will collect and dispose of the waste.

SHARPS

Blades, glass ampoules, syringes and needles, which should be kept as one unit once assembled, should all be disposed of into a special 'sharps' box for general sharps use. A separate sharps box used for the disposal of cytotoxic drugs should be appropriately labeled and have a black lid. This is because these drugs are very toxic. The following points must be remembered:

- The box should be out of the reach of children
- Do not force or overfill a box
- Do not try to retrieve anything from inside it once deposited
- The box should be closed and sealed when three-quarters full. Each box should have the practice post code and an I.D number on it

Once sharps boxes are sealed they are disposed of in the same way as the yellow clinical waste sacks. These should all be stored in a locked cupboard or room, to which the public have no access, until the contractor collects the rubbish. Sharps boxes should not be put inside any bags. Each practice should nominate a procedure for the regular changing of yellow bags and boxes.

GENERAL WASTE

This should be placed in disposable bags and put into the local authority waste bin. Remember to check which is your designated day for collection. Local authorities have rules about how they will collect and empty bins, arrangements for bank holidays, etc. – it is a good idea to check these should you move to a new area. It is important that cleaning staff regularly empty bins from all areas as well as re-stocking items such as paper towels in cloakrooms. Remember that cleaning staff must be carefully protected from any potential injury or contamination.

STERILISATION PROCEDURES

Part of a comprehensive infection control system must include the methods by which articles used in general practice, whether for treatment or diagnosis, are rendered safe for use. Although the practice nurse will be the main professional concerned in this area, the informed medical secretary should also have a working knowledge of accepted protocols and the methods used in each practice.

PRE-CLEANING

Each practice must develop safe practice for the collection of dirty/used instruments from consulting rooms. One procedure may be to provide a named collection box, containing soapy water to soak articles, in each consulting room or treatment area. The disposal of these articles is usually the responsibility of the practice nurse on a daily/twice daily basis. In any event, used instruments must be thoroughly cleaned before they can be sterilised. Instruments may be put through a special high performance washer. This type of machine will be a requirement in general practice in the future. When cleaning instruments, remember that the following points should be observed as routine.

- To use a separate 'dedicated' sink for the cleaning process – a dirty area

- To wear household rubber gloves
- To wear a plastic apron, used for that job only and disposed of after use
- To use detergent and hot water to clean instruments, taking care to remove blood or other organic matter and paying particular attention to the joints, hinges and serrations of instruments
- To rinse carefully
- Not to use a brush unless you protect your face, especially your eyes.

If these points are not observed properly, not only will staff put themselves at risk of contamination, but the instruments may not be in a fit state to be sterilised. If contaminants are left on instruments, those areas will fail to be sterilised properly and microorganisms could then survive the sterilising process.

STERILISATION

As discussed in Chapter 10, autoclaves are considered to be the most efficient method of sterilisation, and this is the method most safely used in general practice. It is necessary to understand how each machine works and to follow the manufacturer's instructions for use and packing. Separate instruments need to be placed open in the autoclave so that each surface is exposed to the sterilising process. Gallipots and receivers should be put on their sides.

Health and safety note: leave instruments to cool down in the autoclave once the cycle is complete.

Following completion of the cycle, sterilised instruments can be laid inside a sterilised bowl or pack for a limited amount of time prior to a procedure. Ideally, instruments should be sterilised immediately before use. Instruments which are clean but un-sterile should be stored in a dust-free environment.

CHEMICAL DISINFECTANT

This method of rendering articles safe for use may have to be used on some occasions, but only when an autoclave is unsuitable. This is because the heat or pressure used in the autoclave may damage a piece of equipment made from material which cannot withstand the process. These may include leads, thermometers, nebuliser masks and mouthpieces.

In these instances the following may be used:

- Milton tablets used as a soaking solution.
- 70% alcohol wipes which may also be supplied for consulting rooms to clean hard surfaces or to wipe low risk items such as ear syringe nozzles.

The use and regular changing of these substances will probably be the responsibility of the practice nurse.

Lotions used for cleaning skin before an invasive procedure such as with minor surgery or IUCD fittings come in sterile 'one use' sachets. Chlorhexadine or normal saline are the lotions commonly used.

SAFE HANDLING OF SPECIMENS

It goes without saying that specimens of any kind will only be taken by trained staff with experience. These are performed to aid diagnosis and to help with the management of disease. However, there are some principles to be observed in the case of any member of staff who might receive a specimen or be required to deal with the dispatch of a specimen at any time. First and foremost are the health and safety considerations we have already looked at such as:

- Wearing protective gloves and aprons
- Ensuring that the tops of containers are tightened and secure to prevent spillage.

Because samples of all kinds are dealt with in general practice, it is necessary for a well ordered system to be organised, in many cases with cooperation with the local laboratory staff. Many general practices have a computer networked system with the local laboratory, enabling them to receive information and test results much faster and more efficiently than previously, when postal systems were the only resource. In addition to this, some hospitals and laboratories have a collection system organised with many general practices, enabling specimens to be transported on a daily basis at a known time. This is of great benefit, especially in more rural areas, where transport can be a problem and normal postal services would take too long.

However, some specimens may still need to be sent by other means, in which case a courier service may be used. It may also be necessary to use a 'Biohazard' sticker on any specimen sent for testing, whether to a laboratory or through a courier. All specimens should be considered to be a potential risk but some may be known to be a high risk, for example those which may be carrying potentially infectious diseases such as hepatitis B or HIV. In these cases the specimen should be labelled as 'high risk' both on the specimen and on the accompanying form.

When specimens are to be sent for analysis:

- Accompanying forms must be completed accurately – check that the correct date and time of collection is filled in and that it has been signed
- Check that the specimen container is labelled with the correct patient details
- Check that the form's details and the patient details match.

You may find that some practices ask patients to put their own specimens into the transporting bag, thus making it unnecessary for staff to touch anything which may constitute a hazard. Marsupial bags are used in some areas – this is a polythene bag which is designed to take a laboratory form, which has a smaller sealable bag attached to it for the specimen. This is to lessen the risk of forms and specimens being parted and lost, which is not only dangerous but extremely annoying to both patient and staff.

Specimens which are to be collected by internal transport systems will be put together in a marked box ready for collection at a stated time.

Some specimens are analysed in the practice. These should also have a proper collection point. This will probably be organised by the practice nurse.

Specimens which are spilt should be dealt with as described in the section on spillage. Any glass involved or bits of containers should be removed into a sharps container using forceps. Always wear gloves for your protection.

It is important that adequate stocks of both forms and the corresponding containers are kept in all the relevant consulting and treatment rooms, so that tests may be performed immediately without the need for another appointment.

It is also important that medical secretaries have a working knowledge of how tests are carried out in their particular practice, who collects them, whether patients are expected to transport a sample to the laboratory themselves and how long one might expect a test to take. This will vary not only from one practice to another but from one area to another. Rural practices may do many more tests on the premises than inner city practices, who may use hospital facilities more readily.

Some specimens require special storage until they are dispatched. They should all be kept in a cool place to lessen the likelihood of deterioration. Some samples may even change in some way, which could produce a false result. If a sample has to be kept for a longer period of time it should be refrigerated. If there is any doubt, the laboratory should be consulted for their advice on safe storage.

Reflection Point 3

What do you think are the most common types of samples likely to be sent from general practice? When you go on work experience make a point of finding out how your practice organises these investigations.

TEST RESULTS

It is most important that any test taken in the practice is recorded in the patient's notes. Some practices also keep a record of tests taken so that late or mislaid results may be traced. This form of log or record may also be used to audit the number of tests for the practice.

Just as important as sending the results is how the results are dealt with on return to the practice. Increasingly test results will be returned to the practice via computer link, which means that the practice can access the patient's results quicker than if waiting for the post. However if this is not possible then results will come either by telephone or by post. Facsimile machines may also be used for sending results quickly but all staff should remember that this could be sensitive or confidential material and that they must therefore take great care with how they receive this information and how they dispose of it. In an increasingly 'paper free' environment, the filing or disposal of results is an issue to think about very carefully.

Staff should be aware of the time lapse that may be involved between sending and receiving a test result, so that patients can be accurately advised. Many practices have a firm policy on processing test results and may use a stamp to summarise the possible actions, which the secretary should use. Care should be taken so that the actual results are not obliterated by the stamp! Test results, once stamped, should be circulated around the medical staff, who will tick the appropriate box for action. They may also give information to staff on instructions to be given to the patient. These may be:

- To make a further appointment – this may be urgent or as soon as possible
- To pick up a prescription
- To make an appointment for further tests with the practice nurse.
- No action necessary.

If a test result has been found to be very abnormal the laboratory staff may telephone the practice immediately to advise them of this. In this case, the patient's notes should be extracted straight away and the appropriate doctor informed. It might be a good idea to have relevant telephone numbers ready as well, should the doctor wish to speak to the laboratory and the patient.

Remember, too, that test results which are obtained in hospital will go firstly to the hospital doctors who requested them, and then to the general practice by letter. It is always possible to speed this up by speaking either to the consultant's secretary or to the laboratory directly. It may be important to know a test result before a patient keeps an appointment with a doctor, as treatment may well depend upon that result.

It is also important that each practice has a policy on giving the test results over the telephone. Obviously, staff must be conversant with the practical considerations as described in this section, but there are other issues to consider. Some practices will not give test results to patients over the telephone.

Scenario

A patient, whose name you do not recognise, telephones for her test result. How would you guarantee that you are talking to the person they say they are?

How would you differentiate between patients with the same surname, or between members of the same family with the same initials?

This chapter has demonstrated the need for cooperation both within the primary health care team and with other professional staff working in other areas. Remember, patient care is at the centre of the activity here, not just the efficient circulation of paper!

TESTS AND INVESTIGATIONS

This section provides a summary of the more usual tests that may be encountered while working in general practice. From time to time there will be others which you will need to find out about.

BLOOD TESTS

Haematology

- Full blood count (FBC). This will include:
  Hb – haemoglobin, to check for anaemia
  RBC – red cell count, to check for abnormalities
  WBC – white cell count, patients on certain drugs need regular checks. Also used for the investigation and treatment of disease such as leukaemia
- ESR – erythrocyte sedimentation rate, indication of infection or inflammation.
- Plasma viscosity is also used in the same way as ESR
- International normalised ratio (INR) – for the management of patients on anticoagulant therapy
- Platelet count – to aid the diagnosis of infection, inflammation, malignancy and trauma
- Clotting times – to check the clotting system. Used in the diagnosis of haemophilia and obstructive jaundice
- Prothrombin times – used in the treatment of haemorrhagic disease
- Paul-Bunnell – for the diagnosis of glandular fever (mononucleosis); also the Monospot test
- Rose-Waaler ⎤ both used in the diagnosis
- Latex fixation ⎦ of rheumatoid arthritis.
- Antinuclear fact/antibody (ANF/ANA) – for lupus erythematosus.

Bacterial blood tests

- VDRL (Venereal disease reference laboratory)

- TPHA (Treponema pallidum haemoglutin assay)
- WR (Wasserman reaction)
- GCFT (Gonococcal complement fixation test)
- Widal reaction – to test for typhoid, paratyphoid and brucellosis

Biochemical blood tests

- Blood sugar – for the diagnosis and management of diabetes
- Glycosylated haemoglobin (HbA1) also for the management of diabetes
- Cardiac enzymes – to diagnose myocardial infarction (heart attack)
- Urea and electrolytes (U & Es) + creatinine – for the management of kidney disease and to monitor patients on diuretics. If potassium levels are particularly required this will need to be from a fresh sample, and may only be taken in the morning
- Liver function tests (LFTs) – to measure enzymes and salts for a number of conditions
- Thyroid function (TFTs) – for the diagnosis and management of thyroid disease and to check on the dosage of thyroxine needed for treatment
- Cholesterol and lipid profile – to screen for cholesterol problems, especially hypercholesterolaemia
- Serum lithium – patients who are on lithium treatment require 3-monthly tests to check that levels are correct

Other tests

- Guthrie test – a test performed on infants between the 6th and 14th day after birth to diagnose phenylketonuria
- Serum electrophoresis – to analyse different proteins present in the blood
- Hormone levels – e.g. oestrogen in pregnancy
- Screening for drug abuse.

URINE TESTS

Stix tests are simple tests performed commonly in general practice, these may be:

- Glucose – for glucosuria found in diabetes and sometimes in pregnancy
- Albumin/protein – for albuminuria/protein-

uria, found in pregnancy and in renal disease
- Blood – for haematuria, found in infection and renal disease
- Ketones for diabetic patients.

LABORATORY TESTS

Microbiology

One of the most common tests performed in this laboratory is culture and sensitivity. This is used to identify an infection and to find out which antibiotic will treat any identified infective organisms. These are said to be 'sensitive' to that particular antibiotic. If antibiotics appear to have no effect on an organism it is said to be 'resistant'. Culture and sensitivity is used to identify infections in specimens from the following sources:

- Urine
- Faeces
- Sputum
- Throat
- Nose
- Ears
- Urethra
- Vagina
- Wounds.

Histology

This laboratory studies tissue microscopically. One of the most common areas of study used in general practice is *cytology*. Specimens are examined for abnormal cells and the following tests will be performed:

- Cervical smears – to screen for carcinoma of the cervix. This process is subject to the achievement of targets for general practitioners to encourage high attendance from patients and to obtain adequate smears.
- Sputum analysis – to diagnose disease, especially malignant, usually taken in the early morning before eating or drinking.

Other specimens sent to histology may be

- Urine – to test for abnormal cells
- Oral – to diagnose abnormal cells from the oral mucosa
- Semen analysis – after vasectomy to ensure successful surgery, or for investigation of infertility.

INVESTIGATIONS

X–ray

Many investigations will have to be performed in hospital, usually in the outpatient department. These are often within the X-ray department which now performs many new and different investigations (Box 17.3).

Endoscopy

This is an examination using an instrument made of flexible tubing, which is lit and is able to inspect hollow organs. A list of some of the endoscopic examinations follows:

- Gastroscopy
- Bronchoscopy
- Oesophagoscopy
- Endoscopic retrograde cholangiopancreatography.

Box 17.3 X-ray

- Plain film, e.g. chest and limb
- Using radio-opaque dye – intravenous pyelogram (IVP), for kidney function or damage
- Barium meal, to investigate the oesophagus, stomach and small intestine
- Barium swallow, to investigate the oesophagus
- Barium enema, to investigate the large bowel
- Ultrasound scan, to examine soft tissue. This process gives a structural image .e.g foetus, gall bladder and venous flow in the lower leg.
- Computed tomography scan (CT scan), to scan soft tissue in cross-sections of whole areas of the body being scanned, e.g. brain
- Nuclear magnetic resonance imaging (NMRI), uses the magnetic field in tissue to create 3D images of whole areas of the body, e.g. brain, abdomen
- Radioisotope – nuclear medicine, uses radioactive tracers injected into the body to measure the function of an organ, e.g. thyroid function
- Mammography, infrared or radiographic examination of the breast
- Bone mineral density, to measure the loss or gain of bone density over time, e.g. osteoporosis

Sigmoidoscopy, colonoscopy, proctoscopy

These are all used to investigate the lower bowel. Proctoscopy may be performed in general practice.

Cardiology

- ECG – electrocardiogram – this shows the electrical activity of the heart, and may be performed either in hospital or general practice.
- Echocardiography – this uses ultrasound to show the movements of the heart.
- Angiography/arteriography – this also uses radio-opaque contrast medium to examine blood vessels.

Neurology

- Lumbar puncture (LP) – a procedure to withdraw cerebrospinal fluid from the lumbar spine for diagnostic purposes.

Respiratory

- Spirometer, to measure the air capacity of the lungs. This may also be measured using a peak

flow meter, and is often used in general practice.

CONCLUSION

After reading this chapter, medical secretaries should be more aware of the dangers which may be involved in medical practice and will be better prepared to cope with some of the important health and safety issues. Understanding of physiological tests should also be improved. Make sure you understand any instructions you have been given when you have to deal with any of the issues discussed in this chapter, so that danger is minimised, and the working environment is as safe as possible for all staff and patients.

Exercises

Make a list of all Health and Safety issues you might find in general practice. Some may be specifically medical, others may be of a more general nature.

Further reading

Hampson GD 1994 Practice nurse handbook, 3rd edn. Blackwell Scientific Publications, Oxford

Richardson A 1995 Preparation to care: A foundation NVQ text for health care assistants. Baillière Tindall, London

Simons P, Quinn B 1996 The GP receptionist's handbook. Baillière Tindall, London

Internet www.healthandsafety.co.uk/safpol.htm

Chapter 18

Managing medicines (drugs)

Tracy Sweet, Helen Mortimer

OBJECTIVES

- To consider the difference between generic and proprietary names for drugs
- To identify the reference sources on drugs used to access information relevant to the role of the medical secretary
- To increase understanding of major legislation governing the supply of medicines to the public
- To examine the documentation in common use when prescribing and supplying drugs, and the need for its accurate completion
- To identify the procedures for running manual and computerised repeat prescribing systems efficiently and accurately
- To outline the possible functions of a medical secretary in a dispensing practice
- To increase knowledge of prescription charges and exemptions.

INTRODUCTION

The medical secretary needs to understand the range of responsibilities that is involved in the management of prescribing and supply of medicines to patients, including:

- the ordering and storage of drugs
- the writing or printing of repeat prescriptions

- the submission of prescriptions to the Prescription Pricing Authority (PPA)
- advising patients on prescription charges, exemption categories and related costs.

Before reading this chapter, it is advisable to obtain up-to-date copies of the following reference sources:

- the *British National Formulary* (BNF)
- the *Monthly Index of Medical Specialities* (MIMS)
- the *Drug Tariff*
- the *ABPI Compendium*.

DRUG NAMES – GENERICS AND PROPRIETARIES

It is important that the medical secretary understands the difference between generic and proprietary names for drugs.

THE GENERIC NAME

When a pharmaceutical company discovers a new compound, it is allocated a 'chemical' name, giving a technical description. The patent is registered using the drug's chemical name, giving the company 20 years of exclusive use.

The drug is also given a *generic* name. The generic name is the drug's official medical name, and often indicates the therapeutic class to which a drug belongs. The generic name is sometimes referred to as the 'approved name'. It is the name used in most medical literature.

THE PROPRIETARY NAME

The drug is marketed using a *proprietary* name. The proprietary name is a brand name or trademark. The name is designed to sell, and is usually easy to remember.

Companies hope that when the drug is manufactured by other firms, GPs will continue to prescribe the drug by its original brand name. Other firms may use the generic name with their firm's endorsement on the packaging and tablets, or market the generic under their own proprietary name.

A well-known example is the generic drug ibuprofen. *Ibuprofen* was originally produced by Boots as Brufen, but is now manufactured by many other suppliers under a variety of proprietary names (e.g.

Nurofen) as well as in a generic form.

When typing drug names, it is usual to write the proprietary name with an initial capital letter, but not the generic name e.g. Brufen, ibuprofen; Calpol, paracetamol mixture.

ADVANTAGES OF GENERIC PRESCRIBING

Economy. Companies that manufacture generic medicines have not incurred development costs, and are, therefore, able to produce the drug at much lower cost. The Department of Health is encouraging GPs and other groups able to prescribe, to increase their use of generic prescribing to cut costs.

Recognition. Medical students are taught pharmacology using generic names; most prescribing in hospitals is by generic name and scientific journals use generic names.

DISADVANTAGES OF GENERICS

Compliance. The pharmacist may supply any producer's generic when dispensing a generic prescription. The patient may, therefore, be confused by receiving medication which varies in size, shape, taste, colour or format. This may undermine the patient's confidence with their medication, eventually affecting compliance. (NB: There are plans to standardise the appearance of generics in the future.)

Naming. The names of generics are overall less memorable than proprietary names – and harder to spell!

Reduced investment. The pharmaceutical industry may invest less on research and development as a reduction in profits occurs.

The average level of generic prescribing in the UK was approximately 63% in September 1998, with a government target of 72%.

REFERENCE SOURCES

In order to work efficiently, the medical secretary must have the ability to *access* further information or check spellings of drug names, as and when required. **The basic references should be easily accessible to the medical secretary, and they should be up to date at all times.** Out-of-date information could be dangerous.

Information on medicines can be obtained from a variety of sources. The more important texts are unbiased and non-promotional. The basic texts the medical secretary should be using, and keeping up to date, are:

- the *British National Formulary* (BNF)
- the *Monthly Index of Medical Specialities* (MIMS)
- the *Drug Tariff*.

BRITISH NATIONAL FORMULARY (BNF)

All doctors and pharmacists receive, free of charge, copies of the BNF. The Department of Health publishes it and arranges distribution within the NHS. The publication is the most widely used primary reference source for information on medicines and prescribing in the UK.

It is published twice yearly, so it is always reasonably up to date.

The main text consists of notes on all the preparations that are available in the UK, divided into numbered chapters on the important organ systems (e.g. the gastrointestinal system) and other main topics (e.g. infections).

Common over-the-counter preparations are now also included. This information is useful for the GP when checking interactions with prescribed medication.

The BNF is written using generic names. Where proprietaries are available, they are summarised after the notes on the generic drug.

The main text is supplemented by several useful appendices, including recommended wording for labelling medicines, which will be particularly relevant to medical secretaries working in dispensing practices. The addresses and telephone numbers for all of the pharmaceutical companies with products detailed in the BNF are listed. The medical secretary may occasionally be asked to contact one of the companies with an enquiry regarding a product.

Inside the back cover is a table giving common Latin abbreviations with their recognised translation. This may be useful to a medical secretary faced with a handwritten prescription containing an unfamiliar abbreviation.

Exercise

What is the difference between q.d.s. and q.d.h.? Check your BNF.

A computerised version of the BNF is now available on subscription to health care professionals. The computer screen format is identical to the pages of the pocket book version of the BNF, but provides additional facilities. For example, a click on an entry in the contents list or index immediately accesses the required page.

Exercise

Click onto 5.1 and list five of the antibacterial sections identified.

MONTHLY INDEX OF MEDICAL SPECIALITIES (MIMS)

This commonly used prescribing guide is published by an independent company, and sent free to all GPs every month. It is, therefore, always up to date. MIMS contains details of all prescribable proprietary drugs, including prices. The index includes both proprietary and generic names for products.

Like the BNF, MIMS is arranged into therapeutic categories (e.g. cardiovascular system), and includes the names, addresses and telephone numbers of all the pharmaceutical companies with products entered in MIMS.

DRUG TARIFF

The *Drug Tariff* is an essential reference source, particularly for dispensing practices. It is compiled by the Prescription Pricing Authority (PPA) for the Department of Health, and is updated each month. A copy is sent to all GPs.

Examples of the information it provides include:

- the information to be added to prescriptions (the 'endorsements') to enable the correct payments to be made to dispensing doctors and community pharmacists
- an up-to-date list of items which cannot be prescribed on an NHS prescription (the 'blacklist')
- prescription charge details
- a list of prescribable appliances (e.g. catheters and stoma bags).

ABPI COMPENDIUM OF DATA SHEETS AND SUMMARIES OF PRODUCT CHARACTERISTICS

Data Sheets and Summaries of Product Characteristics (SPCs) are documents prepared by pharmaceutical companies on their products. They are non-promotional, factual information sheets, conforming to a standard format.

The ABPI Compendium is a compendium of data sheets and SPCs containing the majority of products made by companies in the UK. It is issued free to all doctors and pharmacists by the Association of British Pharmaceutical Industry (ABPI).

Much more detailed information is available on drugs from this reference source, including storage requirements, legal category, treatment of over-dosage.

PHARMACEUTICAL REPRESENTATIVES

Pharmaceutical representatives have access to a large database of up-to-date technical information and literature maintained by the companies for whom they work. Representatives can, therefore, be a valuable source of information, particularly on a new drug.

Some representatives provide resources and information for the practice, e.g.:

- posters for the waiting room (e.g. for flu vaccination campaigns)
- specialised record cards, printed by the company, e.g. for recording blood pressure checks, diabetic clinic attendances.
- advice on storing vaccines.

The medical secretary may be responsible for making appointments for the representatives to see GPs to discuss new drug developments and products. Appointments may also be made with practice or dispensary managers to discuss discounts on bulk orders, or new products.

THE MEDICINES ACT 1968

The Medicines Act 1968 is concerned with the manufacture, sale, supply, packaging, labelling, advertising, safety and use of medicines.

The Medicines Act requires each drug to be licensed before marketing. Product licences are considered on the basis of their safety, quality and efficacy.

Thalidomide was first marketed in 1956 for the treatment of insomnia and vomiting in early pregnancy. In 1961 there was a marked increase in the incidence of congenital birth defects, typically an absence or reduction of the long bones of the limbs. Unfortunately, the association with thalidomide was not recognised for several years with the result that thousands of babies were born worldwide with these deformities.

The legal framework governing the licensing of drugs results from the recommendations of a committee set up as a direct result of the thalidomide disaster. (Before the Medicines Act came into effect, there was no legal requirement for approval or control of the development of new medicines on the grounds of their safety.)

Under the Act, the Committee on the Safety of Medicines (CSM) advises on the safety, quality and effectiveness of new medicines and collects and investigates reports on adverse reactions to all medicines on the market, issuing warnings about any newly identified hazards.

THE YELLOW CARD SYSTEM

Under a voluntary scheme, introduced in 1964, GPs are requested to report suspected adverse drug reactions to the Committee on the Safety of Medicines on yellow, pre-paid report forms, found at the back of the BNF, as well as the back of prescription forms. In recent years, there have been several examples of drugs being withdrawn by the CSM as a result of adverse reaction reporting. The CSM may, alternatively, modify either the indications for use, contraindications to use or the recommended dose. At present nurse prescribers have to inform either a GP or a consultant of adverse reactions, who complete a yellow card. Adverse reactions to over-the-counter treatments and complementary treatments are also included in the yellow card scheme.

'BLACK TRIANGLE' REQUIREMENT

Drugs annotated with an inverted black triangle in the BNF and MIMS carry a requirement to report all adverse reactions to the CSM, however minor. The symbol is used for the first two years of a product's life.

MEDICINES CLASSIFICATION

The sale and supply of medicines is controlled by the Medicines Act 1968 and Directive 2001/83/EC. All medicines are classified according to one of three following categories:

- Prescription only Medicines (POM) – available only on prescription. e.g. Augmentin.
- Pharmacy (P) – available under the supervision of a pharmacist. e.g. paracetamol packs containing more than 24 tablets.
- General Sales List (GSL)- available in general retail outlets such as supermarkets. e.g. paracetamol packs containing fewer than 24 tablets.

Exercise

Identify four medicines under each of the three categories.

As prescription charges increase, more and more prescriptions cost less over the counter than the actual prescription charge. The medical secretary may, therefore, be asked by some patients whether their prescription can be purchased over the counter. The legal classification of each drug is shown in the ABPI Compendium of Data Sheets and SPCs. The retail cost is shown in MIMS.

SUPPLY OF MEDICINES

A Prescription Only Medicine (POM) prescribed by a GP on a prescription must be provided in accordance with the Medicines Act 1968. For example, the drug must be supplied in a suitable container (as listed in the *Drug Tariff*).

The Medicines Act requires all medicine labels to include the following information:

- the patient's name
- the date on which the medicine is dispensed
- the dispensing GP or pharmacist's name, address and telephone number
- a reminder that medicines should be kept out of the reach of children.

Some warning labels, such as 'for external use only', if appropriate, are also a legal requirement.

Although not a legal requirement, labels also usually show:

- the name of the product
- the quantity
- directions regarding use.

DISPENSING OF MEDICINES

The Medicines Act 1968 gives GPs the right to dispense medicines when certain conditions are met.

Practice and community nurses with health visiting or district nursing qualifications are also able to prescribe a limited range of drugs, once they have undergone a programme of training.

THE LIMITED LIST

In an attempt to control the cost of prescribed drugs, on 1 April 1985 the Department of Health created a 'blacklist' of products in certain therapeutic groups which should not be prescribed by GPs at NHS expense. Some drugs are barred from NHS prescribing completely, whilst others are excluded as proprietaries but accepted in their generic form. For example, Valium is blacklisted, but its generic version, diazepam, can still be prescribed.

Should GPs prescribe blacklisted products the community pharmacist or dispensing doctor would not receive payment. The BNF shows blacklisted items with the symbol N̶H̶S̶. The *Drug Tariff* has a totally up-to-date list. (As the list occasionally changes, it is important to access an up-to-date list of blacklisted products.) Should a patient insist on a blacklisted drug, the GP could issue a private prescription and the patient would have to pay the full cost of the drug.

DRUGS TO BE PRESCRIBED IN CERTAIN CIRCUMSTANCES UNDER THE NHS

A small number of drugs can only be prescribed under the NHS for *certain patients* for the treatment of *specific conditions*, as detailed in the *Drug Tariff*. The GP must add SLS (meaning selected list scheme) to the prescription form to confirm that the patient is being treated for the specified condition.

BORDERLINE SUBSTANCES

In certain circumstances some foods and preparations have the characteristics of drugs. The Advisory Committee on Borderline Substances advises on the circumstances when such substances may be regarded as drugs, i.e. for the treatment of specified conditions. When prescribing borderline substances for an approved condition, the prescription must be endorsed 'ACBS'. Without this endorsement, the GP is likely to be questioned on the prescribing of the item.

The BNF and *Drug Tariff* list borderline substances.

MISUSE OF DRUGS ACT 1971

The Misuse of Drugs Act 1971 provides comprehensive control to prevent the misuse of *controlled drugs*.

THE SCHEDULES AND CLASSES OF DRUGS

Controlled drugs are classified into five *schedules*, beginning with the most heavily controlled drugs. The schedules dictate the requirements with regard to import, export, production, supply, possession, prescribing and record-keeping.

Schedule 1 drugs (e.g. LSD) are not used medicinally. The possession and supply of such drugs is prohibited.

Schedule 2 drugs include diamorphine, morphine and pethidine, and are subject to the full drug requirements relating to:

- prescription writing
- safe custody
- entries in controlled drugs register
- destruction.

Many Schedule 2 drugs are available in injection form, and are personally administered by GPs. All medical secretaries, whether working in an urban or rural dispensing practice, are, therefore, likely to be required to order controlled drugs and be responsible for maintaining an accurate controlled drugs register. It is important that the medical secretary knows the laws related to such functions.

Schedule 3 drugs are subject to special prescription writing requirements only.

Schedule 4 drugs include most benzodiazepines,

which are subject to minimal controls.

Schedule 5 drugs include those, which because of their strength, are exempt from virtually all the controlled drugs requirements.

Preparations contained in Schedules 2 and 3 are marked CD in the BNF and MIMS. The ABPI Compendium of Data Sheets and SPCs gives the schedule for all controlled drugs.

SECURITY OF CONTROLLED DRUGS

All controlled drugs in Schedule 2 must be kept in a locked safe or cabinet, with nothing on the outside to indicate its use. The number of people with access to the key should be limited. It is sensible to

---

Box 18.1 Information that should be included on a prescription

- The date
- The full name and address of the patient
- The age of the patient (this is a legal requirement for children under 12 years of age)
- The name of the drug (preferably in capital letters) and its strength
- The form (e.g. tablets, capsules, syrup)
- The frequency (the number of doses in a day)
- The dose (how many are to be taken at each frequency)
- The quantity to be dispensed
- The name, surgery address, telephone number, national index code and the name of the Health Authority of the prescriber – GP or nurse
- The signature of the GP/nurse.

Box 18.2 Information required in the Controlled Drugs Register

For drugs received	*For drugs supplied*
The date received	The date supply made
The name and address of supplying person/firm	The name and address of person supplied
The amount received	The name of the GP authorised to hold and
The form in which the drugs are supplied	supply
	The amount supplied

avoid fitting the cabinet where it can be seen by members of the public, for example opposite a reception hatch or window.

Safe custody requirements also apply to the following Schedule 3 drugs:

- buprenorphine (e.g. Temegesic)
- diethylpropion
- temazepam.

PRESCRIBING CONTROLLED DRUGS – PRESCRIPTION REQUIREMENTS

In addition to the usual information required when writing prescriptions, for drugs listed in Schedules 2 and 3 the prescription must also comply with the following legal requirements:

- be handwritten by the GP
- include the total quantity or number of dosage units written in words and figures.

Temazepam is the only Schedule 3 drug which is exempt from all the special prescription writing requirements. Phenobarbitone, another Schedule 3 drug, is exempt from the handwriting requirements only (except in relation to the date).

If the prescription given to the patient is incomplete, or incorrectly written, it cannot be dispensed, and will be returned to the GP for clarification.

INVOICES

All invoices for Schedule 3 and 5 controlled drugs must be retained for 2 years.

THE CONTROLLED DRUGS REGISTER

Every transaction, in relation to Schedule 2 drugs *received* and *dispensed*, must be recorded in the controlled drugs register. A separate register must be kept for each surgery.

The register must include the entries shown in Box 18.2. The register must:

- be a bound book with ruled and headed columns
- be written in ink or indelible pen
- have separate sections for each class of drug
- have entries made on the day of transaction, or the following day
- have no cancellations or alterations (corrections must be made in the margin or as a footnote, and must be signed and dated)
- be kept on the premises to which the register relates
- be available for inspection at any time, e.g. by the Home Office drugs inspector
- be kept for 2 years from the date of the last entry.

Whilst not legal requirements, the following are considered to be good practice:

- A column to record the balance of stock. (This allows the actual stock to be reconciled with the entry recorded in the register, thus enabling any stock shortages to be identified and investigated.)
- Separate registers for each GP's bag.

DESTRUCTION OF CONTROLLED DRUGS

Once drugs have passed their expiry date, they must be destroyed. Controlled drugs in Schedule 2 may only be destroyed in the presence of a person authorised by the Secretary of State, e.g. a police officer or Home Office inspector.

Details including the name of the drug, the amount and date must be entered in the controlled drugs register, and signed by the person in whose presence the drug was destroyed.

This legal requirement does not apply to controlled drugs returned to a GP by a patient. The 'audit trail' of controlled drugs leads from their import, through every stage, and ends with supply to the patient.

SECURITY

The Misuse of Drugs Act covers security measures to help prevent users unlawfully obtaining supplies of drugs and prescription pads.

SECURITY OF PRESCRIPTIONS

There are detailed instructions regarding writing prescriptions for controlled drugs in a way that reduces the opportunity to make unauthorised alterations. It is obviously good practice to apply the same procedures to all prescriptions.

Prescriptions should be regarded as security stationery. To improve security, in line with the requirements of the Misuse of Drugs Act, prescription forms now include serial numbers. Practice staff are required to record the serial numbers of prescription forms received from the NHS Support Services. In the event of a loss or suspected theft, the practice must inform the police and the NHS Support Services immediately of the missing serial numbers. Stolen prescription forms may then be detected if they are subsequently presented for dispensing.

Prescriptions also now have a coloured background to make photocopying more difficult, and contain anti-tampering devices within the ink and paper to make forgeries detectable. Forms also have a message which can be seen under UV lights to aid detection of counterfoiled forms.

However, to avoid losses or thefts, blank prescription forms:

- must not be pre-signed
- must be locked away when not in use
- must not be left unattended at a reception desk or in the consulting room
- must not be left in a car, particularly if displaying a DOCTOR ON CALL sign
- must not be used as notepads.

Prescriptions given to patients should have an oblique line below the last item to prevent the addition of items. A circle around the quantity to be supplied also helps avoid unauthorised alterations. The prescription must only be completed by the person whose name and personal identification number appears on it. They must not be shared.

SECURITY OF PREMISES

It is important, particularly in the case of dispensing practices, that security for the whole premises is good. Addicts may break into a surgery if they feel able to obtain money, prescription forms or drugs. Good security measures will, therefore, act as a deterrent.

Measures can include:

- window locks for all windows
- window bars, particularly for dispensaries
- an intruder alarm system, preferably connected to the police station
- security lighting which activates when someone approaches the building.

Dispensing practices should consider storing their medicines other than alphabetically, as an addict would then have more difficulty in finding the drugs required.

Only limited amounts of cash should be kept on the premises, in a lockable metal container, preferably in a locked drawer. Dispensing practices should ensure that the prescription charges collected are banked regularly.

DOCUMENTATION

There are a variety of standard forms necessary for prescribing and dispensing. Most of them are available from the NHS Support Services. Many practices have also devised their own forms.

The medical secretary is often responsible for maintaining adequate stocks of both the standard forms and those that are devised by the practice. They should be easily accessible in drawers and cupboards, e.g. prepayment certificates in the reception area.

The medical secretary should be familiar with the forms, and know how to use them.

STANDARD DOCUMENTATION

NHS prescription forms

Prescriptions are produced by doctors as a request to a pharmacist or dispenser to supply specific items. NHS prescription forms in dispensing practices then become a record of supply, which are used as a request for payment to the Prescription Pricing Authority (PPA).

NHS prescriptions are:

- an order for medication
- an invoice for submission to the PPA.

The back of the prescription form provides a checklist for the patient to tick and sign if eligible for free prescriptions.

The vast majority of prescriptions in general practice are issued on a FP10C computerised prescription form or a FP10NC for handwritten prescriptions (Figure 18.1). Both of these forms are green.

Prescriptions are valid for 6 months.

Prescriptions for controlled drugs are valid for 13 weeks.

Prescription writing requirements

The prescription form provides all of the informa-

NAME

Age if under
12 years

yrs.   mths.   Address

Pricing
Office
use only

Pharmacy Stamp

Pharmacist's
pack & quantity
endorsement

No. of days treatment
N.B. Ensure dose is stated

NP

CANCELLED

Signature of Doctor   Date

For
phar-
macist
No. of
Prescns.
on form

IMPORTANT:- Read the notes overleaf before going to the pharmacy

Form FP10 (Comp.)(D)
(Rev 96)

IMPORTANT NOTES FOR PATIENTS

- Before getting the item(s) overleaf dispensed you must mark ✗ in a box at Part A, then complete either **Part B** or **Part C** or **both** as appropriate.
- If you think you might be entitled to a refund of the money you have paid, you must get an NHS receipt (FP57) when you pay. *You cannot get one later.*
- If you need a lot of medication you may want to buy a prepayment certificate.
- To find out more about prescription charges, get leaflet HC11 *"Are you entitled to help with health costs?"* from your pharmacist.

Part A   I am   ✗   the patient named overleaf
                    ✗   the patient's parent/guardian/representative   *(delete as appropriate)*

Part B   for the item(s) overleaf
I have paid the sum of £
Signed   Date

Part C   I do not have to pay the charge because the patient: (✗ *in the appropriate boxes*)

IS EXEMPT ON AGE GROUNDS:
M ✗ under 16 years of age
N ✗ 16-18 *and* in full time education
O ✗ 60 years or over

HOLDS AN EXEMPTION CERTIFICATE:
P ✗ maternity or medical exemption (FP92)
Q ✗ prepayment certificate (FP96)
R ✗ War/MoD pensioner   Ref. no:
        exemption certificate
        - *and the items overleaf are for the pensionable disability.*

RECEIVES OR IS THE PARTNER OF SOMEONE RECEIVING:
S ✗ Income Support
T ✗ Family Credit
U ✗ Disability Working Allowance and (*until 7 October 1996*) had capital of
        £8,000 or less on the date the claim was made
V ✗ Income-based Jobseeker's Allowance (*from 7 October 1996*)
W ✗ a current NHS charges   HC2/AG2 no:
        certificate for full help

OR:
X ✗ is being given no-charge contraceptives

Signed   Date
Name
Address
*(if different
from overleaf)*

WARNING   **TO GIVE FALSE INFORMATION MAY LEAD TO PROSECUTION**
This form is the property of the National Health Service

Figure 18.1 Prescription form FP10. (Reproduced by permission of the Department of Health)

```
        Drs. A. B. Smith & C. D. Jones.
             Tel: 01579 337744

     Qty 21 AMOXYCILLIN CAPS 250MG (AAH)
     ONE to be taken THREE TIMES daily

   TAKE AT REGULAR INTERVALS-FINISH COURSE

     Date: 00-00-0000   Mr Percy Patient

          Keep out of children's reach
```

```
        Drs. A. B. Smith & C. D. Jones.
             Tel: 01579 337744

   Date: 00-00-0000        One item enclosed
               Mr Percy Patient
                 19 The Road
           St. Stephen St. Austell
                  PL26 1ZZ

          Keep out of children's reach
```

Figure 18.2 Computer printed labels

```
When requesting or collecting
repeat prescriptions please call
after 11 am.

As from Date 00-00-0000,
Saturday surgeries will only be
held at the Mile Road surgery.

Telephone No. PLEASE TICK BOX
FOR THE MEDICINE YOU REQUIRE

Date:00-00-0000

- - - - - - - - - - - - - - - - - -
THYROXINE TABLETS    60 [ ]
100mcg, ONE TO BE TAKEN DAILY
- - - - - - - - - - - - - - - - - -


Review is due before
Date:00-00-0000
```

Figure 18.3 A repeat prescription form

tion on which the prescription will be dispensed. It is important, therefore, that the patient and the medication are clearly identified with sufficient information to enable the correct drug to be dispensed with an accurate label to the correct patient (Figure 18.2). The medical secretary is often involved in the printing of repeat prescription forms (Figure 18.3). However, to be able to check computerised prescriptions include sufficient and appropriate detail, and to enable a service to be maintained when the practice computers are out of action, the medical secretary also needs to be familiar with the recommendations for prescription *writing*.

The prescription form should include the information shown in Box 18.1

Handwritten prescriptions should be written in ink (legibly).

Special markings

The name and strength of the drug should always appear on the label of a dispensed medicine unless the GP deletes the letters NP (nomen propium – Latin for proper name) from the prescription form. The name of the preparation will not then appear on the label. Instead, wording such as 'the sleeping tablets' would be used. The use of NP is a rare event, but occasionally the GP may not want the patient to know what is being prescribed, for example if the patient is able to relate the drug name to a particular disease.

Abbreviations

All of the instructions on a prescription form should be written or printed in English and in full. The only acceptable exceptions to this rule are the commonly used Latin abbreviations, e.g.

bd	twice a day
mane	in the morning
nocte	at night

In addition, the following 'rules' should be observed:

- print/write quantities of less than 1 gram in milligrams, e.g. 500mg, not 0.5g
- print/write quantities of less than 1 mg in micrograms, e.g. 100 micrograms, not 0.1mg

- add a zero in front of a decimal point when there is no other figure and decimals are unavoidable, e.g. 0.5ml, not .5ml.

Computerised prescriptions

Computerised prescription forms (FP10C) are available from the NHS Support Services in continuous stationery form. They are double the width of a prescription, perforated between the two halves – the left side comprising the prescription, and the right side blank.

Computer software usually leaves it to the practice to decide on the content of the blank side. This tear-off section can provide a very useful source of information for the patient, and is often used to list current repeat prescriptions, thereby doubling as a repeat prescription request form. A practice message may be added – either on a prescribing matter or some other administrative function, e.g.

- a reminder that a review of repeat drugs is due
- simple health advice
- information on new appointment arrangements.

It is illegal to computer print a prescription for a Schedule 2 or 3 controlled drug (except temazepam and phenobarbitone).

Nurses' prescription forms

Practice nurses with a district nursing or health visitor qualification, community nurses and specialist hospital nurses, are allowed to prescribe from a limited list of drugs once they have undergone an approved nurse prescriber training. The items which nurses are entitled to prescribe are published in the *Drug Tariff* and the BNF, *Nurse Prescribers' Formulary* (NPF) and *Nurse Prescribers' Extended Formulary* (NPEF). The prescription form used is a lilac FP10P and clearly annotated District Nurse/Health Visitor Prescriber. The prescription form includes the nurse's NMC PIN number, the practice identification number and the full address of the practice. The same guidelines apply for completion, security and accountability for nurse prescribers as for GPs. Nurses cannot prescribe controlled drugs

Form FP10 (MDA)

This form is used by GPs to prescribe controlled drugs for the treatment of drug addiction for dispensing in instalments (usually on a daily basis). Supplies are obtainable from the Support Services

Exercise

A community nurse asks to borrow the practice nurse's prescription pad as he has forgotten his pad. What would you do?

in pads of 10 numbered forms. The form is a light blue, double-sided, prescription form.

Application for dispensing services

Form GMS1, the form used by patients to register with a GP, is also used to apply for dispensing services at dispensing practices, usually at the time of registration or following a change of address to a dispensing area of the practice.

Invoice for drugs and appliances supplied – Form FP34D

Form FP34D is completed at the end of each month, and sent with prescription forms to the PPA to claim reimbursement of drug expenditure and dispensing fees.

Receipt form – FP57

Form FP57, a receipt of prescription charges paid, should be issued to any patient seeking a refund. The form is only relevant to dispensing practices.

Patients requesting receipts include those on a low income, and those who have applied for, but not yet received, an exemption certificate.

Prepayment certificates – Form FP95

Patients who need frequent prescriptions and who pay prescription charges can save money by purchasing a prepayment certificate (often referred to as a 'season ticket'). A prepayment certificate is cost-effective for patients who need more than five items in four months. The medical secretary can help patients by drawing their attention to the availability of prepayment certificates.

The application form is available from practices, the Post Office and Benefit Agency offices. The application form and payment are sent to the Support Services by the patient, and a prepayment certificate is then issued.

NHS prescriptions – How to Get Your Prescriptions Dispensed – leaflet HC11

It is important that patients who might be entitled to exemption from charges or to help with costs on grounds of low income are informed accordingly. The HC11 leaflet should be displayed prominently for patients, as it explains who is eligible for free prescriptions, as well as information on prepayment certificates and refunds. When a patient claims exemption the form must be shown and it is recorded on the prescription that it has been seen, this is to prevent fraud. Exemption certificates are now issued in the form of swipe cards by the PPA.

PRACTICE-SPECIFIC DOCUMENTATION

Private prescriptions

Private prescriptions should be written on headed notepaper, or on specially printed prescription forms. A private prescription has to include the same essential identifying information as an NHS prescription. In addition, it must specify the GP's qualifications.

Unlike NHS prescriptions, private prescriptions can be repeated. Most private prescription forms include a box for 'number of repeats'. The prescription can then be supplied the authorised number of times.

Private prescription forms must be presented and dispensed for the first time within 6 months of issue.

The same rules apply to the writing of both NHS and private prescriptions for controlled drugs. Repeat dispensing of private prescriptions for controlled drugs is not allowed. However, the GP can direct that a prescription be dispensed in instalments.

Private prescriptions are written for:

- medicines solely in anticipation of the onset of an illness abroad, e.g. drugs taken on holiday for possible illnesses such as diarrhoea and vomiting
- malaria prophylaxis
- private patients
- blacklisted substances
- overseas visitors (at the GP's discretion)
- patients unable to produce a medical card, where the GP has reasonable doubts that the patient is registered with the practice.

GPs are entitled to charge a patient for issuing a private prescription in the above circumstances, unless it is for a blacklisted product. The British Medical Association (BMA) publishes a recommended fee each year.

REPEAT PRESCRIPTIONS

A repeat prescription is an order for further supply of medication without a face-to-face contact with the GP. Repeat prescriptions are for patients who need replacement drugs more frequently than they need to see the GP, e.g. patients with hypertension, asthma and diabetes. Up to two-thirds of all prescriptions are issued as repeats.

Not all drug therapy is suitable for inclusion in a repeat prescribing system; some drugs are intended for short-term use only.

GPs differ on the quantity of drug they prescribe for patients on a repeat prescription. However, there is a generally held view that prescribing should be for a maximum of 28 days. This helps control drug misuse and reduce drug wastage, e.g. due to changes in medication, deaths.

Patients may continue to receive medication unnecessarily or be using it inappropriately unless they are regularly reviewed by the GP, or sometimes the practice nurse. The patient may be suffering from a condition, such as hypertension, which needs regular review. The repeat prescription system will, therefore, limit repeats – either by the number of prescriptions or by a time interval. The review period will depend on the drug, the condition being treated and the individual patient. When producing repeat prescriptions, the medical secretary must ensure that the authorised number of repeats is not exceeded.

The medical secretary is often responsible for the production of repeat prescriptions, and should, therefore, be familiar with the following aspects of a repeat prescription system.

ACCEPTING REPEAT PRESCRIPTIONS

Various procedures have been developed for accepting repeat prescriptions, whether requested by letter, over the telephone or in person.

Repeat prescription cards. Listing the authorised repeats are handed in or posted to the surgery. The items requested should be clearly indicated by the patient.

Telephone requests. Some practices accept requests by telephone, particularly for the housebound and elderly, to avoid mistakes over names of medicines, it is important that the person taking the call has access to the patient's records. A separate telephone line for repeat prescription requests may be required to avoid congestion. However, most practices discourage telephone requests and require patients to write or to fax requests.

Right-hand side of FP10C. This can be used to request repeats. The print-out holds an up-to-date record of authorised repeat medication for the patient to tick and post or hand in to the practice.

PRODUCING PRESCRIPTIONS

From the various requests, the medical secretary must produce accurate repeat prescriptions.

By referring to the repeat prescribing records, the medical secretary should check that:

- the patient and the drugs are clearly identified
- the drug, dose and quantity correspond
- the item is authorised as a repeat
- a further issue is authorised
- the interval since the last issue is neither too early nor too late.

In the case of queries, the GP will usually need the medical records as well as the repeat prescribing records.

Each time a repeat prescription is issued, the date and drugs dispensed should be recorded, using manual or computerised records. There are two common systems.

Repeat prescription sheets. Separate record sheets can be tagged to the patients' records or filed alphabetically, separate from the main filing system.

Computerised repeat prescribing records. These are increasingly popular. They provide a fast and efficient recording system. A computerised repeat prescription system has the following advantages:

- The prescription forms are legible, typewritten and accurate.
- The computer gives the patient a printed record of their repeat medication.
- The patient is automatically informed if he/she is due for review before further repeats.
- The computer monitors the interval between prescriptions.

COLLECTION ARRANGEMENTS

Most practices ask for a minimum of 48 hours notice for collection of repeat prescriptions. The secretary will need to ensure that the prescription forms are signed by the GP in time for collection. The forms are often stored alphabetically, awaiting collection. The storage area must be a secure place away from the reception desk, as signed prescriptions are open to abuse if stolen.

Increasingly practices are requesting stamped self-addressed envelopes to post the repeat prescription to the patient.

Prescriptions may be collected by a local pharmacist, so that the medication can be dispensed ready for the patient to collect later that day.

THE ADVANTAGES OF REPEAT PRESCRIBING

An efficient repeat prescribing system gives the patients easy access to medication when needed. The need to consult the GP is reduced, saving time for both the GP and the patient. Patients can plan when to collect their prescriptions or arrange for collection on their behalf.

Patients who are uncomfortable when asked to make frequent contact with health care workers find a repeat prescribing system suits them much better.

DISADVANTAGES OF REPEAT PRESCRIBING

The patient does not see the GP as often. The patient may begin to take their medication incorrectly or may mix drugs inappropriately with over-the-counter medicines.

DISPENSING OF DRUGS

Almost all practices dispense a limited range of drugs to their patients. Some medical secretaries may be required to undertake dispensing duties, but this work requires specialist training and is, therefore, outside the remit of this textbook.

All practices dispense drugs to their patients if needed for their *immediate* treatment, as well as some *personally administered* drugs. The most commonly dispensed items for personal administration include vaccines, injections, intrauterine contraceptive devices and sutures.

Patients in rural areas may obtain all their medicines from a dispensing GP provided they live more than one mile from the nearest pharmacy.

Dispensing GPs can also dispense to all temporary residents (irrespective of where they live).

Reflection Point 1

A 10-year-old girl calls to collect her mother's repeat prescription. How would you manage this situation?

PAYMENTS FOR DISPENSING SERVICES

To obtain payment for NHS prescriptions, each item dispensed must be recorded on an FP10 and sent to the PPA. The PPA then prices the prescriptions, and notifies the Primary Care Trust (PCT) of the payments due to dispensing GPs and community pharmacists.

Remuneration comprises the following elements:

- the **basic price** of the drug (as defined in the *Drug Tariff* for generic preparations and MIMS for proprietary products)
- an **on-cost allowance** (currently 10.5% of the basic price)
- a container allowance, paid whether or not a container, medicine spoon etc. is required
- a **dispensing fee** paid on a sliding scale according to the number of prescription items submitted each month
- a VAT **allowance** to cover VAT on purchases of drugs, appliances and containers – unless the practice is entitled to reclaim VAT from HM Customs and Excise.

Before payments are made to the practice a deduction is made from the basic price to allow for the discount that GPs are assumed to obtain from their suppliers.

The PPA no longer requires separate FP10s for eight high-volume personally administered vaccines, e.g. influenza and tetanus. Instead an Appendix to Form FP34D is completed each month, listing the number of each vaccine administered. (A list of the patients who received each vaccine is retained at the practice.)

SUBMITTING PRESCRIPTION FORMS TO THE PPA

It is often the medical secretary's responsibility to send the prescription forms to the PPA at the end of each month. The following procedure should be followed:

1. Form FP34D should be completed. Each GP's name and national index code is entered, along with the number of prescription forms and items being submitted on their prescription forms. The number of high-volume vaccines administered is recorded in the Appendix.

2. The secretary should check that the prescriptions have been correctly completed and signed. If a prescription form is not clear, the PPA will not be able to price the item, and the form will be returned to the practice for clarification, delaying payment.

3. The prescription forms for the month, along with a completed and signed FP34D, are packed securely, and posted to the PPA. It is recommended that the parcel is sent by recorded delivery. The package must arrive no later than the 5th day of the month after the prescriptions were dispensed. For example, prescriptions dispensed during March should arrive by 5 April. If the secretary misses the deadline, the PPA may delay payment.

COLLECTING PRESCRIPTION CHARGES

Dispensing GPs are responsible for collecting prescription charges for each item supplied to those patients who pay. The total charges collected are either declared to the PCT each month, and deducted from drug payments received, or sent direct to the PCT.

The medical secretary may be required to collect prescription charges from patients. The cash received should be stored securely in a lockable site, and regularly transferred to the bank. Some patients may pay prescription charges by cheque.

PRESCRIPTION CHARGES

Over 80% of items are issued to patients who are exempt from paying prescription charges. The various categories of patients who are eligible for free prescriptions are shown in Box 18.3.

Box 18.3 Criteria for free prescriptions

Automatic exemption on age grounds
- Children under 16
- Students under 19 in full-time education
- Men and women aged 60 and over

Patients holding exemption certificates
- Pregnant mothers
- Women who have given birth in the last 12 months
- Patients suffering from specified medical conditions, e.g. diabetes and epilepsy (the full list is included in the Drug Tariff)
- War and service pensioners (only for prescriptions needed to treat their war disablement)

Patients who have purchased a prepayment certificate (Form FP95)

People with DSS exemption certificates, including people receiving income support or family credit

Free prescriptions
- Prescription charges are not made for items supplied under the personal administration arrangements
- Contraceptive substances and appliances are prescribed free of charge to women
- Bulk prescriptions are not chargeable. A bulk prescription is a single prescription form for two or more patients. It is only valid for schools or institutions of 20 or more people, where the GP writing the prescription is responsible for at least 10 of the residents. The prescription is made out in the name of the institution, instead of a patient's name. Only P and GSL products can be prescribed on a bulk prescription.

PURCHASING DRUGS

Drugs can be obtained from several sources:

- direct from drug companies (usually in bulk)
- through drug representatives
- from a wholesaler.

The majority of practices deal mainly with wholesalers. Bulk purchases from drug companies are usually reserved for drugs, which are frequently prescribed. Some drug companies offer higher discounts than wholesalers, sometimes on a 'special offer' basis. Special offers are usually promoted by the drug representative. Practices occasionally combine their orders to reach the larger quantities required to obtain additional discount.

STOCK CONTROL

Stock control is a key element in the provision of a good dispensing service, as well as affecting profits.

Patients who have to return for some, or all, of their drugs because of inadequate stock are getting a poor level of service.

However, excess stock can be an expensive error as the drug may be superseded by newer versions or become out of date before there is an opportunity for use. The only patient using the drug may have moved out of the area or died. Excess stock also requires additional storage space. GPs are not reimbursed for the cost of drugs until they are dispensed. It is wise, therefore, to make the interval between purchase of drugs and reimbursement as short as possible.

A good system of stock control requires the setting of minimum stock levels and re-order quantities for each drug to ensure that enough of a product is held to meet demand without tying up money unnecessarily or risking wastage.

Appropriate stock levels are determined by:

- the number of prescriptions dispensed
- the average quantity prescribed per prescription
- the delivery intervals
- the shelf-life of drug
- the cost of the drug
- the requirement for immediate availability of some drugs.

Drug usage figures can be estimated by inspecting invoices. Alternatively, a fully computerised practice can access drug usage figures very quickly.

There are several computer packages offering electronic ordering facilities and electronic stock control, saving time spent monitoring stock levels and preparing order lists.

There are also several manual stock control systems, including the following:

1. An *order book* can be used to record the drugs stocked, along with minimum stock levels and re-order quantities. Tight stock control requires daily stock counts of the items used that day, noting where stock is below the minimum set. The supplies required are then ordered.

2. *Stock cards* can be used for each drug, and completed after dispensing each item. Each prescription quantity supplied is deducted from the current stock total, until a minimum is reached. The cards also carry the ordering details. (A file or ring binder could be used to serve the same purpose.)

3. The simplest system is to *label the shelves* with the minimum stock level and re-order quantities for each drug. However, a lot of time can be wasted checking that orders have been placed, particularly when several members of staff are involved in the process.

Adequate supplies of the various tablet and medicine containers, bags for dispensed medicines, prescription forms, labels, also need to be maintained.

STOCK-TAKING

A stock-take is normally carried out at the end of the practice's financial year for inclusion in the practice accounts. A stock-take is also required on partnership dissolution. The drug stock is one of the main financial assets of the dispensing practice, and, therefore, needs to be accurately assessed. Stock-takes enable out-of-date stock to be identified and destroyed, excessive quantities of particular items to be highlighted and any stock shortages to be identified and investigated.

STORAGE CONDITIONS

Storage conditions are detailed, as necessary, on the drug containers. Some drugs need to be kept in lightproof containers, some at certain temperatures and others need to be kept away from moisture. A maximum/minimum thermometer in the dispensary refrigerator is essential.

It is important that the storage instructions are followed. For example, if heat sensitive vaccines, such as polio, are stored at temperatures 6°C above the recommended range for just one day the vaccine would not be effective, and should not be used.

STORAGE SYSTEMS

Storage can be pull-out racks, drawers, open shelving or cupboards. Pull-out racks and drawers are secure, as well as space-saving. However, they are

Exercises

Using MIMS, look up the generic names for these proprietary products:

Adalat

Inderal

Floxapen

Ventolin

Voltarol.

Look up the following drugs in the ABPI Compendium of Data Sheets and SPCs, and enter their legal categories (P, POM or GSL):

Canesten cream

Frusene

Liquid Gaviscon.

You will see that GSL products can be sold with reasonable safety from retail outlets, but self-administration of POM medicines could be dangerous.

Check the price of the GSL and P products in an up-to-date copy of MIMS.

Refer to the Drug Tariff to identify which patients may be prescribed cyanocobalamin tablets under the NHS.

Using the Drug Tariff, research the approved conditions for which sunflower oil may be prescribed.

Find a recent edition of the BNF, and refer to the specimen prescription form for a controlled drug. Take a photocopy and file with your course notes.

expensive. Shelves are more visible, but also more dusty, and difficult to label and keep tidy.

Whichever storage system is used, the drugs should be stocked in a methodical manner. The most common methods are as follows:

1. *Alphabetical* storage ensures that all items are easily found. However, over-stocking in a particular therapeutic group will not be so obvious.

Alphabetical filing can also increase the chance of selecting and dispensing a wrong, but similarly named, item.

2. Storing according to *drug groups* (as set out in MIMS and the BNF) enables the GP to choose a particular type of medication by looking at the range stocked. Over-stocking of a particular drug group is readily seen.

EXPIRY DATES

Drugs deteriorate with time. Stock with the shortest shelf-life should always be at the front, and used first. It is essential to check expiry dates regularly, and to remove and destroy out-of-date drugs promptly. Checks should include drugs in the GPs' bags. Stock should rarely need to be destroyed. Whenever it does, ordering and stock level decisions should be reviewed.

SUMMARY OF KEY ISSUES

The *generic* name is a drug's official medical name, and often indicates the therapeutic class to which a drug belongs. The *proprietary* name is the brand name. When typing drug names, it is usual to write the proprietary name with an initial capital letter, using lower case for the generic name.

The reference sources with which the medical secretary should be familiar are the *British National Formulary* (BNF), the *Monthly Index of Medical Specialities* (MIMS) and the *Drug Tariff*. It is important that information is accessed from up-to-date editions.

The Medicines Act 1968 is concerned with the safety of medicines, and legislates for three classes of medicinal products:

- General Sale List medicines (GSL)
- Pharmacy medicines (P)
- Prescription Only Medicines (POM).

The Medicines Act also controls the supply of medicines, e.g. labelling requirements. It gives certain GPs the right to dispense medicines.

The Misuse of Drugs Act 1971 provides comprehensive control to prevent the misuse of controlled drugs. Schedule 2 and 3 drugs are the most heavily controlled with special requirements relating to prescription writing, safe custody, entries in controlled drugs registers and destruction. Prescriptions for drugs in Schedules 2 and 3 must be handwritten by the GP, with the total quantity or number of dosage units written in words and figures.

NHS prescription forms are an order for medication, and an invoice for submission to the PPA.

Prescriptions are valid for 6 months. Prescriptions for controlled drugs are valid for 13 weeks.

The medical secretary may be responsible for maintaining supplies of prescription forms and other documentation relating to the prescribing and supply of medicines.

The medical secretary is often responsible for producing *repeat prescriptions*. Prescriptions must be accurately prepared – either manually or using a computer. Checks to be made by the secretary include ensuring that the item is authorised as a repeat, that a further issue is authorised and neither too early nor too late. Accurate records of the drugs issued must also be made.

Patients in rural areas may obtain their medicines from a *dispensing practice* provided they live more than one mile from the nearest pharmacy. However, all practices dispense drugs to their patients if needed for their immediate treatment, as well as some *personally administered items*. It is often the medical secretary who is responsible for sending the prescription forms and Form FP34D to the Prescription Pricing Authority (PPA) each month.

The medical secretary may be responsible for ordering drug supplies, and maintaining an efficient stock control system. Manufacturers' storage instructions must be followed, and expiry dates checked regularly.

CONCLUSIONS

The medical secretary is likely to be involved in several aspects relating to the prescribing and supply of medicines to patients, including:

- typing of letters including reference to drugs prescribed
- arranging appointments for pharmaceutical representatives to see the GP or practice manager
- making entries in the controlled drugs register
- arranging for destruction of expired controlled drugs
- maintaining supplies of the various documentation
- advising patients on prescription charges and exemption categories
- producing repeat prescriptions

Exercises

A patient at the reception desk requests a repeat prescription for her 'heart pills'. What procedure would you follow, and to which reference sources may you refer?

As a secretary working at a busy general practice, it is necessary for you to be aware of measures to prevent drug abuse. A new member of staff is joining the practice as a receptionist. Prepare an information sheet for her, explaining the special care that must be taken to prevent drug abuse.

You are a medical secretary working in a dispensing practice. The computer is not working and the GP has written a prescription including the abbreviation prn. Use the BNF to check the meaning of this abbreviation.

A young man calls into the surgery and asks to collect his grannie's repeat prescription for temazepam, he says that it hasn't arrived in the post. What would you do?

Using your BNF, check the entry for Analgesics. Identify the groups of patients, who should not be prescribed (contraindicated) Aspirin.

A patient hasn't followed the practice procedure for repeat prescriptions and has called into the surgery to ask for one. He is becoming angry and abusive. How would you manage this situation?

Why is good stock management important?

Who is exempt from prescription charges?

Identify the method used to prevent further items being added to a prescription. What other procedure can help?

Scabies, headlice and impetigo are common infestations / infections, identify the treatments available. What is the first course of treatment for headlice?

- submitting prescription forms to the PPA
- collecting prescription charges from patients
- ordering drugs and maintaining an efficient stock control system.

All of these tasks must be carried out paying due regard to accuracy and security.

Accuracy is particularly important when accepting repeat prescription requests and producing the prescriptions.

Security of blank and signed prescription forms is essential if drug abuse is to be avoided. Complying with the Misuse of Drugs Act also requires practices to ensure that controlled drugs are securely stored.

It is clear that the medical secretary's responsibilities in relation to medicines should be taken extremely seriously to ensure that patients receive accurate prescriptions and drug misuse is minimised.

Useful websites

www.bnf.org British National Formulary site
www.rspgb.org.uk Royal Pharmaceutical Society of Great Britain site
www.patient.co.uk Health Information site
www.emims.net MIMS website

www.npc.co.uk National Prescribing Centre NHS
www.mca.gov.uk Medicine Controls Agency
www.doh.gov.uk Useful Department of Health government site

Appendices

SECTION CONTENTS

Appendix 1

Prefixes and suffixes

A knowledge of the prefixes and suffixes used in medical terminology, and outlined below, will help the medical secretary to understand the meaning of a large number of commonly used words and phrases. In addition, a good medical dictionary is an essential tool.

a-, an- not, without
ab- away from
acr- extremity, peak
ad- towards
aden- gland
adip- fat
-aemia blood
aer- air
-aesthesia sensation
-algia pain
amyl- starch
ana- up
andr- male
angi- (blood) vessel
ante- before, in front
anti- against
apo- away, from
arthr- joint
-asis state of
aut- self
bi-, bis- two
bil- bile
bio- life
blast- bud
blephar- eyelid
brachi- arm
brachy- short
brady- slow
bronch- windpipe
calc- chalk

carcin- cancer
card- heart
carp- wrist
cata-, kata- down, negative
cav- hollow
-cele swelling
cent- hundred
-centesis piercing
cephal- head
cerebr- brain
cervic- neck
cheil-, chil- lip
cheir-, chir- hand
chlor- green
chol- bile
chondr- cartilage
chrom- colour
-cide killing
cine-, kine- motion
-cle small
co-, col-, com-, con- together, with
colp- vagina
contra- against, counter
cortic- bark, rind
cost- rib
cox- hip
crani- skull

cryo- cold
crypt- hidden, concealed
cyan- blue
cyst- bladder
cyt- cell
-cyte cell
dacry- tear
dactyl- finger
de- down, from
dec- ten
demi- half
dent- tooth
derm- skin
-desis binding
dextr- right
di-, diplo- two, double
dia- through
dis- apart, away from
dors- back
dys- difficult, abnormal
ect- outside
-ectasis stretching
-ectomy cutting out
em-, en-, end-, ent- in, inside, within
enter- intestine
epi- upon, over
erythr- red

eu- good, normal
ex-, exo- out of
extra- outside
faci- face
-facient making
flav- yellow
galact- milk
gastr- stomach
-genic producing
ger- old age
gloss- tongue
glyc- sweet
gnath- jaw
-gram tracing
-graph tracing
gynae- female
haem- blood
hemi- half
hepat- liver
hex- six
hist- tissue, web
hom- same, like
hydr- water
hyper- above
hypno- sleep
hypo- below
hyster- womb
-ia, -iasis state, condition
idi- peculiar, distinct

infra- below
inter- between
intra- within
intro- inwards
iso- equal
-itis inflammation of
kary- nut, nucleus
kerat- horn, cornea
-kinesis, -kinetic motion
lact- milk
laryng- windpipe
later- side
leuc-, leuk- white
-lith stone
-lysis destruction
macr- large
mal- bad, abnormal
-malacia softening
mamm- breast
mast- breast
medi- middle
megal- large
-megaly enlargement
melan- black
meso- middle
meta- after
metr- uterus
micr- small
milli- thousand
mono- single
-morph form
muco- mucus
multi- many
myc- fungus
myel- marrow
myo- muscle
narc- numb
naso- nose

necr- corpse
neo- new
nephr- kidney
neur- nerve
ocul- eye
odont- tooth
-odynia pain
-oid like
oligo- few
-ology study
-oma tumour
onc- mass
onych- nail
oo- egg
ophthalm- eye
-opsy looking
or- mouth
orchid- testis
orth- straight
os- mouth
os-, oste- bone
-osis pathological state
-ostomy opening
ot- ear
-otomy cutting
ovi- egg
pachy- thick
paed- child
pan- all
para- beside, beyond
path- suffering, disease
-pathy disease
-penia lack
pent- five
per- through
peri- around
-pexy fixing
-phagia swallowing

pharmac- drug
-phasia speech
phleb- vein
-phobia irrational fear
phon- sound
photo- light
phren- diaphragm, mind
-phylaxis prevention, protection
physi- form, nature
-plegia paralysis
pneum- lung
pod- foot
-poiesis formation
poly- many
post- after
prae-, pre-, pro- before, in front
proct- anus
pseud- false
psych- mind
pyo- pus, matter
pyr- fire, fever
quadr- four
quint- five
radi- ray
re- back, again
ren- kidney
retro- backwards
rhin- nose
-rrhoea discharge
-rrhaphy repair
rub- red
salping- (uterine) tube
sarc- flesh
sclero- hard
-scope viewing instrument

-scopy looking
semi- half
sept- seven
-sonic sound
sphygm- pulse
splen- spleen
spondy- vertebra
steat- fat
sub- below
super-, supra- above
syn- with
tachy- quick
tars- eyelid, instep
-taxia, -taxis arrangement, order
tetra- four
therm- heat
thorac- chest
thromb- clot
-tome cutting instrument
toxic- poison
trans- through, across
tri- three
trich- hair
troph- nourishment
-tropy turning
tympano- middle ear
ultra- beyond
uni- one
uri- urine
-uria urine
vas- vessel
xanth- yellow
xero- dry
zoo- animal

Reproduced with permission from Kasner K, Tindall DH 1984 Baillière's Nurses' Dictionary, 23rd edn. Baillière Tindall, London

Appendix 2

Bones and organs of the human body

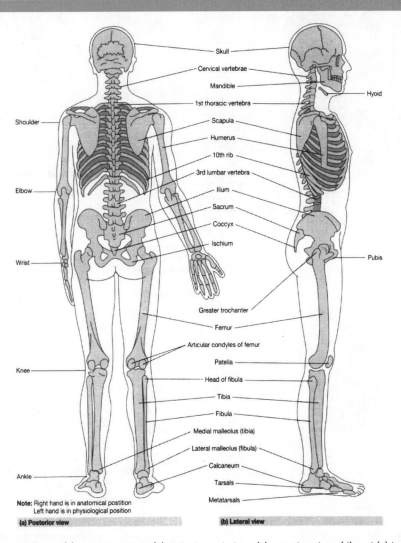

Figure 1 The human skeleton (a) posterior view, (b) right lateral view, (c) anterior view, (d) and (e) bones of the forearm. Reproduced with permission from Hinchliff SM, Montague SE, Watson R 1996 Physiology for nursing practice, 2nd edn. Baillière Tindall, London

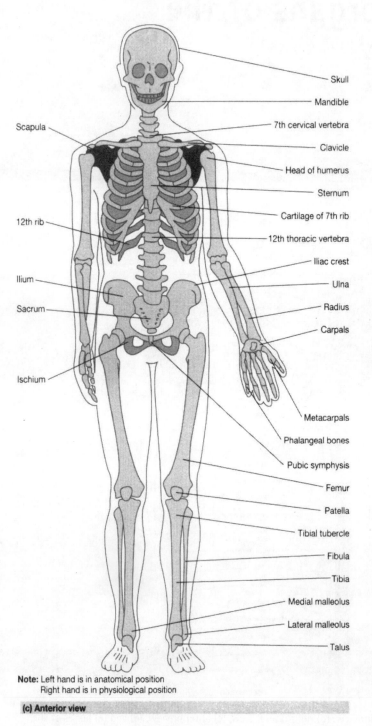

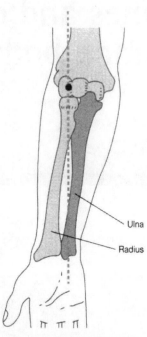

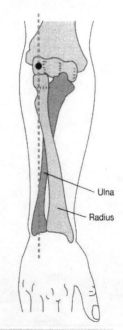

Skull

Mandible

7th cervical vertebra

Clavicle

Head of humerus

Sternum

Cartilage of 7th rib

12th thoracic vertebra

Iliac crest

Ulna

Radius

Carpals

Scapula

12th rib

Ilium

Sacrum

Ischium

Metacarpals

Phalangeal bones

Pubic symphysis

Femur

Patella

Tibial tubercle

Fibula

Tibia

Medial malleolus

Lateral malleolus

Talus

Ulna

Radius

(d) Forearm supinated

Ulna

Radius

(e) Forearm pronated

Note: Left hand is in anatomical position
Right hand is in physiological position

(c) Anterior view

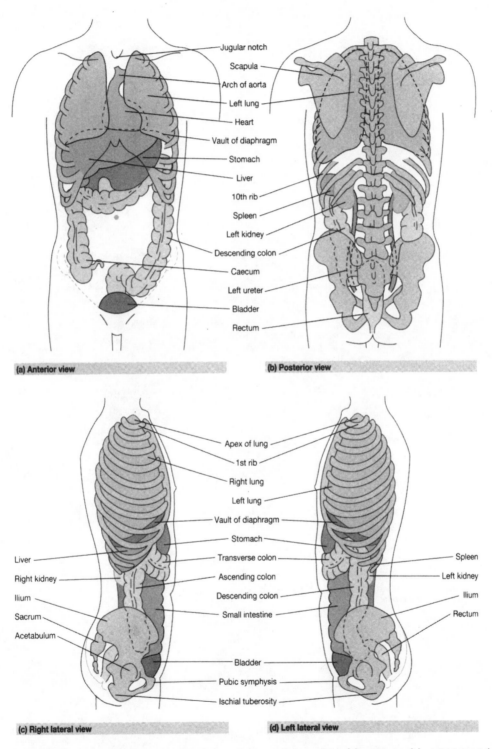

Figure 2 Anatomical relationships between the organs of the trunk in anterior (a), posterior (b), right lateral (c) and left lateral (d) views. Reproduced with permission from Hinchliff SM, Montague SE, Watson R 1996 Physiology for nursing practice, 2nd edn. Baillière Tindall, London

Appendix 3

Useful addresses

Joan Datsun

Action for Sick Children (formerly National
Association for the Welfare of Children in
Hospital)
Argyle House
29-31 Euston Road
London
NW1 2SP

Action for Smoking and Health (ASH)
109 Gloucester Place
London
W1H 4EJ

Age Concern England
60 Pitcairn Road
Mitcham
Surrey
CR4 3LL

Alcohol Concern (National Agency of Alcohol
Misuse)
305 Gray's Inn Road
London
WC1X 8QF

Alcoholics Anonymous
PO Box 1
Stonebow House
Stonebow
York
Y01 2NJ

Alzheimer's Disease Society
3rd Floor Bank Building
Fulham Broadway
London
SW6 1EP

APEX Partnership
22-24 Worple Road
Wimbledon
London
SW19 4DD

Arthritis and Rheumatism Council (ARC)
41 Eagle Street
London
WC1R 4AR

Association for Improvements in the Maternity
Services (AIMS)
163 Liverpool Road
London
N1 0RF

Association of British Paediatric Nurses (ABPN)
PO Box 14
Ashton-under-Lyne
Lancashire
OL5 9WW

Association of Carers
20-25 Glasshouse Yard
London
EC1A 4JS

Association of Community Health Councils
(England and Wales)
30 Drayton Park
London
N5 1PB

Association of Radical Midwives
c/o Haringay Women's Centre
40 Turnpike Lane
London
N8 0PS

Asthma Society (merged with Asthma Research
Council to become National Asthma Campaign)
Providence House
Providence Place
London
N1 0NT

Back Pain Association
31-33 Park Road
Teddington
Middlesex
TW11 0AB

Breast Care and Mastectomy Association
15-19 Britton Street
London
SW3 3TZ

British Association for Cancer United Patients
(BACUP)
3 Bath Place
Rivington Street
London
EC2A 3JR

British Colostomy Association
15 Station Road
Reading
RG1 1LG

British Deaf Association
38 Victoria Place
Carlisle
Cumbria
CA1 1HU

British Diabetic Association
10 Queen Anne Street
London
W1M 0BD

British Dietetic Association
Daimler House
Paradise Circus
Queensway
Birmingham
B1 2BJ

British Epilepsy Association
Anstey House
40 Hanover Square
Leeds
LS3 1BE

British Geriatric Society (BGS)
1 St Andrew's Place
London
NW1 4LB

British Heart Foundation
102 Gloucester Place
London
W1H 4DH

British Nutrition Foundation
High Holborn House
52-54 High Holborn
London
WCIV 6RQ

British Pregnancy Advisory Service
Austry Manor
Wooten
Waven
Solihull
West Midlands
BG5 6DA

British Red Cross Society (BRCS)
9 Grosvenor Crescent
London
SW1X 7EJ

Cancer Link
17 Britannia Street
London
WC1X 9JN

Capability (formerly Spastics Society)
12 Park Crescent
London
W1N 4EQ

Carers' National Association
20-25 Glasshouse Yard
London
EC1A 4JT

Childline
Royal Mail Building
Studd Street
London
N1 0QW

Coeliac Society
PO Box 220
High Wycombe
Buckinghamshire
HP11 2HY

Commission for Racial Equality
Elliot House
10-12 Allington Street
London
SW1E 5EH

Commonwealth Nurses Association
c/o International Department Royal College of
Nursing
20 Cavendish Square
London
W1M 0AB

Community Practitioners' and Health
Visitors' Association
40 Bermondsey Street
London
SEI 3UD

Coronary Prevention Group
Central Middlesex Hospital
Acton Lane
London
NW10 7NS

CRUSE (National Association for the Widowed
and their Children)
Cruse House
126 Sheen Road
Richmond
Surrey
TW9 1UR

Department of Health (England)
Richmond House
79 Whitehall
London
SW1A 2NS

Department of Health (Northern Ireland)
Dundonald House
Upper Newtonwards Road
Belfast
BT4 3SB

Disabled Living Foundation
380-384 Harrow Road
London
W9 2HU

English National Board for Nursing, Midwifery
and Health Visiting (ENB)
Victory House
170 Tottenham Court Road
London
W1T 0HA

Equal Opportunities Commission
Overseas House
Quay Street
Manchester
M3 3HN

Family Planning Association (FPA)
Margaret Pyke House
27-35 Mortimer Street
London
W1N 7RJ

Foresight (Association for the Promotion of
Preconceptual Care)
The Old Vicarage
Church Lane
Witley
Godalming
Surrey
GU8 5PN

Gamblers Anonymous and GAM-ANON
17-23 Blantyre Street
Cheyne Walk
London
SW10 0DT

General Medical Council (GMC)
178 Great Portland Street
London
W1N 6JE

Gerontology Nutrition Unit
Royal Free Hospital
School of Medicine
21 Pond Street
London
NW3 2PN

Haemophilia Society
123 Westminster Bridge Road
London
SE1 7HR

Health Education Authority
Hamilton House
Mabledon Place
London
WC1H 9TX

Health and Safety Executive
2 Southwark Bridge
London
SE1 9HS

Health Service Ombudsman
Church House
Great Smith Street
London
SW1P 3BW

Health Visitors Association
50 Southwark Street
London
SE1 1UN

Help the Aged
16-18 St James's Walk
London
EC1R 0BE

Hospice Information Service
St Christopher's Hospice
51-59 Lawrie Park Road
Sydenham
London
SE26 6DZ

Ileostomy Association (now Ileostomy and
Internal Pouch Support Group)
Amblehurst House
PO Box 23
Mansfield
Nottinghamshire
NG18 4TT

Infection Control Nurses Association (ICNA)
c/o Janet Roberts
Clatterbridge Hospital
Bebington
Wirral
Merseyside
L63 4JY

Institute of Complementary Medicine
PO Box 194
London
SE15 1QZ

International Confederation of Midwives
10 Barley Mow Passage
Chiswick
London
W4 4PH

International Council of Nurses
37 rue Vermont
Geneva
Switzerland

Invalids at Home
23 Farm Avenue
London
NW2 2BJ

King's Fund
11-13 Cavendish Square
London
W1M 0AN

Lady Hoare Trust for Physically Disabled Children
(Associated with Arthritis Care)
7 North Street
Midhurst, West Sussex
GU29 9DJ

Leukaemia Society
14 Kingfisher Court
Venny Bridge
Pinhoe, Exeter
EX4 8JN

Macmillan Cancer Relief
Anchor House
15-19 Britten Street
London
SW3 3TZ

Malcolm Sargent Cancer Fund for Children
14 Abingdon Road
London
W8 6AF

Marie Curie Memorial Foundation
28 Belgrave Square
London
SW1X 8QG

Medic-Alert Foundation
11-13 Afton Terrace
London
N4 3JP

Medicines Control Agency
Market Towers
1 Nine Elms Lane
London
SW8 5NQ

MIND (National Association for Mental Health)
15-19 Broadway
London
E15 4BQ

Multiple Sclerosis Society
25 Effie Road
Fulham
London
SW6 1EE

Narcotics Anonymous
PO Box 246
London
SW12 8DL

National Association of Theatre Nurses
22 Mount Parade
Harrogate
HG1 1BX

National Board for Nursing, Midwifery and
Health Visiting for Northern Ireland
RAC House
70 Chichester Street
Belfast
BT1 4JE

National Board for Nursing, Midwifery and
Health Visiting for Scotland
22 Queen Street
Edinburgh
EH2 1JZ

National Childbirth Trust (NCT)
Alexandra House
Oldham Terrace
London
Q3 6NH

National Council for One Parent Families
255 Kentish Town Road
London
NW5 6NH

National Council for Vocational Qualifications
222 Euston Road
London
NW1

National Federation of Kidney Patients'
Associations
Acorn Lodge
Woodsets
Nr Worksop
Nottinghamshire
S81 8AT

National Institute of Clinical Excellence (NICE)
90 Long Acre
London
W3 6NH

National Schizophrenia Fellowship
79 Victoria Road
Surbiton, Surrey
KT6 4NS

National Society for Epilepsy
Chalfont Centre for Epilepsy
Chalfont St Peter
Gerrards Cross, Buckinghamshire
SL9 0RJ

National Society for the Prevention of Cruelty to
Children
(NSPCC)
67 Curtain Road
London
EC2A 3NH

Neonatal Nurses Association (NNA)
7 Milton Chambers
19 Milton Street
Nottingham
NG1 3EN

NHS Management Executive
Quarry House
Quarry Hill
Leeds
L52 7EU

Nurses Welfare Service
Victoria Chambers
16-18 Strutton Ground
London
SW1P 2HP

Nursing and Hospital Carers Information Centre
121 Edgware Road
London
W2 2HX

Nursing and Midwifery Staffs Negotiating Council
20 Cavendish Square
London
W1M 0AB

Parent's Friend
c/o Voluntary Action
Leeds Stringer House
34 Lupton Street
Hunslet, Leeds
LS10 2QW

Parkinson Disease Society
36 Portland Place
London
W1N 3DG

Pregnancy Advisory Service
13 Charlotte Street
London
W1P 1HD

Primary Nursing Network Nursing Developments
King's Fund Centre
126 Albert Street
London
NW1 7NF

Renal Society
64 South Hill Park
London
NW3 3SJ

Royal Association in Aid of the Deaf and Dumb
27 Old Oak Road
London
W3 7SL

Royal Association for Disability and Rehabilitation
Unit 12, City Forum
250 City Road
London
EC1V 8AF

Royal College of Midwives (RCM)
15 Mansfield Street
London
W1M 0BE

RCM English Board
Kings House
2nd Floor
Kings Street
Leeds LS1 2HH

RCM Northern Ireland Board
Friends Provident Building
58 Howard Street
Belfast
BT1 6PH

RCM Scottish Board
37 Frederick Street
Edinburgh
EH2 1EP

RCM Welsh Board
4 Cathedral Road
Cardiff
CF1 9LJ

Royal College of Nursing of the United Kingdom
(RCN)
20 Cavendish Square
London
W1M 0AB

Royal College of Nursing (Northern Ireland)
17 Windsor Avenue
Belfast
BT9 6EE

Royal College of Nursing (Scottish Board)
42 South Oswald Road
Edinburgh
EH9 2HH

Royal College of Nursing (Welsh Board)
Ty Maeth
King George V Drive
East Cardiff
CF4 4XZ

Royal Commonwealth Society
New Zealand House
Haymarket
London
SW1Y 4TQ

Royal Institute of Public Health and Hygiene
28 Portland Place
London
W1N 4DE

Royal National Institute for the Blind (RNIB)
224 Great Portland Place
London
W1N 6AA

Royal National Institute for the Deaf (RNID)
19-23 Featherstone Street
London
EC1Y 8SL

Royal National Pension Fund for Nurses
Burdett House
15 Buckingham Street
London
W2N 6ED

Royal Society of Health
38a St George's Drive
London
SW1Y 4BH

Royal Society of Medicine
1 Wimpole Street
London
W1M 8RE

Royal Society for the Prevention of Accidents
(ROSPA)
Cannon House
The Priory
Queensway
Birmingham
B4 6BS

St John Ambulance Association and Brigade
1 Grosvenor Crescent
London
SW1X 7ES

Samaritans Incorporated
17 Uxbridge Road
Slough
Berkshire
SL1 1SN

SCOPE
12 Park Crescent
London
W1N 4EQ

Scottish Home and Health Department
St Andrew's House
Regent Road, Edinburgh
EH1 3DE

Sickle Cell Society
54 Station Road
London
NW10 4UA

Society and College of Radiographers
2 Carriage Row
183 Eversholt Green, London
NW1 1BU

Standing Conference on Drug Abuse
1-4 Hatton Place
Hatton Garden
London
EC1N 8ND

Stillbirth and Neonatal Death Society (SANDS)
28 Portland Place
London
W1N 4DE

Stress Syndrome Foundation
Cedar House
Yalding
Kent
ME18 6JD

Sue Ryder Foundation
Cavendish
Sudbury
Suffolk
CO10 8AY

Terrence Higgins Trust
52-54 Gray's Inn Road
London
WC1X 8JU

Twins and Multiple Birth Association
54 Broad Lane
Hampton
Middlesex
TW12 3BG

UNISON (Head Office)
1 Mabledon Place
London
WC1H 9HA

United Kingdom Central Council for Nursing,
Midwifery and Health Visiting (UKCC)
23 Portland Place
London
W1N 3AF

Vegan Society
47 Highlands Road
Leatherhead
Surrey
KT22 8NQ

Welsh National Board for Nursing, Midwifery and
Health Visiting
13th Floor
Pearl Assurance House
Greyfriars Road
Cardiff
CF1 3AG

Welsh Office
Crown Buildings
Cathays Park
Cardiff
CG10 1DX

Women's Health Concern (WHC)
17 Earls Terrace
London
W8 6LP

Women's Royal Voluntary Services (WRVS)
17 Old Park Lane
London
W1Y 4AJ

World Health Organization
Avenue Appia 1211
Geneva 27
Switzerland

Appendix 4

Degrees, diplomas and organisations: Abbreviations in nursing and health care

AA	Alcoholics Anonymous
ABPN	Association of British Paediatric Nurses
AIMSW	Association of the Institute of Medical Social Workers
AOC	Aromatherapy Organisations Council
APEX	Association of Professional and Executive Staffs
ASH	Action on Smoking and Health
BA	Bachelor of Arts
BACUP	British Association of Cancer United Patients
BAON	British Association of Orthopaedic Nurses
BDA	British Dental Association
BDSc	Bachelor of Dental Science
BEd	Bachelor of Education
BITA	British Intravenous Therapy Association
BMAS	British Medical Acupuncture Society
BN	Bachelor of Nursing
BPOG	British Psychosocial Oncology Group
BRA	British Reflexology Association
BRCS	British Red Cross Society
BSc (Soc SC-Nurs)	Bachelor of Science (Nursing)
BSMDH	British Society of Medical and Dental Hypnosis
CATS	Credit Accumulation Transfer Scheme
CCETSW	Central Council for Educational Training in Social Work
CCHE	Central Council for Health Education
CMT	Clinical Midwife Teacher
CNAA	Council for National Academic Awards
CNF	Commonwealth Nurses Federation
CNN	Certificated Nursery Nurse
COSHH	Control of Substances Hazardous to Health
CSP	Chartered Society of Physiotherapists
DCH	Diploma in Child Health
DDA	Dangerous Drugs Act
DipAr	Diploma in Aromatherapy
DipEd	Diploma in Education
DipHyp	Diploma in Hypnotherapy
DipMedAc	Diploma in Medical Acupuncture
Dip NEd	Diploma in Nursing Education
DipPhyto	Diploma in Phytotherapy
DN	Diploma in Nursing
DNA	District Nursing Association
DNE	Diploma in Nursing Education
DoH	Department of Health
DPH	Diploma in Public Health
DPhil	Doctor of Philosophy
DPM	Diploma in Psychological Medicine
DSc	Doctor of Science
DTM&H	Diploma in Tropical Medicine and Hygiene
EN	Enrolled Nurse
ENB	English National Board for Nursing, Midwifery and Health Visiting
FCSP	Fellow of the Chartered Society of Physiotherapists
FETC	Further Education Teaching Certificate
FNIF	Florence Nightingale International Foundation
FNIMH	Fellow of National Institute of Medical Herbalists
FPA	Family Planning Association

FRcn	Fellow of the Royal College of Nursing
FRS	Fellow of the Royal Society
FRSH	Fellow of the Royal Society of Health
GMC	General Medical Council
GNVQ	General National Vocational Qualification
HEA	Health Education Authority
HFEA	Human Fertilisation and Embryology Authority
HSA	Hospital Savings Association
HV	Health Visitor
HVA	Health Visitors' Association
ICN	International Council of Nurses
ICNA	Infection Control Nurses Association
ICW	International Council of Women
IFA	International Federation of Aromatherapists
IHF	International Hospital Federation
INR	Index of Nursing Research
LFHom	Licensed Associate of the Faculty of Homeopathy
MA	Master of Arts
MAACP	Member of Acupuncture Association of Chartered Physiotherapists
MAO	Master of the Art of Obstetrics
MAOT	Member of the Association of Occupational Therapists
MBA	Master of Business Administration
MBAC	Member of British Acupuncture Council
MBIM	Member of the British Institute of Management
MCSP	Member of the Chartered Society of Physiotherapists
MFHom	Member of Faculty of Homeopathy
MIND	National Association for Mental Health
MMAA	Member of Modern Acupuncture Association
MPhil	Master of Philosophy
MRC	Medical Research Council
MRSH	Member of the Royal Society of Health
MRSHom	Member of Royal Society of Homeopaths
MRSS	Member of Register of Shiatsu Society
MSc	Master of Science
MSF	Manufacturing Science and Finance
MSRG	Member of the Society of Remedial Gymnasts
MSR(R)	Member of the Society of Radiographers (Radiography)
MSR(T)	Member of the Society of Radiographers (Radiotherapy)
MTD	Midwife Teachers' Diploma
NAMCW	National Association for Maternal and Child Welfare
NAMH	National Association for Mental Health
NATN	National Association of Theatre Nurses
NAWCH	National Association for the Welfare of Children in Hospital
NHS	National Health Service
NIB	Northern Ireland Board for Nursing, Midwifery and Health Visiting
NIMH	National Institute of Medical Herbalists
NNA	Neonatal Nurses Association
NNEB	National Nursery Education Board
NUMINE	Network of Users of Microcomputers in Nurse Education
NUS	National Union of Students
NVQ	National Vocational Qualification
OHNC	Occupational Health Nursing Certificate
ONC	Orthopaedic Nurses' Certificate
OND	Ophthalmic Nursing Diploma
OT	Occupational Therapist
PhD	Doctor of Philosophy
PMRAFNS	Princess Mary's Royal Air Force Nursing Service
PNA	Psychiatric Nurses' Association
ProfDipAr	Professional Diploma in Aromatherapy
QARANC	Queen Alexandra's Royal Army Nursing Corps
QARNNS	Queen Alexandra's Royal Naval Nursing Service
QIDN	Queen's Institute of District Nursing
QNI	Queen's Nursing Institute
RCM	Royal College of Midwives
RCN	Royal College of Nursing
RGN	Registered General Nurse
RHV	Regional Health Visitor
RM	Registered Midwife
RMN	Registered Mental Nurse
RN	Registered Nurse
RNMH	Registered Nurse for the Mentally Handicapped
RNT	Registered Nurse Tutor
RSCN	Registered Sick Children's Nurse
StAAA	St Andrew's Ambulance Association
StJAA	St John Ambulance Association

StJAB	St John Ambulance Brigade	**ST**	Speech Therapist
SCM	State Certified Midwife	**UKCC**	United Kingdom Central Council for Nursing, Midwifery and Health Visiting
SHHD	Scottish Home and Health Department		
SNB	Scottish National Board for Nursing, Midwifery and Health Visiting	**VSO**	Voluntary Service Overseas
		WFH	Word Federation of Hypnotherapists
SNNEB	Scottish National Nursing Examination Board	**WHO**	World Health Organization
		WNB	Welsh National Board for Nursing, Midwifery and Health Visiting
SRN	State Registered Nurse		
SSStJ	Serving Sister of the Order of St John of Jerusalem	**WRVS**	Women's Royal Voluntary Service

Appendix 5

Professional organisations and trade unions

COMMUNITY AND DISTRICT NURSING ASSOCIATION (CDNA)

The CDNA is a specialist professional association and trade union affiliated to the Trades Union Congress (TUC) and Scottish Trades Union Congress (STUC). For 30 years the Community and District Nursing Association has taken an active role in campaigning on issues affecting its membership.

For nearly 35 years the CDNA (formerly the DNA) has been the only professional body which solely represents the interests of community and district nurses. The CDNA is run by people who have worked in primary health care and nursing education so they are well aware of the issues facing their members.

The Association recognises that, with all the changes and development taking place within health care in the community, a body which represents the sole interests of nurses who practise in the community is needed now more than ever.

For further information: http://www.cdna.tvu.ac.uk.

UNISON

UNISON is the UK's biggest trade union with over 1.3 million members.

UNISON members are people working in the public services, for private contractors providing public services, and in the essential utilities. They include manual and white collar staff working full- or part-time in local authorities, the National Health Service (NHS), colleges and schools, the electricity, gas and water industries, transport and the voluntary sector.

Every member of UNISON belongs to a branch which is made up of people working for the same employer.

Local stewards represent members at work and help find the answers to any problems. They are volunteers and play a vital role in recruiting new members and organising the branches.

The organisation

UNISON has a clear structure to make sure that all members can have their say. The union is divided into 13 regions, each with its own regional council made up of delegates elected from branches in the area.

The governing body of UNISON is the annual national delegate conference, where the union's policy is decided by delegates elected from branches, regions and self-organised groups (see below). Policies decided at conference are carried out by the National Executive Council (NEC) which is elected from the regions and service groups.

Alongside this local structure, UNISON has six service groups which bring together members working in similar areas. These are: local government, health care, higher education, energy, water and transport.

Women make up two-thirds of UNISON's members so care is taken to ensure that their voices are heard through the union. At every level of the union, when people are elected to committees or delegations, women must be elected in fair proportion to their membership. Even the NEC has to elect 44 women out of its 67 seats and 13 are held by low-paid women. UNISON calls this 'proportionality'.

UNISON also has 'self-organised groups' to represent people who are likely to face particular discrimination at work – women, black members, disabled members and lesbians and gay men.

UNISON is the largest union in the TUC and plays an important role in developing policy. It has a big voice too in the Scottish, Welsh and Irish trades union congresses.

For further information:
http://www.unison.org.uk.

ROYAL COLLEGE OF NURSING (RCN)

What is the RCN?

With more than 310,000 members, the RCN is the world's largest professional union of nurses. The RCN is run by nurses for nurses, it campaigns on the part of the profession, and is a leading player in the development of nursing practice and standards of care. It is a provider of higher education and promotes research, quality and practice development through the RCN Institute. It is also a registered charity.

The RCN promotes the interests of nurses and patients by working with government, MPs, other unions, professional bodies and voluntary organisations. It is the voice of British nursing both at home and abroad, with representatives on a number of European, Commonwealth and international bodies. The RCN also represents the United Kingdom on the International Council for Nurses.

The RCN's Royal Charter

The Royal Charter sets out the purposes of the RCN:

- To promote the science and art of nursing and the better education and training of nurses and their efficiency in the profession of nursing.
- To promote the advance of nursing as a profession in all or any of its branches.
- To promote the professional standing and interests of members of the nursing profession.
- To promote the above aims in both the UK and

other countries through the medium of international agencies and other means.
- To assist nurses who, by reason of ill health or other adversity, are in need of assistance of any nature.
- To institute and conduct examinations, and to grant certificates and diplomas to those who satisfy the requirements laid down by the Council of the College.

Working for nurses

For busy professionals and nursing students, the RCN offers its members a wide range of services including:

- Advice and support with problems at work
- Legal representation
- A range of education and continuing professional development activities
- Professional advice
- A counselling and personal advice service
- Immigration advice
- Support and activities for nursing students.
- Free publications on nursing, health-care and employment issues
- The largest nursing library in Europe.

RCN Council

This is the RCN's ruling body, democratically elected by the members. Its 25 representatives include 14 from England and two each from Northern Ireland, Scotland and Wales. Students have two elected representatives. The other three members are the RCN president, deputy president and chair of the RCN Congress. The RCN Council is responsible for the policies of the RCN and the general secretary is responsible for implementing policy. Council takes account of resolutions carried by the RCN Congress and recommendations from its standing committees.

RCN Congress

Congress is the RCN's main annual debating forum. It plays a major part in shaping policy and initiating activity through resolutions and matters of discussion. Congress voters are drawn from branches and national forums but members may also attend as non-voting delegates.

RCN branches, national forums, Council and its

standing committees, the RCN National Boards, the UK Stewards Committee and the UK Safety Representatives' Committee submit resolutions and matters for discussion on a wide range of issues. These are submitted to the Congress Agenda Committee who develop and manage the Congress agenda.

At local level the RCN has board offices in Northern Ireland, Scotland and Wales and offices throughout England. It has over 274 branches throughout the UK, over 70 professional groups covering a wide range of nursing specialisms and special interests, and a network of stewards and safety representatives in the workplace.

For further information: http://www.rcn.org.uk.

INTERNATIONAL COUNCIL OF NURSES (ICN)

The ICN's mission is to represent nursing worldwide, advancing the profession and influencing health policy.

It is a federation of national nurses' associations (NNAs) representing nurses in more than 120 countries. Founded in 1899, the ICN is the world's first and widest-reaching international organisation for health professionals. Operated by nurses for nurses, the ICN works to ensure quality nursing care for all, sound health policies globally, the advancement of nursing knowledge, and the presence worldwide of a respected nursing profession and a competent and satisfied nursing workforce.

The ICN Code for Nurses is the foundation of ethical nursing practice throughout the world. ICN standards, guidelines and policies for nursing practice, education, management, research and socio-economic welfare are accepted globally as the basis of nursing policy.

The ICN advances nursing, nurses and health through its policies, partnerships, advocacy, leadership development, networks, congresses and special projects, and by its work in the arenas of professional practice, regulation and socio-economic welfare. It is particularly active in:

- Professional nursing practice
  - International classification of nursing practice
  - Advanced nursing practice and entrepreneurship
  - HIV/AIDS
  - Women's health
  - Primary health care

- Nursing regulation
  - Continuing education
  - Ethics and human rights
  - Credentialing
- Socio-economic welfare for nurses
  - Occupational health and safety
  - Remuneration
  - Human resources planning
- Career development.

Partnerships and strategic alliances include links with governmental and non-governmental agencies, foundations, regional groups, national associations and individuals assisting the ICN in advancing nursing worldwide.

ICN goals and values

Three goals and five core values guide and motivate all ICN activities.

The goals are:

- To bring nursing together worldwide
- To advance nurses and nursing worldwide
- To influence health policy.

The five core values are:

- Visionary leadership
- Inclusiveness
- Flexibility
- Partnership
- Achievement.

The ICN is based in Geneva, Switzerland. For further information on ICN structure, publications and activities: http://www.icn.ch.

ROYAL COLLEGE OF MIDWIVES (RCM)

The RCM represents over 96% of the UK's practising midwives and is the world's largest and oldest professional midwifery organisation. It works to advance the interests of midwives and the midwifery profession – and, by doing so, enhances the wellbeing of women, babies and families.

The RCM is governed by an elected Council of practising midwives. Each of the four UK countries – Scotland, Northern Ireland, England and Wales – has its own RCM Board, which provides services to midwives in those countries and advises the Council on strategic issues. In addition, the London-based headquarters provide a range of UK-wide functions and services.

Over 200 RCM branches hold regular meetings where members can give and receive support and discuss professional and workplace issues.

Working for midwifery, working for midwives

The vast majority of UK midwives belong to the RCM because of the combined professional, trade union and educational benefits that only the RCM can offer. These include:

- Education and research
  - A range of training and professional development courses, to promote clinical excellence and to develop the midwifery leaders of tomorrow
  - Active promotion of research, evidence-based practice and the development of midwifery as a learning profession
  - The largest midwifery library in the world. The RCM collection, which reflects more than a century of change for midwifery and women, includes journals, theses and over 5000 books.

- Professional affairs
  - An extensive range of publications and policy papers, providing guidance and comment on the challenges facing mothers and midwives
  - The RCM Midwives' Journal, devoted exclusively to midwifery matters, delivered direct to each member every month
  - A voice for midwifery in national policy forums.

- Industrial relations
  - Regional officers through the UK, who are all practising midwives. Only the RCM provides field-based staff who combine expertise in both midwifery and industrial relations
  - Over 600 workplace-based stewards and health and safety representatives, themselves midwives working in the NHS
  - Medical malpractice insurance, giving cover against legal liability to the sum of £3 million.

Working for women

The RCM is committed to developing a maternity service that truly meets women's and babies' physical, psychological and emotional needs throughout pregnancy, labour and the postnatal period. The RCM sees this as a vital contribution to public health and an essential investment in the wellbeing of tomorrow's citizens. In partnership with service users themselves, the RCM has fought for a maternity service which treats women as partners in their own care, which respects the power of normal childbirth, and which puts both research evidence and the women's own wishes centre-stage.

The RCM also uses its expertise to help improve the wider issues affecting women's and infants' health. It has campaigned for better support for women who are pregnant in prison, or suffering domestic violence or female genital mutilation (FGM). It works to promote breastfeeding, to improve neonatal care, and to help new parents feel confident and supported. It advises the Government, the NHS and others on how maternity care can help women enjoy not just a healthy pregnancy but increased quality of family life and wellbeing.

Working internationally

As the only World Health Organization (WHO) Collaborating Centre for Midwifery, the RCM works with the Safe Motherhood Initiative (SMI) to promote maternal and infant health across the globe. It also works with a range of partners overseas, providing support and resources to help improve midwifery education and practice and maternal and infant health. The College is a founder member of the International Confederation of Midwives (ICM) and works with midwives worldwide, assisting with midwifery development by providing advice on legislation, research, education and practice.

For further information see RCM addresses in Appendix 8, Useful Addresses.

COMMUNITY PRACTITIONERS' AND HEALTH VISITORS' ASSOCIATION (CPHVA)

The Community Practitioners' and Health Visitors' Association (CPHVA) is the UK professional body that represents registered nurses and health visitors who work in primary or community health settings. The CPHVA is an autonomous professional section of Manufacturing Science and Finance (MSF). MSF represents 65,000 professionals working in the NHS and altogether represents

400,000 members employed in the manufacturing, science and finance sectors.

With 18,000 members, the CPHVA is the third largest professional nursing union and is the only union which has public health at the centre of its activities and parliamentary lobbying. It campaigns to protect the status of community practitioners and the services they deliver, and influences policy decisions by the production of reports and consultation documents as well as the staging of conferences and seminars.

Membership includes:

- Access to expert advice on professional and clinical issues
- Expert advice and representation on pay, contracts, and terms and conditions of employment
- A comprehensive annual programme of specialist and professional development, education and training courses, conferences and seminars
- An information resources centre
- The award-winning Community Practitioner journal free every month and the Opportunities job supplement free every fortnight
- Indemnity insurance cover against claims of up to £3 million
- Access to the CPHVA's networks of special interest groups and databases.

As an autonomous section of MSF, CPHVA entitles its members to the range of updated benefits available to all MSF members. These include the MSF First CD-Rom with free Internet access direct to the home as well as the most competitive offers on items ranging from mobile phones to holidays, pensions and financial services.

Appendix 6

Drugs and their control

Chris Evans

The two acts that control the manufacture, supply and use of drugs are the Medicines Act 1968 and the Misuse of Drugs Act 1971.

THE MEDICINES ACT

The Act defines 'medicinal products' as substances sold or supplied for administration to humans or animals for medicinal purposes. Part 3 of the Act, and order made under it, control the manufacture and sale or supply of medicines, and for this purpose broadly classify them into three classes:

- Prescription-only medicines (PoM).
- Pharmacy medicines (P).
- General sales list medicines (GSL).

Different legal requirements apply to the sale, supply and labelling of each class.

In hospitals and other institutions, all medicines should be appropriately and securely stored in order to ensure that they remain safe and effective in use and to deter unauthorised access to them and hence possible misuse (see Department of Health 1988).

THE MISUSE OF DRUGS ACT

This Act designates and defines as Controlled Drugs a number of 'dangerous or otherwise harmful' substances. These substances are all also by definition prescription-only medicines under the Medicines Act. The controls imposed by the Misuse of Drugs Act are therefore additional to those

under the Medicines Act. The main purpose of the Misuse of Drugs Act is to prevent abuse of Controlled Drugs by prohibiting their manufacture or supply except in accordance with various regulations made under the Act. Other regulations govern requirements for safe custody, destruction and supply to addicts.

For these purposes, under the current (1985) Regulations, Controlled Drugs are classified into five Schedules, each representing a different level of control. For practical purposes Schedule 2 is the most relevant to hospital and community nursing practice. It includes: cocaine; the major opioids such as diamorphine, methadone, morphine, papaveretum and pethidine; and the major stimulant amphetamine (and related drugs). (Amendments to this list and the list of drugs in the other Schedules may be made from time to time.)

Prescriptions for Schedule 2 drugs (and for those in Schedules 1 and 3) must:

- Be handwritten, signed and dated by the prescriber.
- Be in ink or be otherwise indelible.
- Include the name and address of the patient.
- State (in words and figures) the total quantity of the drug to be supplied.
- State the dose to be taken.

(Some of these requirements may be relaxed for the prescription of some Controlled Drugs to addicts, for the treatment of their addiction, by doctors who hold a special Home Office licence.)

In hospitals, ordering, supply and storage of Controlled Drugs is subject to tight control:

- They are stored separately in a locked cupboard (which may be within a second outer cupboard) to which access is restricted. The key to the cupboard is held by a first level nurse.
- Supply from the pharmacy is made to a ward or department only on receipt of a written order signed by a responsible nurse.
- A record is kept of stock held and details of doses given. A special register is used for this and no other purpose, and it is usually the case that each entry is countersigned by two nurses. The records should be regularly checked by the nurse in charge and by a pharmacist, according to health authority policy.

Abbreviations used in prescriptions

Abbreviations of Latin are being replaced by English versions, which are considered safer; however, the nurse may still meet the Latin abbreviations given in Appendix 7.

Self-administration of drugs by hospital inpatients

For the inpatient approaching discharge, there are obvious benefits to be gained from the opportunity to assume responsibility for self-administration of prescribed medicines while access to professional support and advice is still readily available (UKCC 1992). Schemes to allow self-administration of their medicines by various groups of hospital inpatients have been established in several National Health Service (NHS) hospitals. Self-administration shifts the balance of responsibility for this part of their care further towards patients. The nurse's fundamental professional duty of care is, however, undiminished and it is essential that local policies and procedures are adequate to ensure that this responsibility is, and can be shown to be, discharged.

ADMINISTRATION OF MEDICINES: UKCC ADVISORY PAPER

The United Kingdom Central Council (UKCC), in an advisory paper on the administration of medicines, clearly states the role and responsibility of the nurse, midwife and health visitor in the administration of prescribed drugs. This paper is reproduced below.

1. This standards paper replaces the Council's advisory paper *Administration of medicines* (UKCC 1986) and the supplementary circular *The administration of medicines* (UKCC 1988). The Council has prepared this paper to assist practitioners to fulfil the expectations which it has of them, to serve more effectively the interests of patients and clients and to maintain and enhance standards of practice.

2. The administration of medicines is an important aspect of the professional practice of persons whose names are on the Council's register. It is not solely a mechanistic task to be performed in strict compliance with the written prescription of a medical practitioner. It requires thought and the exercise of professional judgement which is directed to the following:

2.1 Confirming the correctness of the prescription.

2.2 Judging the suitability of administration at the scheduled time of administration.

2.3 Reinforcing the positive effect of the treatment.

2.4 Enhancing the understanding of patients in respect of their prescribed medication and the avoidance of misuse of these and other medicines.

2.5 Assisting in assessing the efficacy of medicines and the identification of side-effects and interactions.

3. To meet the standards set out in this paper is to honour, in this aspect of practice, the Council's expectation (set out in the Council's Code of professional conduct (UKCC 1992), that: As a registered nurse, midwife or health visitor you are personally accountable for your practice and, in the exercise of your professional accountability, must:

    (a) Act always in such a manner as to promote and safeguard the interests and wellbeing of patients and clients.

    (b) Ensure that no action or omission on your part, or within your sphere of responsibility, is detrimental to the interests, condition or safety of patients and clients.

    (c) Maintain and improve your professional knowledge and competence.

    (d) Acknowledge any limitations in your

knowledge and competence and decline any duties or responsibilities unless able to perform them in a safe and skilled manner.

4. This extract from the Code of professional conduct applies to all persons on the Council's register irrespective of the part of the register on which their name appears. Although the content of pre-registration education programmes varies, dependent on the part or level of the register involved, the Council expects that, in this area of practice as in all others, all practitioners will have taken steps to develop their knowledge and competence and will have been assisted to this end. The word 'practitioner' is, therefore, used in the remainder of this paper to refer to all registered nurses, midwives and health visitors, each of whom must recognise the personal professional accountability which they bear for their actions. The Council therefore imposes no arbitrary boundaries between the role of the first level and second level registered practitioner in this respect.

Treatment with medicines

5. The treatment of a patient with medicines for therapeutic, diagnostic or preventative purposes is a process which involves prescribing, dispensing, administering, receiving and recording. The word 'patient' is used for convenience, but implies not only a patient in a hospital or nursing home, but also a resident of a residential home, a client in her or his own home or in a community home, a person attending a clinical or a general practitioner's surgery and an employee attending a workplace occupational health department. 'Patient' refers to the person receiving a prescribed medicine. Each medicine has a product licence, which means that authority has been given to a manufacturer to market a particular product for administration in a particular dosage range and by specified routes.

Prescription

6. The practitioner administering a medicine against a prescription written by a registered medical practitioner, like the pharmacist responsible for dispensing it, can reasonably expect that the prescription satisfies the following criteria:

6.1 It is based, whenever possible, on the patient's awareness of the purpose of the treatment and consent (commonly implicit).

6.2 The prescription is either clearly written, typed or computer-generated, and the entry is indelible and dated.

6.3 Where the new prescription replaces an earlier prescription, the latter has been cancelled clearly and the cancellation signed and dated by an authorised registered medical practitioner.

6.4 Where a prescribed substance (which replaces an earlier prescription) has been provided for a person residing at home or in a residential care home and who is dependent on others to assist with the administration, information about the change has been properly communicated.

6.5 The prescription provides clear and unequivocal identification of the patient for whom the medicine is intended.

6.6 The substance to be administered is clearly specified and, where appropriate, its form (for example, tablet, capsule, suppository) stated, together with the strength, dosage, timing and frequency of administration and route of administration.

6.7 Where the prescription is provided in an outpatient or community setting, it states the duration of the course before review.

6.8 In the case of controlled drugs, the dosage is written, together with the number of dosage units or total course if in an outpatient or community setting, the whole being in the prescriber's own handwriting.

6.9 All other prescriptions will, as a minimum, have been signed by the prescribing doctor and dated.

6.10 The registered medical practitioner understands that the administration of medicines on verbal instructions, whether she or he is present or absent, other than in exceptional circumstances, is not acceptable unless covered by the protocol method referred to in paragraph 6.11.

6.11 It is understood that, unless provided for in a specific protocol, instruction by telephone to a practitioner to administer a previously unprescribed substance is not acceptable, the use of facsimile transmission (fax) being the preferred method in exceptional circumstances or isolated locations.

6.12 Where it is the wish of the professional staff concerned that practitioners in a particular setting be authorised to administer, on their own authority, certain medicines, a local protocol has been agreed between medical practitioners, nurses and midwives and the pharmacist.

Dispensing

7. The practitioner administering a medicine dispensed by a pharmacist in response to a medical prescription can reasonably expect that:

7.1 The pharmacist has checked that the prescription is written correctly so as to avoid misunderstanding or error and is signed by an authorised prescriber.

7.2 The pharmacist is satisfied that any newly prescribed medicines will not dangerously interact with or nullify each other.

7.3 The pharmacist has provided the medicine in a form relevant for administration to the particular patient, provided it in an appropriate container giving the relevant information and advised appropriately on storage and security conditions.

7.4 Where the substance is prescribed in a dose or to be administered by a route which falls outside its product licence, unless to be administered from a stock supply, the pharmacist will have taken steps to ensure that the prescriber is aware of and has chosen to exceed that licence.

7.5 Where the prescription for a specific item falls outside the terms of the product licence, whether as to its route of administration, the dosage or some other key factor, the pharmacist will have ensured that the prescriber is aware of this fact and, mindful of her or his accountability in the matter, has made a record on the prescription to this effect and has agreed to dispense the medicine ordered.

7.6 If the prescription bears any written amendments made and signed by the pharmacist, the prescriber has been consulted and advised and the amendments have been accepted.

7.7 The pharmacist, in pursuit of her or his role in monitoring the adverse side-effects of medicines, wishes to be sent any information that the administering practitioner deems relevant.

Standards for the administration of medicines

8. Notwithstanding the expected adherence by registered medical practitioners and pharmacists to the criteria set out in paragraphs 6 and 7 of this paper, the nurse, midwife or health visitor must, in administering any medicines, in assisting with administration or overseeing any self-administration of medicines, exercise professional judgement and apply knowledge and skill to the situation that pertains at the time.

9. This means that, as a matter of basic principle, whether administering a medicine, assisting in its administration or overseeing self-administration, the practitioner will be satisfied that she or he:

9.1 Has an understanding of the substances used for therapeutic purposes.

9.2 Is able to justify any actions taken.

9.3 Is prepared to be accountable for the action taken.

10. Against this background, the practitioner, acting in the interests of the patient, will:

10.1 Be certain of the identity of the patient to whom the medicine is to be administered.

10.2 Ensure that she or he is aware of the patient's current assessment and planned programme of care.

10.3 Pay due regard to the environment in which that care is being given.

10.4 Scrutinise carefully, in the interests of safety, the prescription, where available, and the information provided on the relevant containers.

10.5 Question the medical practitioner or pharmacist, as appropriate, if the prescription or container information is illegible, unclear, ambiguous or incomplete or where it is believed that the dosage or route of administration falls outside the product licence for the particular substance and, where believed necessary, refuse to administer the prescribed substance.

10.6 Refuse to prepare substances for injection in advance of their immediate use and refuse to administer a medicine not placed in a container or drawn into a syringe by her or him, in her or his presence, or prepared by a pharmacist, except in the specific circumstances described in paragraph 40 of this paper and others where similar issues arise.

10.7 Draw the attention of patients, as appropriate, to patient information leaflets concerning their prescribed medicines.

11. In addition, acting in the interests of the patient, the practitioner will:

11.1 Check the expiry data of any medicine, if on the container.

11.2 Carefully consider the dosage, method of administration, and route and timing of administration in the context of the condition of the specific patient at the operative time.

11.3 Carefully consider whether any of the prescribed medicines will or may dangerously interact with each other.

11.4 Determine whether it is necessary or advisable to withhold the medicine pending consultation with the prescribing medical practitioner, the pharmacist or a fellow professional colleague.

11.5 Contact the prescriber without delay where contraindications to the administration of any prescribed medicine are observed, first taking the advice of the pharmacist where considered appropriate.

11.6 Make clear, accurate and contemporaneous record of the administration of all medicines administered or deliberately withheld, ensuring that any written entries and the signature are clear and legible.

11.7 Where a medicine is refused by the patient, or the parent refuses to administer or allow administration of that medicine, make a clear and accurate record of the fact without delay, consider whether the refusal of that medicine compromises the patient's condition or the effect of other medicines, assess the situation and contact the prescriber.

11.8 Use the opportunity which administration of a medicine provides for emphasising, to patients and their carers, the importance and implications of the prescribed treatment and for enhancing their understanding of its effects and side-effects.

11.9 Record the positive and negative effects of the medicine and make them known to the prescribing medical practitioner and the pharmacist.

11.10 Take all possible steps to ensure that replaced prescription entries are correctly deleted to avoid duplication of medicines.

Applying the standards in a range of settings

Who can administer medicines?

12. There is a wide spectrum of situations in which medicines are administered, ranging, at one extreme, from the patient in an intensive therapy unit who is totally dependent on registered professional staff for her or his care to, at the other extreme, the person in her or his own home administering her or his own medicines or being assisted in this respect by a relative or another person. The answer to the question of who can administer a medicine must largely depend on where within that spectrum the recipient of the medicines lies.

Administration in the hospital setting

13. It is the Council's position that, at or near the first stated end of that spectrum, assessment of response to treatment and speedy recognition of contraindications and side-effects are of great importance. Therefore prescribed medicines should only be administered by registered practitioners who are competent for the purpose and aware of their personal accountability.

14. In this context it is the Council's position that, in the majority of circumstances, a first level registered nurse, a midwife, or a second level nurse, each of whom has demonstrated the necessary knowledge and competence, should be able to administer medicines without involving a second person. Exceptions to this might be where:

14.1 The practitioner is instructing a student.

14.2 The patient's condition makes it necessary.

14.3 Local circumstances make the involvement of two persons desirable in the interests of the patients (for example, in areas of specialist care, such as a paediatric unit without sufficient specialist paediatric nurses or in other acute units dependent on temporary agency or other locum staff).

15. In respect of the administration of intravenous drugs by practitioners, it is the Council's position that this is acceptable, provided that, as in all other aspects of practice, the practitioner is satisfied with her or his competence and mindful of her or his personal accountability.

16. The Council is opposed to the involvement of persons who are not registered practitioners in the administration of medicines in acute care settings and with ill or dependent patients, since the requirements of paragraphs 8 to 11 inclusive of this paper cannot then be satisfied. It accepts, however, that the professional judgement of an individual practitioner should be used to identify those situations in which informal carers might be instructed and prepared to accept a delegated responsibility in this respect.

Administration in the domestic or quasi-domestic setting

17. It is evident that in this setting, on the majority of occasions, there is no involvement of registered practitioners. Where a practitioner engaged in community practice does become involved in assisting with or overseeing administration, then she or he must observe paragraphs 8 to 11 of this paper and apply them to the required degree. She or he must also recognise that, even if not employed in posts requiring registration with the Council, she or he remains accountable to the Council.

18. The same principles apply where prescribed medicines are being administered to residents in small community homes or in residential care homes. To the maximum degree possible, though related to their ability to manage the care and administration of their prescribed medicines and comprehend their significance, the residents should be regarded as if in their own home. Where assistance is required, the person providing it fills the role of an informal carer, family member or friend. However, as with the situation described in paragraph 17,

where a professional practitioner is involved, a personal accountability is borne. The advice of a community pharmacist should be sought when necessary.

Self-administration of medicines in hospitals or registered nursing homes

19. The Council welcomes and supports the development of self-administration of medicines and administration by parents to children wherever it is appropriate and the necessary security and storage arrangements are available.

20. For the hospital patient approaching discharge, but who will continue on a prescribed medicines regimen following the return home, there are obvious benefits in adjusting to the responsibility of self-administration while still having access to professional support. It is accepted that, to facilitate this transition, practitioners may assist patients to administer their medicines safely by preparing a form of medication card containing information transcribed from other sources.

21. For the long-stay patient, whether in hospital or a nursing home, self-administration can help foster a feeling of independence and control in one aspect of life.

22. It is essential, however, that where self-administration is introduced for all or some patients, arrangements must be in place for the appropriate, safe and secure storage of the medicines, access to which is limited to the specific patient.

The use of monitored dosage systems

23. Monitored dosage systems, for the purpose of this paper, are systems which involve a community pharmacist, in response to the full prescription of medicines for a specific person, dispensing those medicines into a special container with sections for days of the week and times within those days and delivering the container, or supplying the medicines in a special container of blister packs, with appropriate additional information, to the nursing home, residential care home or

domestic residence. The Council is aware of the development of such monitored dosage systems and accepts that, provided they are able to satisfy strict criteria established by the Royal Pharmaceutical Society of Great Britain and other official pharmaceutical organisations, that substances which react to each other are not supplied in this way and that they are suitable for the intended purpose as judged by the nursing profession, they have a valuable place in the administration of medicines.

24. While, to the present, their use has been primarily in registered nursing homes and some community or residential care homes, there seems no reason why, provided the systems can satisfy the standards referred to in paragraph 25, their use should not be extended.

25. In order to be acceptable for use in hospitals or registered nursing homes, the containers for the medicines must:

25.1 Satisfy the requirements of the Royal Pharmaceutical Society of Great Britain for an original container.

25.2 Be filled by a pharmacist and sealed by her or him or under her or his control and delivered complete to the user.

25.3 Be accompanied by clear and comprehensive documentation which forms the medical practitioner's prescription.

25.4 Bear the means of identifying tablets of similar appearance so that, should it be necessary to withhold one tablet (for example, digoxin), it can be identified from those in the container space for the particular time and day.

25.5 Be able to be stored in a secure place.

25.6 Make it apparent if the containers (be they blister packs or spaces within a container) have been tampered with between the closure and sealing by the pharmacist at the time of administration.

26. While the introduction of a monitored dosage system transfers to the pharmacist the responsibility for being satisfied that the container is filled and sealed correctly so as to comply with the prescription, it does not alter the fact that the practitioner administering the medicines must still consider the appropriateness of each medicine at the time administration falls due. It is not the case, therefore, that the use of a monitored dosage system allows the administration of medicines to be undertaken by unqualified personnel.

27. It is not acceptable, in lieu of a pharmacist-filled monitored dosage system container, for a practitioner to transfer medicines from their original containers into an unsealed container for administration at a later stage by another person, whether or not that person is a registered practitioner. This is an unsafe practice which carries risks for both practitioner and patient. Similarly it is not acceptable to interfere with a sealed section at any time between its closure by the pharmacist and the scheduled time of administration.

The role of nurses, midwives and health visitors in community practice in the administration of medicines

28. Any practitioner who, whether as a planned intervention or incidentally, becomes involved in administering a medicine, or assisting with or overseeing such administration, must apply paragraphs 8 to 11 of this paper to the degree to which they are relevant.

29. Where a practitioner working in the community becomes involved in obtaining prescribed medicines for patients, she or he must recognise her or his responsibility for safe transit and correct delivery.

30. Community psychiatric nurses whose practice involves them in providing assistance to patients to reduce and eliminate their dependence on addictive drugs should ensure that they are aware of the potential value of short-term prescriptions and encourage their use where appropriate in the long-term interests of their clients. They must not resort to holding or carrying prescribed controlled drugs to avoid their misuse by those clients.

31. Special arrangements and certain exemptions apply to occupational health nurses. These are described in Information Document 11 and the appendices of A guide to an occupational health nursing service: a handbook for employers and nurses (Royal College of Nursing 1991).

32. Some practitioners employed in the community, including in particular community nurses, practice nurses and health visitors, in order to enhance disease prevention, will receive requests to participate in vaccination and immunisation programmes. Normally these requests will be accompanied by specific named prescriptions or be covered by a protocol setting out the arrangements within which substances can be administered to certain categories of persons who meet the stated criteria. The facility provided by the Medicines Act 1968, for substances to be administered to a number of people in response to an advance 'direction', is valuable in this respect. Where preventive treatment has not been possible and there is no relevant protocol or advance direction, particularly in respect of patients about to travel abroad and requiring preventive treatment, a telephone conversation with a registered medical practitioner will suffice as authorisation for a single administration. It is not, however, sufficient as a basis for supplying a quantity of medicines.

Midwives and midwifery practice

33. Midwives should refer to the current editions of both the Council's Midwives rules (UKCC 1991a) and A midwife's code of practice (UKCC 1991b), and specifically to the sections concerning administration of medicines. At the time of publication of this paper, Midwives rules sets out the practising midwife's responsibility in respect of the administration of medicines and other forms of pain relief. A midwife's code of practice refers to the authority provided by the Medicines Act 1968 and the Misuse of Drugs Act 1971, and regulations made as a result, for midwives to obtain and administer certain substances.

What if the Council's standards in paragraphs 8 to 11 cannot be applied?

34. There are certain situations in which practitioners are involved in the administration of medicines where some of the criteria stated above either cannot be applied or, if applied, would introduce dangerous delay with consequent risk to patients. These will include occupational health settings in some industries,

small hospitals with no resident medical staff and possibly some specialist units within larger hospitals and some community settings.

35. With the exception of the administration of substances for the purpose of vaccination or immunisation described in paragraph 32 above, in any situation in which a practitioner may be expected or required to administer 'prescription-only medicines' which have not been directly prescribed for a named patient by a registered medical practitioner who has examined the patient and made a diagnosis, it is essential that a clear local policy be determined and made known to all practitioners involved with prescribing and administration. This will make it possible for action to be taken in patients' interests while protecting practitioners from the risk of complaint which might otherwise jeopardise their position.

36. Therefore, where such a situation will or may apply, a local policy should be agreed and documented which:

36.1 States the circumstances in which particular 'prescription-only medicines' may be administered in advance of examination by a doctor.

36.2 Ensures the relevant knowledge and skill of those to be involved in administration.

36.3 Describes the form, route and dosage range of the medicines so authorised.

36.4 Wherever possible, satisfies the requirements of Section 58 of the Medicines Act 1968 as a 'direction'.

Substances for topical application

37. The standards set out in this paper apply, to the degree to which they are relevant, to substances used for wound dressing and other topical applications. Where a practitioner uses a substance or product which has not been prescribed, she or he must have considered the matter sufficiently to be able to justify its use in the particular circumstances.

The administration of homeopathic or herbal substances

38. Homeopathic and herbal medicines are subject to the licensing provisions of the Medicines Act 1968, although those on the

market when that Act became operative (which means most of those now available) received product licences without any evaluation of their efficacy, safety or quality. Practitioners should, therefore, make themselves generally aware of common substances used in their particular area of practice. It is necessary to respect the right of individuals to administer to themselves, or to request a practitioner to assist in the administration of substances in these categories. If, when faced with a patient or client whose desire to receive medicines of this kind appears to create potential difficulties, or if it is felt that the substances might be either an inappropriate response to the presenting symptoms or likely to negate or enhance the effect of prescribed medicines, the practitioner, acting in the interests of the patient or client, should consider contacting the relevant registered medical practitioner, but must also be mindful of the need not to override the patient's rights.

Complementary and alternative therapies

39. Some registered nurses, midwives and health visitors, having first undertaken successfully a training in complementary or alternative therapy which involves the use of substances such as essential oils, apply their specialist knowledge and skill in their practice. It is essential that practice in these respects, as in all others, is based upon sound principles, available knowledge and skill. The importance of consent to the use of such treatment must be recognised. So, too, must the practitioner's personal accountability for professional practice.

Practitioners assuming responsibility for care which includes medicines being administered which were previously checked by other practitioners

40. Paragraph 10.6 of this paper referred to the unacceptability of a practitioner administering a substance drawn into a syringe or container by another practitioner when the practitioner taking over responsibility for the patient was not present. An exception to this is an already established intravenous infusion, the use of a syringe pump or some other kind of

continuous or intermittent infusion or injection apparatus, where a valid prescription exists, a responsible practitioner has signed for the container of fluid and any additives being administered and the container is clearly and indelibly labelled. The label must clearly show the contents and be signed and dated. The same measures must apply equally to other means of administration of such substances through, for example, central venous, arterial or epidural lines. Strict discipline must be applied to the recording of any substances being administered by any of the methods referred to in this paragraph and to reporting procedures between staff as they change and transfer responsibility for care.

Management of errors or incidents in the administration of medicines

41. In a number of its annual reports, the Council has recorded its concern that practitioners who have made mistakes under pressure of work, and have been honest and open about those mistakes to their senior staff, appear often to have been made the subject of disciplinary action in a way which seems likely to discourage the reporting of incidents and therefore be to the potential detriment of patients and of standards.

42. When considering allegations of misconduct arising out of errors in the administration of medicines, the Council's Professional Conduct Committee takes great care to distinguish between those cases where the error was the result of reckless practice and was concealed and those which resulted from serious pressure of work and where there was immediate, honest disclosure in the patient's interest. The Council recognises the prerogative of managers to take local disciplinary action where it is considered to be appropriate but urges that they also consider each incident in its particular context and similarly discriminate between the two categories described.

43. The Council's position is that all errors and incidents require a thorough and careful investigation which takes full account of the circumstances and context of the event and

the position of the practitioner involved. Events of this kind call equally for sensitive management and a comprehensive assessment of all of the circumstances before a professional and managerial decision is reached on the appropriate way to proceed.

Arrangements for prescribing nurses

44. In March 1992 the Act of Parliament entitled the Medicinal Products: Prescription by Nurses, etc. Act 1992 became law. This legislation came into operation in October 1993. It permits nurses with a district nursing or health visiting qualification to prescribe certain products from a Nurse Prescriber's Formulary. The statutory rules specify the categories of nurses who can prescribe under this limited legislation.

45. A nurse prescriber can be defined as a community nurse or practice nurse who is identified as a nurse prescriber on the UKCC register, writing a prescription for an item in the Nurse Prescriber's Formulary using form FP10(CN) or FP10(PN), within a Nurse Prescribing Demonstration Scheme or within a health authority or trust that has implemented nurse prescribing. Nurse prescribing can therefore only be undertaken in community or primary care settings. All other schemes, e.g. in hospitals, whereby nurses are able to supply or administer medicines cannot accurately be termed 'nurse prescribing', and should be retitled if necessary.

46. Statutory Instrument 1994 No 2402 sets out the necessary training and qualifications for nurses to prescribe. It states that nurses who are able to prescribe must:

46.1 Be registered on parts 1 to 12 of the UKCC register.

46.2 Have a district nurse qualification and be employed by a health authority, trust or fundholding practice.

46.3 Be registered in part 11 as a health visitor and be employed by a health authority, trust or fundholding practice.

46.4 Be named on the professional register and marked as qualified to prescribe. Amendments to this Statutory Instrument have been made to allow eligible nurses employed in Primary Care Act pilots to prescribe.

47. Nurse prescribers may only prescribe from the items listed in the Nurse Prescriber's Formulary.

48. Useful address: Association for Nurse Prescribing, Porters South, 4 Crinan St, London N1 9SQ (tel 0207 843 4517).

49. Enquiries in respect of this Council paper should be directed to the Registrar and Chief Executive, United Kingdom Central Council for Nursing, Midwifery and Health Visiting, 23 Portland Place, London W1N 3AF.

References

DoH 1988 Guidelines for the safe and secure handling of medicines: the Duthie Report. Department of Health, London

DoH 1999 Review of prescribing, supply and administration of medicines: final report. Department of Health, London

Medicinal Products: Prescription by Nurses, etc. Act 1992. HMSO, London

Medicines Act 1968 (reprinted 1986). HMSO, London

Misuse of Drugs Act 1971 (reprinted 1985). HMSO, London

National Health Service Executive 1998 Nurse prescribing – a guide for implementation. NHSE, Leeds

Nurse Prescriber's Formulary 1998 British Medical Association and Royal Pharmaceutical Society of Great Britain, London

Royal College of Nursing 1991 A guide to an occupational health nursing service: a handbook for employers and nurses, 2nd edn. RCN, London

UKCC 1986 Administration of medicines. A UKCC advisory paper: a framework to assist individual professional judgement and the development of local policies and guidelines. UKCC, London

UKCC 1988 The administration of medicines, PC88/05. UKCC, London

UKCC 1991a Midwives rules. UKCC, London

UKCC 1991b A midwife's code of practice. UKCC, London

UKCC 1992 Code of professional conduct for the nurse, midwife and health visitor, 3rd edn. UKCC, London

Appendix 7

Prescription abbreviations

These are abbreviations that are used extensively in writing prescriptions.

a.c. before meals
Amps. Ampoules
b.d. twice daily
b.i.d. twice daily
c. with
Caps capsules
Gtt Drops
Liq Solution
mitte dispense
mane in the morning
mcg micrograms
(there are 1000mcg in one milligram)
mg milligram(s)
(there are 1000mg in one gram)
Mist mixture
ml millilitre(s) (there are 1000ml in one litre)

nocte at bed-time
o.d. once daily
o.m. each morning
o.n. each night
o.p. original pack
p.c. after meals
prn as required
q.i.d. four times daily
q.d.s. four times daily
Rx supply
Sig let it be labelled
s.o.s. when required
stat to be taken immediately
Syr Syrup
Tabs tablets
t.d.s three times daily
t.i.d. three times daily
Ung ointment
ut dict as directed

Appendix 8

Medical abbreviations

In order to produce concise notes and instructions quickly, doctors and other health care practitioners are forced to use a large number of abbreviations. This can cause problems for medical secretaries as there is little standardisation of medical abbreviations and they are easy to misinterpret. Care should be taken in their use.

The following list contains only those abbreviations which are widely used and are not specific to one hospital or practice. Where abbreviations have a Latin origin they appear in italics with the Latin words following in brackets.

aa (ana) of each
a.c. (ante cibum) before meals
ad to; up to
ad lib. (ad libitum) as much as needed
aet. (aetas) aged
A/G ratio albumin/globulin ratio
alb. albumin
alt. dieb. (alternis diebus) every other day
alt. hor. (alternis horis) every other hour
alt. noct. (alternis noctibus) every other night
AN antenatal
ante (ante) before
AP anteroposterior
APH antepartum haemorrhage
APT alum-precipitated toxoid
aq. (aqua) water
aq.-dist. (aqua distillata) distilled water
ARM artificial rupture of membranes
Ba.E barium enema
Ba.M barium meal
BBA born before arrival
BCG Bacille Calmette-GuÈrin
b.d. or b.i.d. (bis in die) twice daily
BI bone injury
bib. (bibe) drink
BID brought in dead
BMR basal metabolic rate

BNF British National Formulary (with date)
BO bowels opened
BP blood pressure or British Pharmacopoeia (with date)
BPC British Pharmaceutical Codex (with date)
BS breath sounds
C (centum gradus) centigrade
c. (circa) about
c. (cum) with
Ca. carcinoma
caps (capsula) capsule
CCF congestive cardiac failure
cf. compare
circ. circumcision
CF cystic fibrosis
cm centimetre
CNS central nervous system
c.o. complains of
Crem (cremor) cream
CSF cerebrospinal fluid
CSOM chronic suppurative otitis media
CSU catheter specimen of urine
CVS cardiovascular system
Cx cervix
D&C dilatation and curettage
dil. (dilutus) dilute
DNA did not attend

DOB date of birth
DT delirium tremens
D and V diarrhoea and vomiting
DU duodenal ulcer
DXR deep X-ray
ECG electrocardiogram
ECT electroconvulsive therapy
EDC expected date of confinement
EDD expected date of delivery
EEG electroencephalogram
ENT ear, nose and throat
e.s. (enema saponis) soap enema
ESN educationally subnormal
ESR erythrocyte sedimentation rate
EUA examination under anaesthesia
ext. (extractum) extract
F Fahrenheit
FB foreign body
FH fetal heart or family history
FHH fetal heart heard
FHNH fetal heart not heard
Fib. fibula
fl. (fluidum) fluid
FMF fetal movements felt
ft. (fiat) let there be made
FTM fractional test meal
g gram
GA general anaesthetic
G and O gas and oxygen
GB gall bladder
GC gonorrhoea
GCFT gonorrhoea complement fixation test
GI gastrointestinal
GP general practitioner
GPI general paralysis of insane
GTT glucose tolerance test
GU gastric ulcer
gt. (gutta) drop (eye-drops)
Gyn. gynaecology
h. (hora) hour
Hb haemoglobin
HP house physician
HS house surgeon
h.s. (hora somni) at bed-time
HV health visitor
id. (idem) the same
i.e. (id est) that is
in d. (in dies) daily
IP inpatient
IQ intelligence quotient
ISQ (in statu quo) without change

IV intravenous
IVP intravenous pyelogram
IZS insulin zinc suspension
KJ knee jerk
KP keratitis punctata
l litre (should be written in full)
LA local anaesthetic or local authority
Lab. laboratory
LE cells lupus erythematosus cells
LIF left iliac fossa
LIH left inguinal hernia
liq. (liquor) a solution in water
LMP last menstrual period
LOA left occipitoanterior
LOP left occipitoposterior
LSCS lower segment caesarean section
LV left ventricle
M. (misce) mix
m. minim
mCi millicurie
MCD mean corpuscular diameter
MCH mean corpuscular haemoglobin
MCHC mean corpuscular haemoglobin concentration
MCV mean corpuscular volume
mEq milliequivalent
mist. (mistura) mixture
mm. millimetre
mmHg millimetres of mercury
MMR mass miniature radiography
MS multiple sclerosis
MSU midstream urine
NAD no abnormality detected
NBI no bone injury
neg. negative
NG new growth
no. (numero) number
noct. (nocte) at night
n.p. (nomen proprium) give proper name
NPU not passed urine
OA osteoarthritis
Ob. obstetrics
OE on examination
Omn. hor. (omni hora) every hour
Omn. noct. (omni nocte) every night
Op. operation
OP outpatient
PA pernicious anaemia
Path. pathology
PBI protein bound iodine
p.c. (post cibum) after meals

PCO patient complains of
PID prolapsed intervertebral disc
PMH previous medical history
PN postnatal
POP plaster of Paris
PP private patients
PPH postpartum haemorrhage
p.r. (per rectum) rectal examination or by the rectum
p.r.n. (pro re nata) whenever necessary
PY physiotherapy
PU passed urine
PUO pyrexia of unknown origin
p.v. (per vaginam) vaginal examination or by the vagina
PZI protamine zinc insulin
q. (quaque) every
q.h. (quaque hora) every hour
q.i.d. (quater in die) four times a day
quotid. (quotidie) daily
q.s. (quantum sufficiat) sufficient quantity
Rx (recipe) take
RA rheumatoid arthritis
RBC red blood corpuscle
Rh. rhesus factor
RIF right iliac fossa
RIH right inguinal hernia
RLL right lower lobe
ROA right occipitoanterior
ROL right occipitolateral
ROP right occipitoposterior
RS respiratory system

s. (sine) without
SB stillborn
SG specific gravity
sig. (signetur) let it be labelled
SMR submucous resection
sol. (solutis) solution
s.o.s. (si opus sit) if necessary
sp. gr. specific gravity
ss. (semis) half
stat. (statim) at once
SWD short wave diathermy
syr. (syrupus) syrup
T and A tonsils and adenoids
TAB typhoid and paratyphoid A and B
TB tuberculosis
TCA to come again
TCI to come in
t.i.d. (ter in die) three times a day
TPR temperature, pulse and respiration
tr. (tinctura) tincture
Ung. (unguentum) ointment
VD venereal disease
vi (virgo intacta) virgin
Vin. (vinum) wine
VV varicose vein
Vx vertex
WBC white blood corpuscle
WR Wasserman reaction
wt weight
XR X-ray
YOB year of birth

Symbols that are commonly used include: ♂male; ♀female; # fracture; -ve negative; +ve positive; Δ diagnosis.

Appendix 9

Personal profiles

Personal profiles or portfolios have become a recognised method of summarising personal achievement, interests and progress. These were brought into the school environment through the National Record of Achievement. This is in order to give you an individual record of experience and achievements to which you can add personal statements, examination results and records, which may provide valuable material for a future CV. You will no doubt remember that your school record of achievement was presented in a special folder with space allocated to different aspects of development. It is useful to consider how this can be extended for future use.

PERSONAL STATEMENT

This is expected to contain information about activities you have been involved in, whether they are clubs, sports, musical activities, drama, etc. It should include activities which you took part in out of college or school hours. Once you have left training, interests may change or even be extended; there is every reason to update your personal statement in this area from time to time.

QUALIFICATIONS AND EXAMINATION RESULTS

It is most useful to keep an accurate and up-to-date record of qualifications gained and when these were achieved. It is very easy to forget the year that

particular examinations were taken, especially when many secretarial examinations take place at several points during each year. To keep a track on these, there should be space allowed to record all successes or re-takes accurately, so that a true record is always there for reference. Whether you wish to include examination slips within the plastic wallets provided is up to you, but it should be stressed that actual certificates and examination slips should be kept together carefully for future reference. Some places of employment may require actual evidence of your success and ask to see official documents.

When making a record of results, always state:

- the type of qualification, e.g. Medical Secretarial Diploma
- the subject area
- the awarding body, e.g. AMSPAR
- the level / result / grade, e.g. Diploma or Certificate
- the date of achievement.

ACHIEVEMENT AND EXPERIENCE

You may have copies of tutors' reports or work placement evidence you would like to include in this section. Other experience you may like to add here are those recognised today as 'key skills'. These are:

- Planning and presentation of information. This may be through listening, reading and using it to present ideas to others whether by speaking, writing or using images.

- Using information technology to process, prepare and present material in different contexts.
- Using application of number to enable calculation and presentation of data.
- Effective personal skills when working as a team or in a one to one situation.
- Problem solving.
- Personal skills, developing and improving skills in order to improve personal performance.

You may also like to add some thoughts of your own on what you think your particular strengths or qualities are. These may be things such as determination or an ability to work under pressure. You may like to include evidence from particular employment to illustrate this.

EMPLOYMENT HISTORY

This is an important section to keep updated. Again, it is all too easy to forget exact dates of jobs you have taken in the past. Keep a record here of:

- job title
- name of employer
- address and telephone number.

It might also be useful to keep a note of any other details connected to work, such as:

- National Insurance number
- Pay roll number.

INDIVIDUAL ACTION PLANS

From time to time it might be useful to sit back and assess where your career is taking you, whether you envisage any change or progress in your job, or indeed, do you want a change at all! A change might be inevitable at some time as circumstances change. In order to develop plans or to just assess where you are at the moment, it might be useful to think in terms of

- a review
- long- or short-term goals – and therefore ...
- targets to achieve
- methods to achieve them.

It is always useful to ask someone else whom you trust and respect to read your personal statements and letters first. Always compose them in a rough form first, before producing a well word-processed version. Whatever you choose to include in your personal profile, try to make sure that the statements and records will create a positive picture of you.

Appendix 10

Career prospects for the qualified medical secretary

Dilys Jones

The medical secretary needs a wide range of skills and abilities. She requires compassion and a concern for people, and the ability to prioritise and to work with great accuracy. She must apply the rules of confidentiality and be aware of the legal aspects. If she makes a mistake, a patient's health may suffer.

AMSPAR stands for the Association of Medical Secretaries, Practice Managers, Administrators and Receptionists. It was established in 1964 and is recognised by the Qualifications and Curriculum Authority and the BMA. It is the largest association for administrative staff in the field of health care and exists to promote, encourage and support the education and maintenance of high standards.

For the medical secretary AMSPAR offers Diploma and Certificate training courses. A list of colleges offering these qualifications is available from head office*. In addition to full training courses, some colleges offer short courses in one or more subject areas aimed at the medical secretary. If you do not possess any AMSPAR qualifications you are still eligible to apply for membership. If you have worked in a health care environment for at least 10 years you are eligible for full membership; 5 years you are eligible to become an associate member and under 5 years you are eligible for affiliate membership. Some of the benefits of membership are: a free legal helpline, participation in local and national conferences, free subscription to the AMSPAR Journal and use of designated letters, e.g. MAMS.

Most medical secretaries find their first job in an NHS hospital, a private hospital, health centre or a general practice. However, there are many other organisations keen to employ qualified medical secretaries, for example in clinical audit, the various medical research bodies, pharmaceutical companies, social services, community-based agencies and medical publishers.

The range of job opportunities in these organisations should not be overlooked. In the largest hospitals, for example, in addition to the whole range of medical specialties, there may be a great deal of education and training in the attached medical school, schools of nursing, physiotherapy and radiography, etc., in which a medical secretary could support a teaching team. The names and addresses of all hospitals in England, Scotland, Wales and Northern Ireland can be found in the back of the Medical Directory (published annually) with details of the consultants in the various specialties. The Medical Directory is available in the reference section of public libraries.

Most of the medical specialties are supported by a college offering information, training and publications, for example The Royal College of Physicians and The Royal College of Surgeons. All these colleges would be interested in employing a qualified medical secretary... though you will find that most have their headquarters in the London area.

Many of the voluntary and community-based agencies advertise medical secretarial posts. A particularly good example is the hospice providing care for the terminally ill. There are a great many charities such as the British Red Cross, Help the Aged, MIND, Save the Children Fund, Shelter and SCOPE. Details of these and many others are in *The Voluntary Agencies Directory* published annually by NCVO

Publications and *Charities Digest* published annually by The Family Welfare Association and available in the reference section of public libraries. Details of research organisations are also included, for example British Heart Foundation, Imperial Cancer Research Fund, Institute of Cancer Research and Medical Research Council.

Some newly qualified medical secretaries may be unsure in which area of the medical field their future lies. Temping can be an interesting way of looking inside a number of organisations and might help you decide on your career path. For those returning to work after a long family break, temping can provide some flexibility before committing to a permanent appointment. Contacting your local hospital can be a good starting point as hospitals like to have a 'bank' of secretarial staff to call on to cover holidays and periods of sickness.

The AMSPAR Advanced Diploma for Medical Secretaries course requires full-time students to spend a period of time on field work. Work experience placements should be in hospital departments and general medical practice. Group visits to the Support Services and community-based agencies can also be included. A work placement is a unique opportunity to observe the routine procedures and the communication links between staff and between the different departments. However, work experience is not provided for observation only, but for the student to learn and assist with a variety of duties. If this role is carried out successfully and the student fits in well with the other members of the team, it is worth bearing in mind that there may be the possibility of a job offer as a result of the work placement.

If you think you might be interested in medical publishing, you will find that the Royal Colleges publish weekly and monthly medical journals, pamphlets and books, and there are several medical publishers.

Recent changes in the structure of the health service have resulted in new administrative posts, and a motivated medical secretary willing to undertake further training may progress to a supervisory or management role.

*AMSPAR
Tavistock House North
Tavistock Square
London   WC1H 9LN
Tel: 020 7387 6005
Fax: 020 7388 2648
www.amspar.co.uk

Appendix 11

Applying for a job

Dilys Jones

JOB ADVERTISEMENTS AND WHERE TO LOOK FOR THEM

Outside of London jobs for medical secretaries will be published in local newspapers. In the London area jobs may be advertised in local as well as national daily and evening newspapers. *The Times*, *The Guardian*, *The Daily Telegraph*, *Daily Express* and *The Mail* advertise relevant posts in their weekly jobs section.

If you are not finding that suitable jobs are being advertised you may decide to use an employment agency. These organisations are paid by employers to find suitable candidates for specific jobs and some agencies specialise in particular fields such as nursing or secretarial work. Make sure you choose an agency that will work for you in a field relevant to the type of job you want or you may find yourself attending interviews which are unsuitable. Look at the AMSPAR website for the details of recruitment sites that specialise in jobs within the health industry (www.amspar.co.uk).

If you are out temping, keep a close eye on any staff notice boards. Whole careers have been founded on information stumbled across in such a manner.

When you see a job advertised in which you are interested, there is likely to be a contact name and address for you to write and obtain an application form and/or job description. Alternatively, there may be only a name and telephone number, and you are invited to telephone for a job description. If you have to telephone at this stage, plan what you want to say before making the call as your telephone manner will be important.

A job description will usually include:

- the job title
- where the vacancy occurs
- the duties and responsibilities of the job, listed in some detail
- who the job holder reports to
- any special conditions of the job.

Study the job description carefully. If you decide to apply you will need to prepare a letter of application, to be accompanied by either a completed job application form or a curriculum vitae. Follow any instructions exactly; if you are asked to handwrite the covering letter, you must do so.

Consider the job advertisement on page 334.

CURRICULUM VITAE

The letters CV are an abbreviation of curriculum vitae, which is Latin for 'course of life'. A CV is a summary of your career, educational and personal life relevant to the job you are applying for.

There is no single 'correct' way of writing a CV. Presenting a good CV is an opportunity to shine over the opposition, and it is worth spending some hours preparing your first one. Your CV must be word processed and printed on the best paper and printer available to you.

When you use your CV, it is important to tailor it to an advertised position or organisation. It may be just a matter of emphasising some experience or qualities you have that are particularly relevant to the job you are applying for. If you are already working, your CV

South London NHS Trust
FULL-TIME MEDICAL SECRETARY
required in the Orthopaedic Department

*The ideal candidate will be well organised and possess good
communication skills and excellent medical secretarial skills.
Shorthand desirable but not essential.
Would suit AMSPAR qualified college leaver.*

*Good interpersonal skills needed for liaising with 2 consultants,
nursing staff and other members of the team. Up-to-date
hardware and software packages – training provided.*

*Hours: 37 per week. Salary: Grade 3 plus proficiency allowances.
For further details and a job description please contact
Sally Lang, Human Resources Department,
South London NHS Trust,
Fulham Road, Chelsea, London SW3 6LJ. Tel: 020 7352 8111*

---

should show your present duties and responsibilities. Better still, also try to show evidence of your achievements in your current post. By keeping your CV on disk, it is easy to make a few amendments and keep it up to date.

It is usual to supply the names, addresses and telephone numbers of two referees at the end of your CV. If you are a college leaver one of your referees should be your course tutor. In addition, consider asking:

- a leader of a club you belong to
- a professional person who knows you well
- your supervisor at your Saturday job.

Do check with these people first that they are willing to write a reference for you.

If you are already employed and do not want your manager to know that you are applying for other jobs, you can mention this in your letter of application by saying something like 'Please do not contact my employer for a reference unless a job offer is to be made'.

On the CV itself, the guidelines are clear:

- No more than two pages

- Well laid out, with clear headings and plenty of white space
- A well chosen typeface (not too fancy)
- Make sure essential information is included (address, telephone no., etc.)
- Previous posts in reverse date order, focusing on achievements.

If you are just completing your college training course and are applying for your first job, your CV may look something like the example on page 335

If you have held previous jobs, then your CV should list these with the latest or present job first. If you are now looking for a full-time job after taking a family break, your CV might look something like the example on page 336.

JOB APPLICATION FORMS

Some organisations ask you to complete a printed job application form. These forms vary as each organisation designs its own.

Some advantages to completing forms are:

CURRICULUM VITAE

ALISON SMITH

14 Stuart Rise	Date of Birth: 12 April 1978
Burgess Hill	Marital Status: Single
West Sussex	Nationality: British
BN12 2RX	
Tel: 01444 871452	

EDUCATION AND QUALIFICATIONS

1987-1994	Fairways Comprehensive School, Burgess Hill
GCSE	English (B), Mathematics (C), Biology (C), Geography (C), Art (D), French (D)
1994-1996	Brighton College
	AMSPAR Medical Secretarial Diploma
	RSA Medical Word Processing Stage II
	RSA Medical Audio Transcription Stage II
	RSA Medical Shorthand Speed 80 wpm

WORK EXPERIENCE

1996	2 weeks assisting the medical secretaries in the Surgical Unit at Brighton Hospital (as part of my course)
	2 weeks assisting the medical secretary/receptionists at the Thorpe Medical Centre, Burgess Hill (as part of my course)
1995/96	Saturday job – cashier at J Sainsbury plc, Burgess Hill

INTERESTS

Bronze Duke of Edinburgh Award – I enjoyed the physical challenges and planning for the expedition

Computers – I am enthusiastic about computers and enjoy looking at software packages with my friends

Tennis – I play regularly at my local club and take part in local competitions

Riding – I help at sessions of Riding for the Disabled

REFEREES

Mrs Jane Adams	Mr John Williamson
Business Department	Practice Manager
Brighton College	Thorpe Medical Centre
Southern Road	High Street
Brighton	Burgess Hill
East Sussex BN3 4RE	West Sussex BN16 2EY
Tel: 01273 644644	Tel: 01273 532288

CURRICULUM VITAE

ROSEMARY BROWN

50 Hyde Road
Brighton
East Sussex
BN3 6BX
Tel: 01273 660342

Date of Birth: 20 June 1962
Marital Status: Married
Nationality: British

EDUCATION AND QUALIFICATIONS

1971-1978	St Mary's School, Brighton
GCSE	English (C), Mathematics (C), Biology (C), History (C), Art (D)
1978-80	Brighton College
	AMSPAR Medical Secretarial Diploma
	RSA Medical Audio Transcription Stage II
	RSA Medical Shorthand 100 wpm
	RSA Typewriting Stage III
1995	Brighton College – Evening Class
	RSA Word Processing Stage II

WORK EXPERIENCE

1995-1996	Medical Receptionist (part-time, 20 hours per week) Burgess Hill Health Centre
1985-1995	Family break to care for my 2 children
1982-1985	Senior Medical Secretary to the Director of the Paediatric Unit, Guy's Hospital, London. Duties included providing secretarial support to the consultants, maintaining the Director's diary, servicing committees, organising staffing rotas and recording statistical and financial information.
1980-1982	Medical Secretary to Consultant Surgeons. Responsible for providing efficient secretarial support to the surgical team, and dealing with patients and relatives in a friendly and reassuring manner.

INTERESTS

Sailing – this is a hobby enjoyed by all the family
Reading – I enjoy a variety of books, but particularly biographies
School Governor at Mannington School since 1994

REFEREES

Mr Anthony Bryden
Practice Manager
Burgess Hill Health Centre
High Street
Burgess Hill
West Sussex BN19 6ST
Tel: 01444 678954

Mr Robert White
Headmaster
Mannington School
West Road
Brighton
East Sussex BN10 8XX
Tel: 01273 882365

- the form tells you what information to provide
- the amount of space provided may indicate how much you are expected to write.

Some disadvantages are:

- it is very difficult to complete an application form using a word processor
- some organisations use the same form for all appointments so it may be difficult to give the information you feel is important.

When you receive an application form, read the instructions very carefully. It is likely that you will be asked to write in your own hand. A useful hint: photocopy the form before you start and draft your answers on the copy, remembering to match what you say to the job description. When you feel you have presented the information about yourself as effectively as possible you can copy your answers clearly and neatly on to the original.

LETTERS OF APPLICATION

There are several types of letter that you may need to send when applying for a job. For example:
a simple letter asking for an application form

- a letter of application to accompany a CV
- a covering letter with a completed application form
- a speculative letter.

You may put your letter of application on the word processor unless instructed otherwise. Whether typing or handwriting your letter, the advice is the same:

- use good quality white paper – it may have to be photocopied
- use size A4 so that it matches your CV
- use 1 inch margins
- the letter should be neat and well spaced
- quote the job reference number
- check for errors in spelling and grammar
- make sure the beginning and ending are correct for each other (e.g. Yours faithfully with Dear Sir, and Yours sincerely with Dear Mrs Williams).

Your letter is as important as your CV. It is an opportunity to further sell yourself as a person, as well as to highlight skills or experience that are particularly relevant to the job. Remember – your application may need to catch the reader's attention in the first 20 seconds in order to ensure that you are shortlisted for a job you really want.
Consider the following:

> *Dear Sir*
>
> *I would like to apply for the post of Medical Secretary you are advertising.*
>
> *I have just passed the Medical Secretarial Diploma at College. I enclose a copy of my CV.*
>
> *Yours faithfully*

This is a poor example of a letter of application. Even though the candidate has the right qualification for the job, the letter does not catch the reader's attention and encourage him/her to read the CV. Also, try and avoid the use of 'I' as the first word of each sentence!
A good letter of application needs to include:

- a heading – quoting the job reference number if there is one
- an introductory paragraph which says what the letter is about and what documents you are enclosing
- one or more paragraphs
  - drawing attention to any skills, qualifications or work experience particularly relevant to the job
  - giving additional details about yourself which are pertinent to the job
- a closing paragraph rounding off the letter.

As a college leaver who has just achieved the Medical Secretarial Diploma, your letter of application for the above post might look something like the example on page 338.

SPECULATIVE APPLICATION LETTERS

As well as replying to advertisements, you may decide to approach organisations directly. Large organisations are bound to have vacancies from time to time.
If you have good qualifications and/or experience, you have every reason to be hopeful. You may be lucky and be offered an interview quickly. More likely the organisation will write and tell you that they are holding your details on file until a suitable vacancy occurs.

4 South Drive
BRIGHTON
East Sussex
BN1 4TW

5 July 1996

Mrs Ann Williams
Personnel Manager
Brighton Hospital
High Street
BRIGHTON
East Sussex
BN1 6AP

Dear Mrs Williams

Ref JP/476 – Medical Secretary in the Paediatric Unit

I would like to apply for the above post advertised in the Brighton Gazette of 2 July 1996. I attach my CV.

For the last 2 years I have been attending a full-time AMSPAR Medical Secretarial Diploma Course at Brighton College. I am optimistic that I have achieved the full qualification.

The course was very interesting and enjoyable. It has given me a broad picture of the structure of the health service and a good working knowledge of medical terminology, communication and office skills.

During my course I visited your hospital for 2 weeks in March 1996. I was attached to the medical secretaries in the Surgical Unit and assisting with the routine administrative procedures was a valuable learning experience.

I think of myself as hardworking and cheerful and look forward to achieving my aim to be part of a health service team.

If you wish to call me for interview I am available at any time.

Yours sincerely

Angela Smith

Enc

Before writing your speculative letter, find out who would be the best person to address your letter to. Phone the organisation and ask for the correct spelling of the person's name and his or her job title.

Your speculative letter is similar to your covering letter of application:

- a short opening paragraph explaining why you are writing
- specify your qualifications and experience for this kind of job
- give a reason for wanting to work with this organisation
- enclose your CV.

LETTER OF ACCEPTANCE

Having been offered a job it is very important to conclude the process with a letter of acceptance straight away. You should reply by return of post.

A suitable letter of acceptance might be:

Dear Mrs Williams

Ref JP/476 – Medical Secretary in the Paediatric Unit

Thank you for your letter of 25 July concerning the above post. I write to confirm that I shall be delighted to accept the offer made in that letter.

As requested I will report to your office at 9.00 a.m. on Monday 2 September.

Yours sincerely

Further reading

Stoyell S & Edwards L 2001 How to write your first CV. Foulsham, London

Houston K 1998 Creating winning CVs and Applications. Trotman and Co Ltd, London

Appendix 12

How to present yourself at interview

Dilys Jones

If you have submitted a good letter of application and an effective CV for a specific job, you will be hoping that you are going to be shortlisted.

If you are shortlisted for a job the next stage is the interview. Most interviewees would confess to feeling nervous about the interview. The best way to combat nervousness is to prepare as thoroughly as possible.

Consider the following in relation to the job you have applied for.

- What are the employers looking for?
- What form will the interview take?
- What should you expect to be asked?
- What questions should you ask?

It is important that you go to the interview with a 'picture' of the organisation. If the interview is to take place in a hospital, visit the reception area and look for leaflets that might give you background information on the work of the hospital. If there do not appear to be any suitable leaflets, then the personnel department may be able to help with information on the structure of the organisation. Ask the reception staff how to get to the exact location of your interview so that you can feel confident of finding the room in good time on the interview day. This visit will also have given you the opportunity to check your route and travelling arrangements.

If your interview is in a general practice, you could visit the premises and ask the reception staff for a copy of the practice leaflet. This will give you a good day-to-day picture of the work of the practice.

Any information you have about the organisation will assist you to answer questions with more understanding and with more confidence.

PLANNING FOR THE INTERVIEW

- Check your route and travelling arrangements.
- Decide what you are going to wear at least 3 days ahead of time. A suit would give a serious and professional first impression. Ensure that all accessories are clean. You will want to be comfortable in your outfit and to feel you look right for the interview.
- Prepare some questions that you may wish to ask at the end of the interview.
- Rehearse your answers to the most common questions beforehand.
- Remember to let your referees know that you have been shortlisted. You might want to give them some details so that they understand what the employer is looking for.

QUESTIONS YOU MIGHT BE ASKED

If an initial interview is being set up by the personnel department, it is likely that a standardised list of criteria will be used to assess the candidate. Be prepared to talk about some or all of the following:

- Why you want the job
- Work experience, including your last job and previous jobs
- Your training and qualifications relevant to the job
- Flexibility
- Long-term career plans
- Leisure interests.

WHAT TO TAKE TO THE INTERVIEW

- A copy of your CV, record of achievement, certificates, portfolio
- Any information supplied about the job
- Name and telephone number of the interviewer in case of delays
- A list of questions to ask at the end of the interview
- A notepad and pen
- Everyday things:
  - glasses – if you need them
  - money
  - any travel or parking instructions
  - handkerchief or clean tissues
  - umbrella – if it looks like rain
  - women might want to carry a spare pair of tights.

Find something appropriate to carry things in. Try and borrow an envelope file or briefcase. Avoid using a plastic bag.

THE INTERVIEW

Arrive well before the interview time. Nothing looks more unprofessional than being late.

Remember that you are there because you have impressed the person who is hiring. Whether you have a good CV, wrote a good letter of application or spoke well on the phone, you have made a positive first impression.

At interview it is your task to show that you can do the job effectively. You must be positive and show you can communicate well verbally. Use active words to describe your skills, experience and achievements. You might find it helpful to think about the following active words to use in some of your responses:

achieve	coordinate	improve
capable	create	manage
control	develop	organise

If asked a general opening question such as 'Tell me something about yourself', you might give the best impression by enquiring what aspects the interviewer would like to know about other than those mentioned in your CV.

Asked why you want this job, you do not have to go into great detail. Something about your interest in the job, the service or the people, and the fact that you feel you have the necessary skills will often suffice.

Self motivation equals enthusiasm. If you want a job, and know why you want it, it is not difficult to show it. Your enthusiasm should shine through, and if you follow this by asking interesting questions, you will leave a favourable impression in the interviewer's mind. You should be able to demonstrate your motivation to achieve. If you have succeeded in achieving all the examinations for the Medical Secretarial Diploma your self motivation is evident.

QUESTIONS YOU MIGHT WANT TO ASK

- Who would I be working with?
- What computer software do you use?
- What is the most demanding aspect of the job?
- Are there opportunities for further training and development?
- Are you able to tell me when a decision will be made?

There are many observers of the recruitment field who suggest that interviewers make up their minds about a candidate in the first four minutes of the interview, so first impressions of your appearance, manner, facial expression and attitude are most important.

It is likely that your interview is with more than one person. Greet each panel member with a firm handshake and smile. When asked to take a seat, sit well back in the chair and place your legs together, not crossed. Look the interviewer in the eye when you are speaking. Experienced interviewers appreciate that almost all candidates will be slightly nervous. Do not be surprised if the beginning of the interview is made up of small talk to break the ice.

Concentrate on the questions you are being asked. If necessary, pause to think before you answer. It is unlikely that a simple 'yes' or 'no' will suffice. Be prepared to expound on any question to the best of your ability. It may be that 30 seconds is the average length of your answers. Stop when you have said all you want to – do not ramble on in order to fill the silence.

Do not criticise any past employers. One of the things you have got to prove is that you are loyal. Find something good to say about previous jobs. You gained additional skills, but now you are looking for more responsibility.

Let the interviewer discuss salary first. The salary can be negotiated at a later stage. It is important to be offered the job first.

The interviewer will indicate that the interview is over. It is acceptable to ask when a decision is likely to be made. On leaving, smile and thank the interviewer(s) for seeing you. It is not necessary to shake hands again.

KEY POINTS TO REMEMBER

Do not:

- interrupt the interviewer
- criticise past employers
- answer with a simple yes or no
- be jokey/flippant/sarcastic – not everybody has the same sense of humour

- smoke
- accept a cup of coffee – unless you can see somewhere to put it down.

Do:

- dress appropriately
- allow plenty of time to reach the interview in comfort
- look at the interviewer(s)
- smile occasionally – it relieves the tension
- think about likely questions and decide on your answers
- have questions ready beforehand – it does not go down well if you have none!

Index

The Essential
MEDICAL SECRETARY

About the CD

Should you wish to keep your records electronically, the CD-ROM that accompanies *The Essential Medical Secretary* contains copies of useful forms in two digital formats.

The forms are available as PDF files, which can be accessed and updated using Adobe Acrobat Reader. A copy of this software is available on the CD should you need to install it. The forms are also available in Microsoft Word format, so that they can be tailored to individual use.

The minimum requirements to run the CD are:

Windows
Intel Pentium processor
Microsoft Windows 95 OSR 2.0, Windows 98 SE, Windows ME, Windows NT1 4.0 with Service Pack 5, Windows 2000 or Windows XP
64MB of RAM
24MB of available hard-disk space
Internet Explorer 4 or later
Flash Player

Macintosh
PowerPC processor
Mac OS software version 8.6, 9.0.4 or Mac OS X
64MB of RAM
24MB of available hard-disk space
Internet Explorer 4 or later
Flash Player